Local Anesthesia and Extractions for Dental Students: Simple Notes and Guidelines

Editor

Esam Ahmad Z Omar

Oral & Maxillofacial Surgery, College of Dentistry, Taibah University, Saudi Arabia

Local Anesthesia and Extractions for Dental Students: Simple Notes and Guidelines

Editor: Esam Ahmad Z Omar

ISBN (Online): 978-1-68108-633-0

ISBN (Print): 978-1-68108-634-7

General:

1. Any dispute or claim arising out of or in connection with this License Agreement or the Work (including non-contractual disputes or claims) will be governed by and construed in accordance with the laws of the U.A.E. as applied in the Emirate of Dubai. Each party agrees that the courts of the Emirate of Dubai shall have exclusive jurisdiction to settle any dispute or claim arising out of or in connection with this License Agreement or the Work (including non-contractual disputes or claims).
2. Your rights under this License Agreement will automatically terminate without notice and without the need for a court order if at any point you breach any terms of this License Agreement. In no event will any delay or failure by Bentham Science Publishers in enforcing your compliance with this License Agreement constitute a waiver of any of its rights.
3. You acknowledge that you have read this License Agreement, and agree to be bound by its terms and conditions. To the extent that any other terms and conditions presented on any website of Bentham Science Publishers conflict with, or are inconsistent with, the terms and conditions set out in this License Agreement, you acknowledge that the terms and conditions set out in this License Agreement shall prevail.

Bentham Science Publishers Ltd.
Executive Suite Y - 2
PO Box 7917, Saif Zone
Sharjah, U.A.E.
Email: subscriptions@benthamscience.org

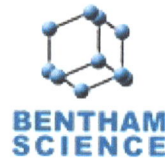

BENTHAM SCIENCE

CONTENTS

FOREWORD

I am pleased to write this foreword of this new book on local anesthesia and exodontia.

The Oral and Maxillofacial Surgery has an extensive body of literature; the dental extraction is one of the essential dentoalveolar procedures and the dentist should be well oriented to it scientifically and technically.

I found this book an excellent and impressive work which has been written in a concise and precise manner. The concept of local dental anesthesia and dental extraction is focused in book.

On reading this book, I have felt, it is not only recommended for undergraduates. It is also highly suitable for postgraduate trainees in their residency program, such as those in the level of Saudi Board of Oral and Maxillofacial Surgery program. It may help in a rapid revision of the management of simple and complicated dental extraction during the pre-exam period.

I dedicate this book to undergraduates and postgraduates trainees with the hope that it fulfills their need in understanding the concepts of dental extraction.

Abdullah Alatal
Oral and Maxillofacial Surgeon
Chief of Saudi Board in Oral and Maxillofacial Surgery (SB-OMS)
Saudi Arabia

PREFACE

The target of this book is the undergraduate dental students to give them the basic concept and outline of the principle of local anesthesia and exodontia in brief short notes form that is easy to understand, remember and to implement clinically.

The local anesthesia and exodontia is the fundamental part of Oral Surgey that should be known well by all dentists, since it is one of the daily surgical procedures in dentistry.

This book is suitable as well for the oral & maxillofacial surgery trainees who are looking for a concise rapid revision of management of simple, complex dental extraction and management of medically compromised patients.

I dedicate this book to my students everywhere, my parent and family. I would like to express sincere thanks to my wife for continuous support, encouraging and help.

ACKNOWLEDGMENTS

I would like to acknowledge **Dr. Fadi Jarab** and **Dr. Wamig Fareed** for their contribution in this work (Chapter 3 and part 2 in chapter 4 written by Fad Jarab and Chapter 6 by Wamiq Fareed).

The figures of this book has been drawn by: **Dr. Omar Mohammad Dad**. I would like to acknowledge him for his help in producing the figures of this book, his help was valuable and appreciated.

This book has been revised by: **Dr. Ghaith Gazal**, and **Dr. Albaraa B. Alolayan**. I would like to acknowledge them for their contribution in this work.

With appreciation and thanks to Instant Anatomy. 10 Summerfield Cambridge, CB3 9HE, UK. http://www.instantanatomy.net, for their permission for using some of their illustration in chapter one (The Outline of the Trigeminal Nerve Anatomy).

CONFLICT ON INTEREST

The authors confirm that this article content has no conflict of interest.

Esam Ahmad Z. Alomar
Oral & Maxillofacial Surgery
College of Dentistry
Taibah University, Madinah
Saudi Arabia

List of Contributors

Esam Ahmad Z Omar   Department of Oral & Maxillofacial Surgery, College of Dentistry, Taibah University, Madinah, Saudi Arabia

Fadi Jarab   Department of Oral & Maxillofacial Surgery, Jordan University of Science and Technology, Jordan

Wamiq Musheer Fareed   Department of Oral & Maxillofacial Surgery, College of Dentistry, Taibah University, Madinah, Saudi Arabia

CHAPTER 1

The Outline of the Trigeminal Nerve Anatomy

Esam Ahmad Z Omar[*]

Department of Oral & Maxillofacial Surgery, College of Dentistry, Taibah University, Madinah, Saudi Arabia

Abstract: The primary sensory nerve of the Oro-facial area is the trigeminal nerve. Understanding the anatomy of this nerve is essential for the dental practitioner to understand the pain mechanism and dental pain pathway. Most of the anatomy books discuss the details of the anatomical relation of Trigeminal nerve instead of an understanding of neural fibers carry by the nerve. This chapter discusses the anatomy, the neural fibers of each branch and the neural connection (nuclei) of the nerve.

Keywords: Anatomy, Central Bathway, Mandibular Nerve, Maxillary Nerve, Nuclie of trigeminal nerve, Ophthalamic Nerve, Sympathatic and Parasympathetic of trigeminal nerve, Trigeminal nerve.

The Trigeminal nerve is mixed Cranial nerve comprises principally of neurons for sensation. It enters the trigeminal ganglion after travelling parallel to the pons surface and exiting the brain. The trigeminal ganglion makes up the spinal nerve by acting as the dorsal root ganglion.

The trigeminal ganglion divides into three major branches, innervating different bone, teeth and facial dermatome. Every branch follows a different path and site to exit the cranium.

The Opthalmic nerve, the primary V1 branch, exits *via* the superior orbital fissure of the cranium, reaching the orbit to innervate the skin existing above the forehead and eye as well as the globe of the eye.

The Maxillary nerve makes the second V2 division, leaving *via* the foramen rotundum, into the pterygopalatine fossa, an area located posterior to the orbit. Thereafter, it again enters the inferior orbital fissure, making its way to the infraorbital foramen on the face, innervating the skin of the nose and cheek and below the eye.

---

[*] **Corresponding author Esam Ahmad Z Omar:** Department of Oral & Maxillofacial Surgery, College of Dentistry, Taibah University, Madinah, Saudi Arabia; Tel: 0569536708; Fax: 00966148494710; E-mail: esamomar@hotmail.com

The Mandibular nerve, the V3 third division, also has a motor component leave with the nerve and joining it at the foramen ovale (the motor root).

The different trigeminal nerve nuclei: Fig. (**1.1**)

- The sensory nucleus is primarily for touch and temperature, present in the pons.
- The spinal nucleus is responsible primarily for temperature and pain, and is a sensory nucleus.
- The sensory nucleus is ventromedial to motor nucleus.

The mesencephalic nucleus is the proprioceptive nucleus for all muscles of mastication.

TRIGEMINAL NERVE (V)
EXTRA NOTES

- Nerve of the first pharyngeal arch
- 3 nuclei in brain stem (see below)
- Somatic but carries parasympathetic and sympathetic
- Mostly sensory but small motor branch in mandibular division
- Motor is branchiomotor (special visceral motor)
- All cell bodies are in the trigeminal ganglion EXCEPT
  for proprioception and these are in the mesencephalic
  nucleus in the brain stem

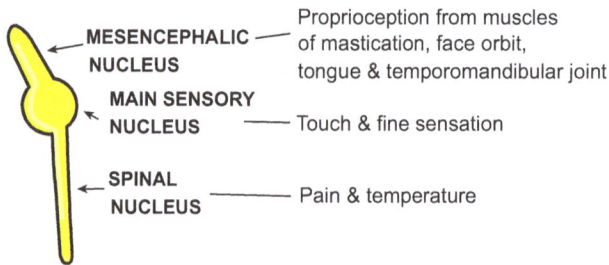

MESENCEPHALIC NUCLEUS — Proprioception from muscles of mastication, face orbit, tongue & temporomandibular joint

MAIN SENSORY NUCLEUS — Touch & fine sensation

SPINAL NUCLEUS — Pain & temperature

- In Meckel's cave
- Motor root inferior
- Blood supply from internal carotid in cavernous sinus & accessory meningeal via foramen ovale
- Nerve supply from nervus spinosus (Vc)

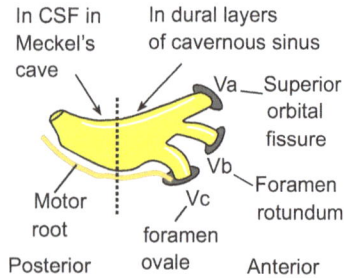

In CSF in Meckel's cave

In dural layers of cavernous sinus

Va — Superior orbital fissure

Vb — Foramen rotundum

Motor root

Vc foramen ovale

Posterior   Anterior

Fig. (1.1). Trigeminal nerve nuclei (Acknowledgment: with appreciation and thanks to Instant Anatomy. 10 Summerfield Cambridge, CB3 9HE, UK. http://www.instantanatomy.net, for their permission for using this illustration).

Nerves supplying parasympathetic fibers in head and neck area:

• Glossopharyngeal nerve (otic ganglion)
• Facial nerve (pterygopalatine ganglion, submandibular ganglion)
• Oculomotor nerve (ciliary ganglion)

The trigeminal nerve receives the parasympathetic and the special sensation (taste) from the following:

The nervus intermedius, or "nerve of Wrisberg" is the intermediate nerve of the facial nerve (cranial nerve VII) situated among the vestibulocochlear nerve (cranial nerve VIII) and the motor of the facial nerve.

The nucleus of nervus intermedius:

• Tractus solitaries (***Taste nucleus***): It contains the sensory taste (from tractus solitarius) which leaves the pons as nervus intermedius as a branch of facial. It gives branch to:
    ○ Chorda tympani nerve travelling towards the submandibular ganglion.
    ○ Greater petrosal nerve travelling towards the pterygopalatine ganglion.
• The superior salivary nucleus: parasympathetic secretory-motor fibers to:
    ○ Submandibular, sublingual salivary gland to sublingual ganglion through the chorda tympani
    ○ And to the minor salivary nucleus of nose and palate through the greater petrosal nerve which joins --- the ptrygo-palatine ganglion. It is made of parasympathetic fibers coming from the superior salivary nucleus and the tractus solitarius' sensory taste and exiting alongside the facial nerve in the facial canal, joining it's motor root at the geniculate ganglion. Parasympathetic axons originate from the superior salivatory nucleus. No synapse is present when these fibers pass the geniculate ganglion. Some of these preganglionic parasympathetic filaments, as they leave the geniculate ganglion, move within the greater petrosal nerve. This way they form a synapse with the pterygopalatine ganglion. These postganglionic neurons provide the lacrimal gland with parasympathetic innervation t through their axons.

The *function* of the tractus solitarius (solitary tract):

1. Solitary tract are structures in the brainstem that receive and carry taste sensation from the visceral sensation from vagus, glossopharyngeal nerve (IX) and facial nerve through it,s fibres to trigeminal nerve (VII).
    ○ Taste from the anterior part of the tongue, more specifically two third (2/3rd) area, through the facial nerve fibers given to the mandibular branch of the

trigeminal nerve by chorda tympani The fibers of the facial nerve when leave the geniculate ganglion at the middle ear, they combine with the mandibular nerve at about one centimeter below the base of the skull by the chorda tympani. The posterior $1/3^{rd}$ general and taste sensation through the glossopharyngeal nerve.

2. Chemoreceptors in the carotid (by means of IX) and aortic body (through X).
3. Stretch receptors from the aorta and carotid supply routes called blood vessel baroreceptors.

Petrosal nerve (Fig. **1.2**) (a nerve going through the temporal bone, specifically the petrous part):

1. Deep petrosal nerve
2. Lesser petrosal nerve (also called the lesser superficial petrosal nerve)
3. Greater petrosal nerve (also called as the greater superficial petrosal nerve)
4. External superficial petrosal nerve

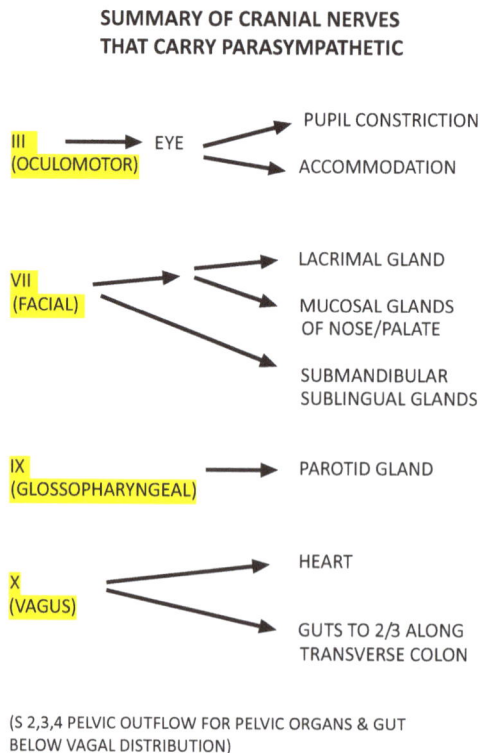

**SUMMARY OF CRANIAL NERVES
THAT CARRY PARASYMPATHETIC**

III (OCULOMOTOR) → EYE → PUPIL CONSTRICTION / ACCOMMODATION

VII (FACIAL) → LACRIMAL GLAND / MUCOSAL GLANDS OF NOSE/PALATE / SUBMANDIBULAR SUBLINGUAL GLANDS

IX (GLOSSOPHARYNGEAL) → PAROTID GLAND

X (VAGUS) → HEART / GUTS TO 2/3 ALONG TRANSVERSE COLON

(S 2,3,4 PELVIC OUTFLOW FOR PELVIC ORGANS & GUT BELOW VAGAL DISTRIBUTION)

Fig. (1.2). Petrosal nerve (Acknowledgments: with appreciation and thanks to Instant Anatomy. 10 Summerfield Cambridge, CB3 9HE, UK. http://www.instantanatomy.net, for their permission for using this illustration).

Deep Petrosal Nerve

Originating from the carotid plexus, the petrosus profundus or deep petrosal nerve travels within a canal positioned lateral to the internal carotid artery, known as the carotid canal.

It contains postganglionic sympathetic filaments supplied by the superior cervical ganglion.

As it passes through the cartilaginous substance of the foramen lacerum, it frames the nerve of the pterygoid canal (Vidian nerve) by combining with the greater petrosal nerve. At that point, without synapsing, it travels through the pterygopalatine ganglion and later joins the postganglionic parasympathetic filaments in supplying the lacrimal gland and nasal cavity.

The parasympathetic part of the large petrosal nerve, known as the greater superficial petrosal nerve rises from the geniculate ganglion of the facial nerve (it's nucleus in tractus solitarius); travelling *via* the hiatus of the facial canal, entering the cranium, and continues underneath the dura mater present in the anterior temporal petrous bone's groove. Afterwards it emerges into the foramen lacerum filling cartilaginous substance and forms the Vidian nerve, the nerve of the pterygoid channel, after attaching with the deep petrosal nerve (sympathetic part).

Nucleus of greater petrosal nerve (Fig. **1.3**):

- Nervus intermedius: leave the cranial cavity *via* the facial nerve
  - Tast sensation
- Superior salivary nucleus: leave the cranial cavity *via* facial nerve
  - Salivation: for the minor the salivary glands at the nose, plate.

Vidian Nerve

Vidian nerve consists of:

- Deep petrosal nerve (sympathetic root)
- And greater petrosal nerve (parasympathetic root)

The nerve present in the pterygoid canal is known as Vidian nerve. It comes to be after the combining of two nerves in the foramen lacerum the deep petrosal nerve, which forms the sympathetic root, and the greater petrosal nerve, which forms the parasympathetic root. These are united by a little rising otic ganglion branch called the sphenoidal branch. Finally, on reaching the pterygopalatine fossa, it combines with the pterygopalatine ganglion.

GREATER PETROSAL NERVE

TEAR AND HAY FEVER GLANDS

Nuclei:
Secretomotor - Superior
                    salivary
Taste - Tractus solitarius

Nervus intermedius

into internal auditory meatus with VII, VIII

Joins VII just before geniculate ganglion

Enters pterygopalatine (hayfever) ganglion in its fossa where parasympathetics synapse; somatic sensory (V) & sympathetics pass through

Distributes to nose, sinuses, palate,naso-pharynx & lacrimal gland

Geniculate ganglion

Cell bodies for taste

Parasympathetics leave VII & pass out of ganglion

Taste returns from palate

Deep pertosal

Pterygoid canal

F.lacerum

Enters pterygoid canal at upper, anterior end of f. lacerum as nerve of pterygoid canal

joined by deep petrosal nerve (sympathetic from plexus on internal carotid artery)

Greater Pertosal nerve

Through roof of petrous temporal, into middle cranial fossa between layers of dura, under V ganglion to reach foramen lacerum

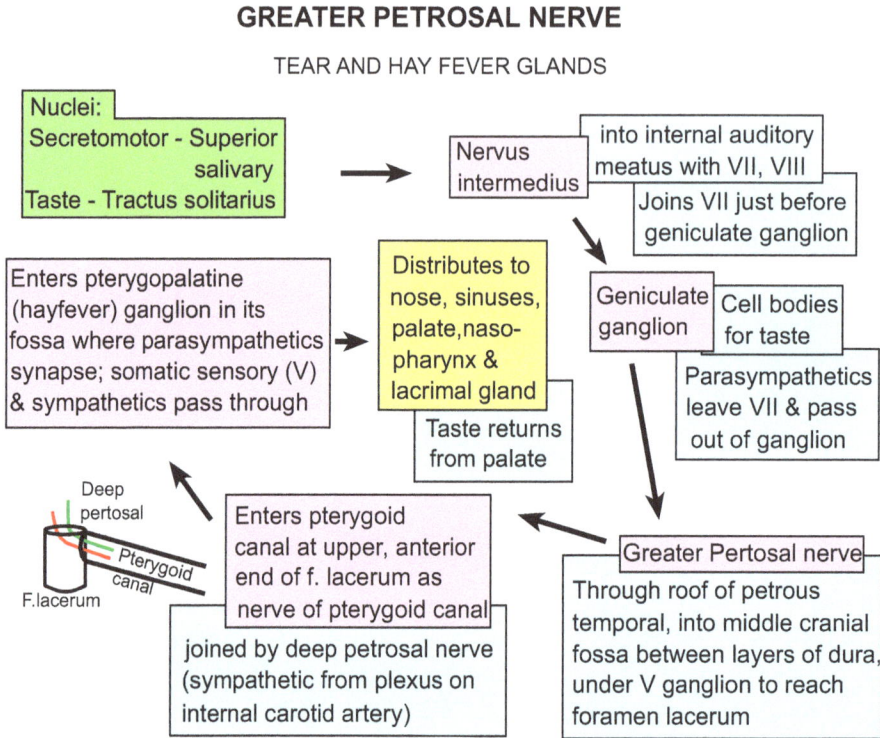

Fig. (1.3). Nucleus of greater petrosal nerve (Acknowledgments: with appreciation and thanks to Instant Anatomy. 10 Summerfield Cambridge, CB3 9HE, UK. http://www.instantanatomy.net, for their permission for using this illustration).

Lesser Petrosal Nerve (Fig. 1.4)

Nucleus of the lesser petrosal:

- Nervus intermedius: leave the cranial cavity *via* the facial nerve
  ○ Tast sensation
- Inferior salivary nucleus: leave the cranial cavity *via* glossopharyngeal nerve (CN IX) *via* Jac1bson's nerve
  ○ Salivation: for the parotid gland.

The lesser petrosal nerve (Fig. **1.4**) conveys parasympathetic (secretory) filaments from both the tympanic plexus (from glossopharyngeal nerve (CN IX) by means of Jacobson's nerve – through the facial nerve from the nervus intermedius and the inferior salivary nucleus and to the parotid gland by means of the otic ganglion. It starts at the geniculate ganglion, advancing through its own particular canal again into the middle cranial fossa, between the two dura mater layers, joining the otic ganglion by leaving the skull through foramen ovale.

LESSER PETROSAL NERVE

TO PAROTID GLAND

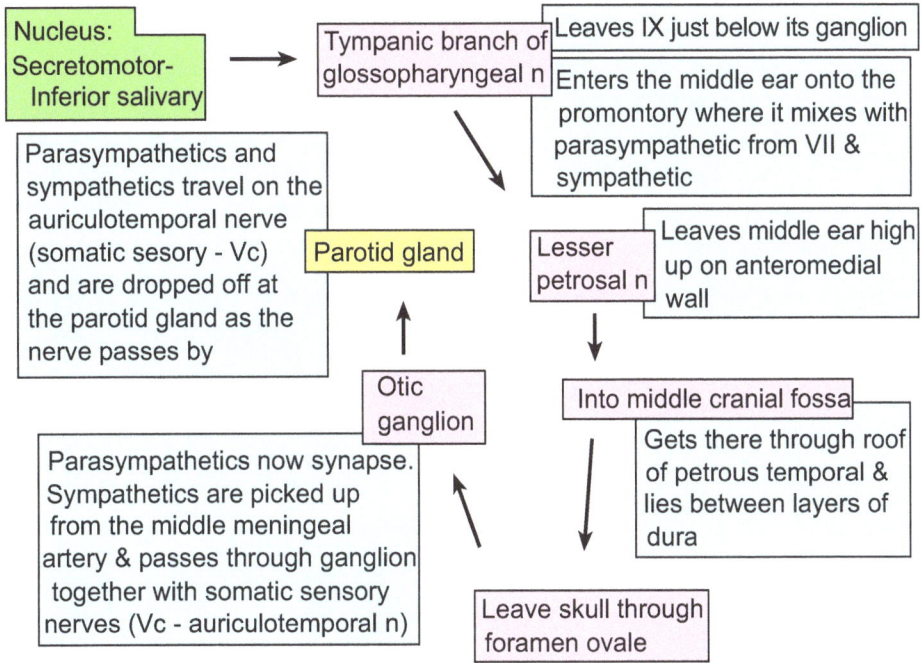

Fig. (1.4). Lesser petrosal nerve (Acknowledgment: with appreciation and thanks to Instant Anatomy. 10 Summerfield Cambridge, CB3 9HE, UK. http://www.instantanatomy.net, for their permission for using this illustration).

The external superficial petrosal nerve is a sympathetic branch, a part of the middle meningeal artery.

Chorda Tympani Nerve

Chorda tympani nerve contains filaments from two two brain stem nuclei.

- Superior salivatory nuclei
- The nucleus of tractus solitarius: Are taste neurons responsible for a taste sensation. Subsequent to synapsing in this nucleus auxiliary axons ascend in the lateral lemniscus to relay in the thalamus. This pathway then goes to the essential gustatory cortex through the posterior limb of internal capsule.

A sensory branch of facial nerve (Nervus intermedius of Wrisberg) joins the facial nerve here. It passes on individual sensory filaments from taste buds present in the anterior 2/3 of the tongue and delicate sense of taste. It additionally contains secretomotor filaments to salivary tissues present the floor of the mouth. Nerves intermedius exits the mind stem disciple to the vestibulocochlear nerve. At the level of inside sound-related meatus, it leaves this nerve, converging with the facial nerve.

Chorda tympani nerve (Fig. **1.5**): exits the facial nerve before it leaves the stylomastoid foramen. It is the facial nerve's biggest branch in its intrabody compartment (intrapetrous - inside the temporal bone's petrous part). It emerges beneath the nerve to stapedius. It navigates anterosuperiorly through the posterior canaliculus typically combined with a posterior tympanic branch of the stylomastoid artery.

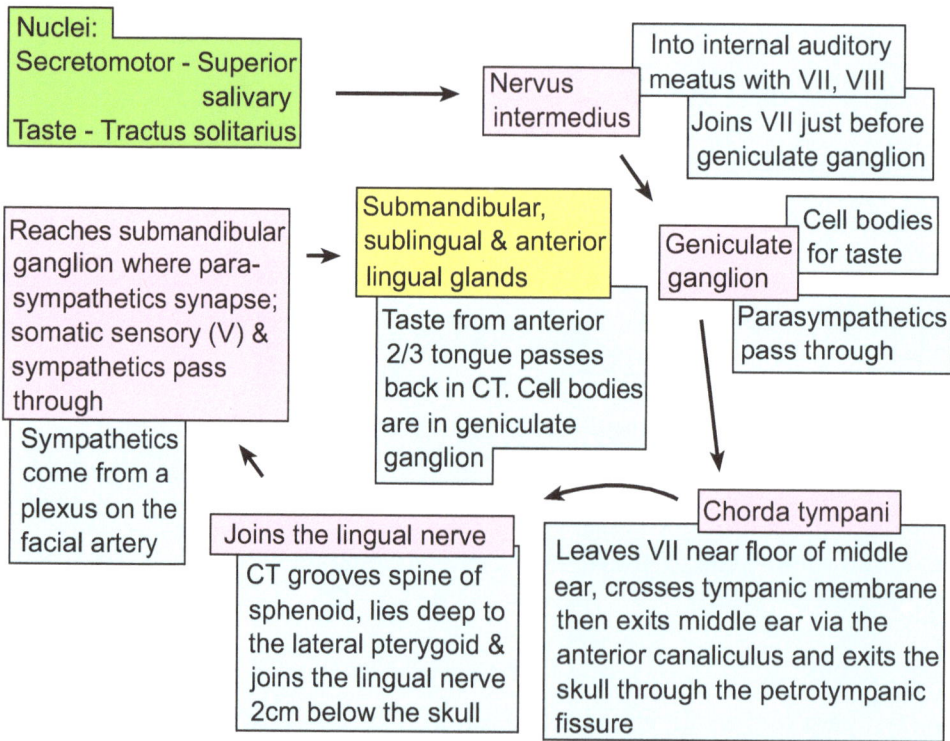

Fig. (1.5). Chorda tympani nerve (Acknowledgment: with appreciation and thanks to Instant Anatomy. 10 Summerfield Cambridge, CB3 9HE, UK. http://www.instantanatomy.net, for their permission for using this illustration).

Chorda Tympani Nerve Function

- It causes the sensation of taste from the anterior part of the tongue, specifically two third (2/3) area
- Supplies secretomotor to the salivary organs (minor and major salivary glands) present in the mouth's floor

- Conveys sensation (general sensation) from the anterior 2/3 area of tongue which includes pain and temperature
- Supplies secretomotor fibers to the submandibular and sublingual salivary glands
- Supplies the tongue with efferent vasodilator fibers.

The Ophthalmic nerve is primarily a sensory nerve (Fig. **1.6**). It is responsible for supplying:

- The cornea
- Iris
- Ciliary body
- Conjunctiva
- The lacrimal gland
- The nasal cavity mucous membrane
- The skin over eyelids, eyebrow,
- The skin over Forehead,
- And The skin over the nose

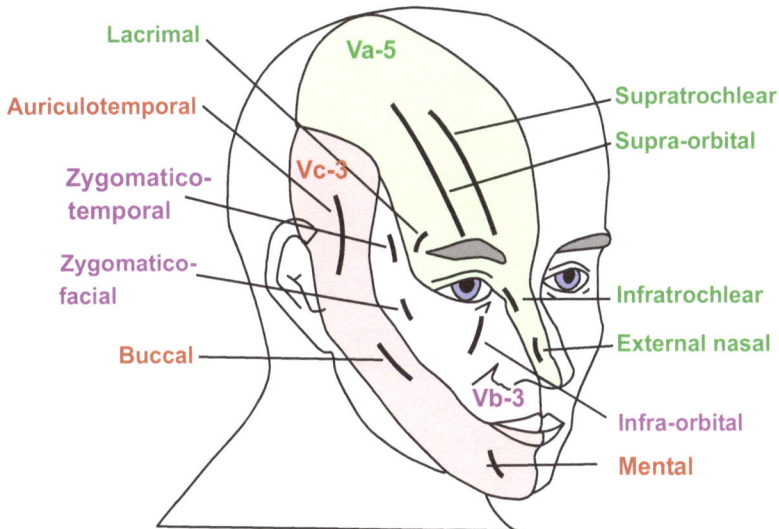

Fig. (1.6). The Ophthalmic nerve is primarily a sensory nerve (Acknowledgment: with appreciation and thanks to Instant Anatomy. 10 Summerfield Cambridge, CB3 9HE, UK. http://www.instantanatomy.net, for their permission for using this illustration).

It is the smallest trigeminal nerve branch, emerging from the ganglion's upper part known as the semilunar ganglion. It is a 2.5 cm long leveled band, travelling beneath the oculomotor and trochlear nerves, along the cavernous' lateral wall. Thereafter it enters the superior orbital fissure making its way to the orbit

- It produces three divisions:

• Nasociliary,
• Frontal,
• and Lacrimal.

The ophthalmic nerve combines with sympathetic filaments of the cavernous that communicate with the abducent, oculomotor, and trochlear nerves.

The smallest branch of the ophthalmic nerve is the lacrimal nerve. In some cases this nerve gets a fiber from the trochlear nerve, however mostly it is obtained from the branch running through the ophthalmic to the trochlear nerve. It forwards towards a separate dura mater tube, entering the orbit through the Rectus lateralis. When here it travels besides the upper surface of the Rectus lateralis, along the lacrimal artery course, and afterwards joins the maxillary nerve's zygomatic branch.

Thereby, it reaches the lacrimal glands and emits a few fibers, which are responsible in supplying the organ and the conjunctiva.

At last, it punctures the orbital septum, and joins with the facial nerve fibers and supplies the skin of the upper eyelid.

Occasionally, the zygomaticotemporal branch from maxillary takes the place of the lacrimal nerve when it is missing. At instances when only the last branch is missing, it is substituted by a continuation of the lacrimal.

The Frontal Nerve

This reaches the orbital cavity *via* the superior orbital fissure (largest branch of the ophthalmic) and keeps running between the Levator palpebrae superiors and the periosteum. As it reached halfway through the base and apex of the orbit it differentiates into, supratrochlear and supraorbital branches.

The smaller branch is the supratrochlear nerve (n. supratrochlear), which goes over the superior oblique muscle. This branch produces descending fibers which connect with the nasociliary nerve's infratrochlear branch of. Thereafter it leaves the orbit through the supraorbital foramen, on the forehead, it ascends beneath the corrugator and frontalis, and pierce these muscles after dividing into branches; it supplies the conjunctiva, upper eyelid skin and the forehead skin near the middle line.

The upper eyelid is supplied by palpebral fibers by the supraorbital nerve (n. supraorbital) which moves between the supraorbital foramen. It then travels to the temple, ending in two divisions, a lateral and medial, supplying the scalp, going till the lambdoidal suture. Initially they are present underneath the Frontalis, with the medial branch passing through the muscle, and the lateral branch through the galea aponeurotica. The pericranium is supplied by little twigs of both branches.

The orbital cavity also has the Nasociliary Nerve (n. nasociliaris; nasal nerve), entering between the lateral rectus muscle's two heads and positioned among the inferior and superior rami of the third cranial nerve. Crossing the optic nerve, it slants underneath the Obliquus and Rectus superior, present at the orbital cavity's medial wall. Thereafter it reaches the anterior ethmoidal foramen, and, travelling to the skull, crosses the lateral edge of the frontal surface of cribriform plate at a groove and the bone of ethmoid. Following its path, it passes through an opening along the edge of the crista galli, finally entering the nasal cavity. It then divides into nasal branches supplying the front part of the septum and mucous membrane of the lateral wall. At the end it forms the external nasal branch, between the lateral nasal cartilage and the lower border of the nasal bone, travelling underneath the Nasalis muscle, thereby supplying the peak of the nose and skin of the ala.

The nasociliary nerve differentiates into accompanying branches, vascularization: the lengthy foundation of the ethmoidal nerves, the ciliary ganglion and the long ciliary.

The radix longa gangili ciliaris which is the long base of the ciliary ganglion originates between the two Rectus lateralis from the nasociliary. It progresses on the optic nerve's lateral side, reaching the postero-superior point of the ciliary ganglion. Occasionally a fiber joins it from the prevalent trochlear nerve ramus or the cavernous plexus of the sympathetic.

The ciliares longi or more commonly called the long ciliary nerves are less in number and begin at the nasociliary, which passes the optic nerve. Travelling alongside the ciliary nerves, short in size, of the ciliary ganglion, they enter the posterior of the sclera, passing through it and the choroid, reach the cornea and iris. These long ciliary nerves also possess sympathetic fibers connecting the superior cervical ganglion with the Dilator pupilae muscle.

Before the nasociliary enters the anterior ethmoidal foramen, it gives rise to the infratrochlear nerve (infratrochlearis). It travels along the Rectus medialis upper surface and is united with a fiber from the supratrochlear nerve when close to the pulley of the Obliquus superior. It then reaches the medial angle of the eye, to supply the eyelids skin, lacrimal sac, conjunctiva, caruncula lacrimalis and nose's side.

The ethmoidal cells are provided by the ethmoidal branches. The branch present posteriorly supplies a few fibers to the sphenoidal sinus and exits the orbital cavity *via* the posterior ethmoidal foramen.

The Ciliary Ganglion (Fig. **1.7**), known as the lenticular or ophthalmic ganglion. The ciliary is basically a sympathetic ganglion that is small, of gray-reddish and pin sized. It is present within adipose tissues lying among the Rectus lateralis muscle and optic nerve, arranged at the back of the orbit. It generally lies on the ophthalmic artery's lateral surface. It has three roots which reach its posterior surface. The nasociliary gives rise to the sensory root. The parasympathetic motor is connected with the nucleus of oculomotor in the brainstem, the Presynaptic parasympathetic fibers derive from the Edinger-Westphal nucleus. Axons from the nucleus of Edinger-Westphal and the nucleus of oculomotor run together in the brainstem and form the oculomotor nerve. Thereafter the motor root reaches the Obliquus inferior after it originates from the branch of the oculomotor nerve. The motor root contains efferent strands of sympathetic nature (preganglionic filaments) emerging from the nucleus of the *oculomotor nerve in the brain (mid-brain) to the ciliary ganglion* where a synapse is formed with filaments of neurons.

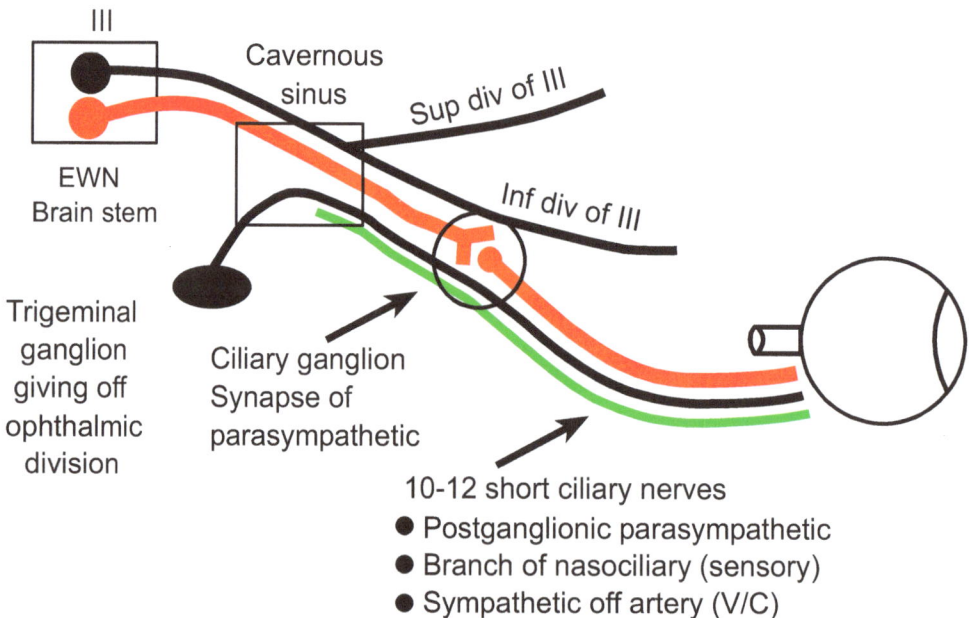

Fig. (1.7). The Ciliary Ganglion (Acknowledgment: with appreciation and thanks to Instant Anatomy. 10 Summerfield Cambridge, CB3 9HE, UK. http://www.instantanatomy.net, for their permission for using this illustration).

The postganglionic travels to the:

• Sphincter muscle of the pupil
• And Ciliary muscle.

The cavernous plexus of the sympathetic gives rise to the sympathetic root which is mostly joined with the long root.

The short ciliary nerves form its branches, which are sensitive in nature and originate from the forepart of the ganglion. They are around six to ten, divided in two groups depending upon their superior and inferior angles. The larger is the lower bundle. They travel ahead with the ciliary arteries in a wave-like course, one present above the optic nerve while the other underneath it. They are also united with the nasociliary long ciliary nerves. They reach the back of the eye glob and enter the sclera, forwarding in delicate depressions on the internal surface. These are further divided into the:

• Iris,
• Ciliary muscle,
• And Cornea.

Maxillary Nerve

• Second division of the trigeminal nerve. The maxillary nerve (Fig. **1.8**) emerges from the middle part of the trigeminal ganglion, moves along the sphenoid bone, passing the Lateral wall of the cavernous sinus, and leaves the cranium to the upper part of the pterygopalatine fossa. It then curves laterally at the infratemporal fossa through the pterygomaxillary fissure. It descends the fossa, moving forward into the infraorbital nerve through inferior orbital fissure.
• The Maxillary nerve branches in the ptrygo-palatine fossa.
• Near its origin gives meningeal branches.
• Two ganglionic branches arise in the pterygopalatine fossa which join the sphenopalatine ganglion.
• Gives off the posterior superior alveolar nerve and the zygomatic nerve while the maxillary nerve is present in the infratemporal fossa.
• The maxillary nerve continues as the infra-orbital nerve.

The infra-orbital nerve is the maxillary nerve's continuation as it reaches the inferior orbital fissure. It proceeds to the roof of maxillary antrum which is the floor of the orbit. It passes first at the infraorbital groove, and is present alongside the infra-orbital branch of the maxillary artery as well as its fellow vein. Then it reaches the infra-orbital canal and finally emerges below the infraorbital rim, through the infra-orbital foramen, into the face. Here it is under cover of the levator labii superioris and orbicularis oculi, and divided into the palpebral, nasal and labial branches.

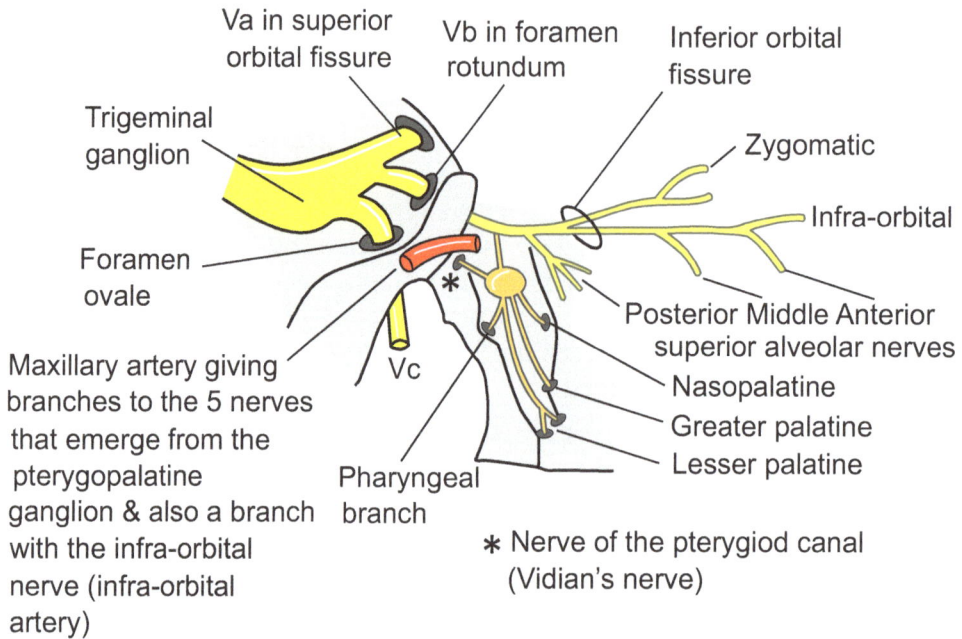

Fig. (1.8). The pterygopalatine ganglion (Acknowledgment: with appreciation and thanks to Instant Anatomy. 10 Summerfield Cambridge, CB3 9HE, UK. http://www.instantanatomy.net, for their permission for using this illustration).

The Pterygopalatine Ganglion (Fig. 1.8) (nasal ganglion, sphenopalatine ganglion)

The head and heck contain four parasympathetic ganglia:

1. The pterygopalatine ganglion,
2. The submandibular ganglion,
3. The otic ganglion,
4. and Ciliary ganglion.

The pterygopalatine is found in sphenopalatine fossa near the sphenopalatine foramen. It is a parasympathetic ganglion. It is heart-shaped, gray to reddish in color, and crosses the pterygopalatine with the maxillary nerve.

The sphenopalatine ganglion (pterygopalatine ganglion) supplies:

- The Paranasal sinuses,
- The lacrimal gland,
- The nasal cavity and nasopharynx mucosa and it,s minor salivary glands,
- The gingiva of the maxilla,
- The hard palate mucous membrane and minor salivary glands,
- It continues anteriorly as nasopalatine nerve,
- Branches of Maxillary nerve.

According to origin it may divide into four branches:

- In the pterygopalatine fossa
- On the face
- In the infraorbital canal
- and In the cranium.

- In the pterygopalatine fossa:
    - Sphenopalatine.
    - Zygomatic.
    - Posterior superior alveolar.
- In the Infraorbital Canal:
    - Anterior superior alveolar.
    - Middle superior alveolar in 28% of cadavers.
- On the Face:
    - External nasal.
    - Inferior palpebral.
    - Superior labial.
- In the cranium: Middle meningeal.
    - The middle meningeal nerve: after it originates from the semilunar ganglion, it originates from the maxillary nerve; it is running with the middle meningeal artery and provides for the dura mater.
    The Zygomatic nerve: emerges from the pterygopalatine fossa's maxillary nerve and reaches the orbital cavity *via* the inferior orbital fissure, and distributes into the following:
    - Zygomaticofacial
    - and Zygomaticotemporal. The zygomaticotemporal branch: is divided around the skin present at the side of the forehead.
    The zygomaticofacial branch: reaches the face *via* the zygomatic bone foramen. It gives supply to the skin of the cheek by perforating the orbicularis oculi.
- The pterygopalatine Branches (Sphenopalatine): two branches exist which reach

the pterygopalatine (sphenopalatine) ganglion (sensory roots).

- The superior posterior alveolar : passes in the infraorbital groove before it arises from the maxillary nerve. Usually two exist in number. They enter the mucosa and send branches to the maxillary sinus mucosa, gums, adjacent parts of the mucous layer of the cheek and all molar teeth except the first molar's mesiobuccal root.
- The middle superior alveolar nerve (*only has been reported in 28% of cadavers*): emerges from the infraorbital canal, and provides supply to two premolar teeth after passing through the maxillary antrum's lateral wall.
- The anterior superior alveolar branch: originates just before the nerve exits the infraorbital foramen; it slips in a channel in the maxillary sinus' front wall and branches to supply the canines and incisors and the 1st and 2nd premolar in 72% of cadavers.

The Inferior orbital nerve as it emerges from the face's infraorbital foramen:

- Inferior palpebral
- The Superior Labial
- The External Nasal

The Pterygopalatine Ganglion (Fig. 1.9)

Roots:

The nervus intermedius which is a part of the facial nerve gives rise to its parasympathetic root *via* the greater petrosal nerve (***it's nuclei are: Tractus Solitarus for taste sensation and Superior Salivary Nucleus as secretory motor***). Afterwards it forms the vidian nerve by joining the sympathetic root which is the deep petrosal nerve. The vidian nerve is a combination of the deep petrosal nerve (sympathetic) and the greater petrosal nerve (parasympathetic).

Sensory root is originated as two sensory branches from the maxillary nerve. The sensory root carries some of the taste fibers from the nervus intermedius to the palates both hard and soft.

Branches of the pterygopalatine ganglion:

- Lesser palatine nerve
- Greater palatine nerve
- Posterior superior lateral nasal branch
- Nasopalatine nerve
- Pharyngeal branch of the maxillary nerve

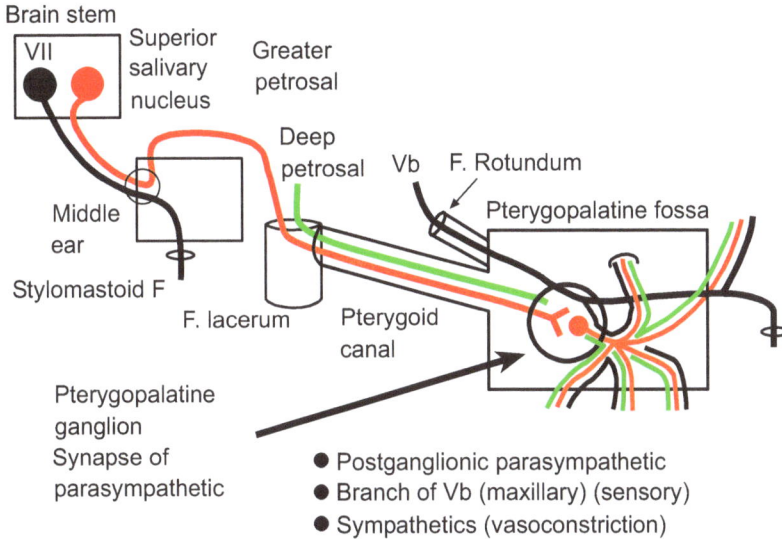

Fig. (1.9). The pterygopalatine ganglion (Acknowledgment: with appreciation and thanks to Instant Anatomy. 10 Summerfield Cambridge, CB3 9HE, UK. http://www.instantanatomy.net, for their permission for using this illustration).

Regional anatomy of maxillary nerve:

- Lateral nasal wall supplied with:
    ○ Posterior superior lateral nasal nerve – maxillary nerve
    ○ Greater palatine nerve – maxillary nerve
    ○ Nasopalatine nerve – maxillary nerve
    ○ Anterior ethmoidal nerve
- Hard palate
    ○ Greater palatine nerve
- Soft palate
    ○ Lesser palatine nerve
- Anterior maxillary teeth
    ○ Anterior superior alveolar nerve
- Maxillary premolars teeth
    ○ Middle superior alveolar nerve
- Posterior teeth except for the mesiobuccal root of 1st molar
    ○ Posterior superior alveolar nerve

The mandibular nerve (inferior maxillary nerve): provides for the:

- The skin of the temporal and auricular areas,
- Gums and teeth of the mandible,

- The lower part of the face,
- The lower lip,
- The anterior mucosa two-thirds of the tongue,
- The muscles of mastication.

Of the three trigeminal divisions, it is the largest. It consists of two roots:

- Large sensory root emerges from the lower surface of the trigeminal ganglion,
- Small motor root emerges from the motor nucleus of the trigeminal. It travels underneath the ganglion, joining the sensory root, just after few millimetres from the exit (the foramen ovale) below the skull base (Fig. **1.10**).

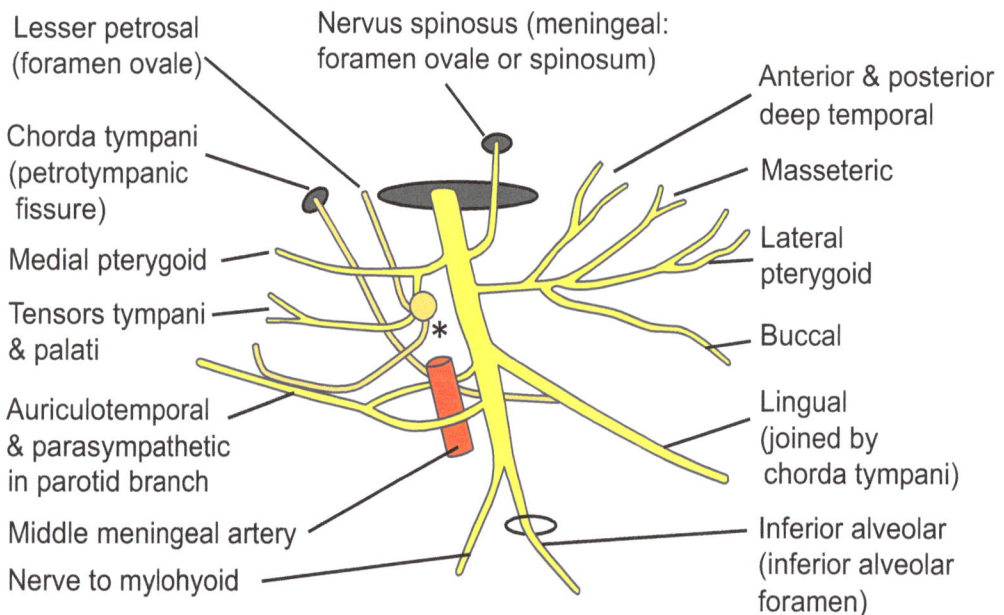

Fig. (1.10). The mandibular nerve (Acknowledgment: with appreciation and thanks to Instant Anatomy. 10 Summerfield Cambridge, CB3 9HE, UK. http://www.instantanatomy.net, for their permission for using this illustration).

Branches:
At nerve is further divided at the base of the skull, giving off:

1. Nervus spinosus (Recurrent branch)
2. The nerve to the medial pterygoid,
3. And after that branched into anterior and posterior trunks.
    1. Nervus spinosus (Recurrent branch): enter the cranium *via* the foramen oval to the foramen spinosum beside the middle meningeal artery. It moves along the main meningeal artery divisions and the dura mater is supplied. It

forms posterior and anterior branches which the posterior branch supplies as well the mastoid cells mucous lining.

2. The medial pterygoid Nerve (pterygoideus internus).

The deep muscle surface is invaded by the nerve to the medial pterygoid muscle. In addition it also sends one or two filaments towards the otic ganglion.

Then the mandibular nerve branches into:

a. Anterior division and
b. Posterior division

The Anterior Division

This division receives almost all of the trigeminal motor root fibers and is the smaller of the two divisions of the mandibular nerve. It further supplies:

• The masticatory muscles (muscles of mastication)
• The mucous membrane and skin of the cheek.

It is divided into:

1. Nerve of lateral pterygoid muscle (motor)
2. The masseteric (motor),
3. Deep temporal (motor),
4. Long buccal nerve (sensory).

The Masseteric Nerve passes the mandibular notch along with the masseteric artery, reaching the Masseter's deep surface; it gives fibers to the temporomandibular joint.

The Deep Temporal Nerves enter the Temporalis' deep surface after turning upward over the lateral pterygoid muscle's upper head.

The long buccal nerve goes through the pterygoid muscle, between its two heads. It descends underneath or through the lower part of the Temporalis; branches on the surface of the Buccinator after rising from under the anterior surface of the Masseter. The buccal nerve supplies the buccal mucous membrane lining of the mouth and the skin over the Buccinator muscle.

The nerve of lateral pterygoid muscle: This nerve frequently arises in conjunction with the long buccal nerve.

The Posterior Division

The larger division on the mandibular nerve is the posterior division. It is basically sensory, yet gets a couple of the motor root fibers. It branches into:

1. Lingual,
2. Auriculotemporal,
3. Inferior alveolar nerves.

The Auriculotemporalis, commonly known as Auriculotemporal Nerve, originates from two roots, present among the middle meningeal course and rises to the foramean ovale. It reaches the neck's medial side of the mandible after running in reverse underneath the lateral pterygoid muscle. Afterwards, it rotates upward along with the superficial temporal artery, located between the mandibular condyle and mandibular auricula, beneath the front of the parotid gland. Passing this gland, it rises above the zygomatic arch, and terminates with superficial temporal branches.

The otic ganglion (Fig. **1.11**) is a small parasympathetic ganglion located in the infratemporal fossa medially to the surface of the mandibular nerve and below the foramen ovale.

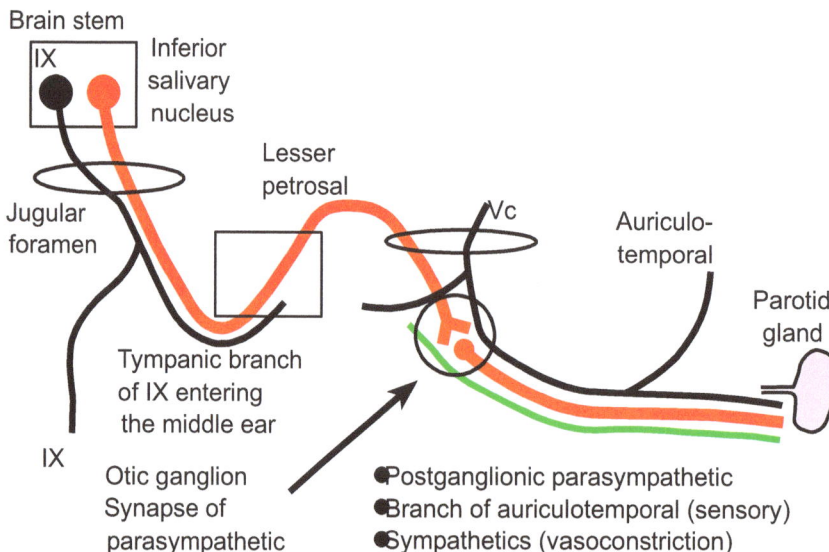

Fig. (1.11). The otic ganglion (Acknowledgment: with appreciation and thanks to Instant Anatomy. 10 Summerfield Cambridge, CB3 9HE, UK. http://www.instantanatomy.net, for their permission for using this illustration).

It receives the fibers that are pre-ganglionic of the glossopharyngeal nerve and innervates the parotid gland for salivation.The parasympathetic pre-ganglionic nucleus of the otic ganglion located at the inferior salivary nucleus.

Pre-ganglionic fibers leave the glossopharyngeal nerve with the tympanic branch and then the lesser petrosal and the tympanic plexus nerve pass to join the otic ganglion, the fibers synapse, and the postganglionic fibers are given to joining auriculotemporal nerve, which supplies the parotid gland. They produce vasodilator and secretomotor effects.

It divides into the following branches:

- Temporal region
- Parotid
- The external acoustic meatus
- Anterior auricular.

The Lingual Nerve, known as the lingualis, reaches:

- The mucosa of the anterior two-third areas of the tongue.
  It passes initially below the lateral pterygoid muscle in the front and medial to the inferior alveolar nerve, it forms an acute angle to join the chorda tympani. The nerve then travels among the ramus of the mandible and medial pterygoid muscle, crossing obliquely over the superior Constrictor muscle present at the tongue's side and the styloglossus. Moving ahead it moves between the areas between the submandibular glands's deep part and the Hyoglossus, finally reaching through the submandibular gland duct, towards the tongue's tip, present beneath the mucous membrane.

Its branches reach to provide supply to:

- The submandibular gland,
- The sublingual gland,
- The gums,
- The mucous membrane of the mouth,
- And the anterior two-thirds tongue's mucous membrane.

The largest division of the posterior part of mandibular nerve is the inferior alveolar nerve. It moves down towards the inferior alveolar artery, initially underneath the lateral pterygoid muscle, and later within the sphenomandibular ligament and the mandibular ramus, reaching the mandibular foramen. Thereafter it moves to the mandibular canal, positioned under the teeth, towards the mental foramen, separating into two terminal divisions, mental and incisive.

Mylohyoid nerve emerges from the inferior alveolar as it reaches the mandibular foramen. It innervates the Digastric muscle's anterior belly and mylohyoid after passing through the medial surface of the ramus of the mandible, and entering the lower surface of the mylohyoid.

The dental branches known as the inferior alveolar nerve provide for the molar and premolar teeth. The incisive branch of the inferior alveolar nerve supplies the incisor teeth and canine.

The mental nerve leaves the mandibular canal through the mental foramen which located in most instances between the 1st and 2nd premolars, and supply:

• The lower lip's mucous membrane and skin,
• The skin of the chin.

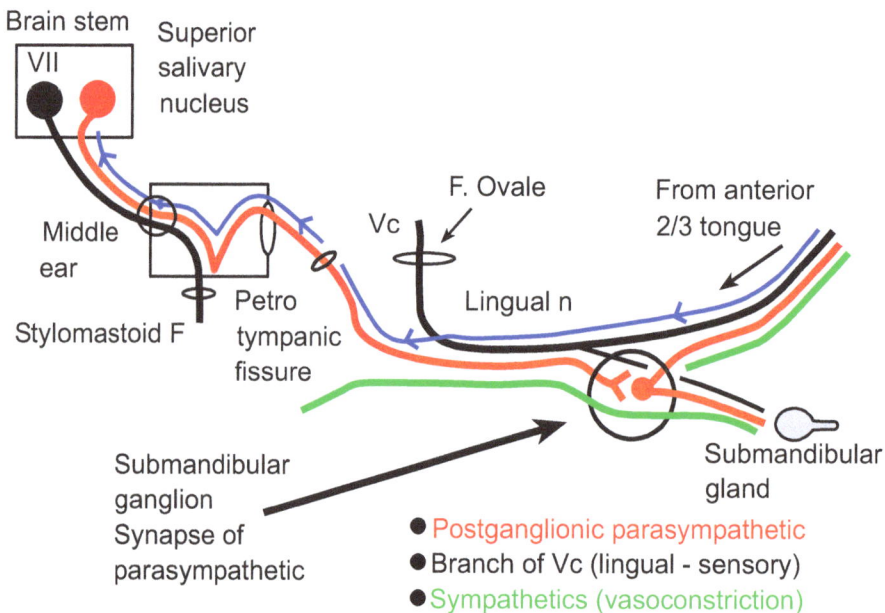

Fig. (1.12). Submandibular Ganglion (Acknowledgment: with appreciation and thanks to Instant Anatomy. 10 Summerfield Cambridge, CB3 9HE, UK. http://www.instantanatomy.net, for their permission for using this illustration).

Submandibular Ganglion (Fig. **1.12**): The submandibular ganglion is fusiform and small in size. It is located on the submandibular gland's medial surface, the hyoglossus, present close to the mylohyoid's posterior border. The anterior and posterior parts of the ganglion are connected with two fibers to the lingual nerve. At the posterior end, it joins the chorda tympani nerve's branch, passing through the lingual sheath. Such are the preganglionic efferent sympathetic filaments of the facial nerve and the superior salivatory nucleus.

Roots of submandibular ganglion:

- Nervus intermedius: leave the cranial cavity *via* the facial nerve
  - Taste sensation
- Superior salivary nucleus: leave the cranial cavity *via* facial nerve
- Salivation: for the minor the salivary glands at the nose, plate

Its branches supply:

- The mucous membrane of the mouth
- The sublingual gland,
- Submandibular gland
- The anterior two-thirds tongue's mucous membrane,
- And the gums.

Summary for sensory dental innervations (Fig. **1.13**):

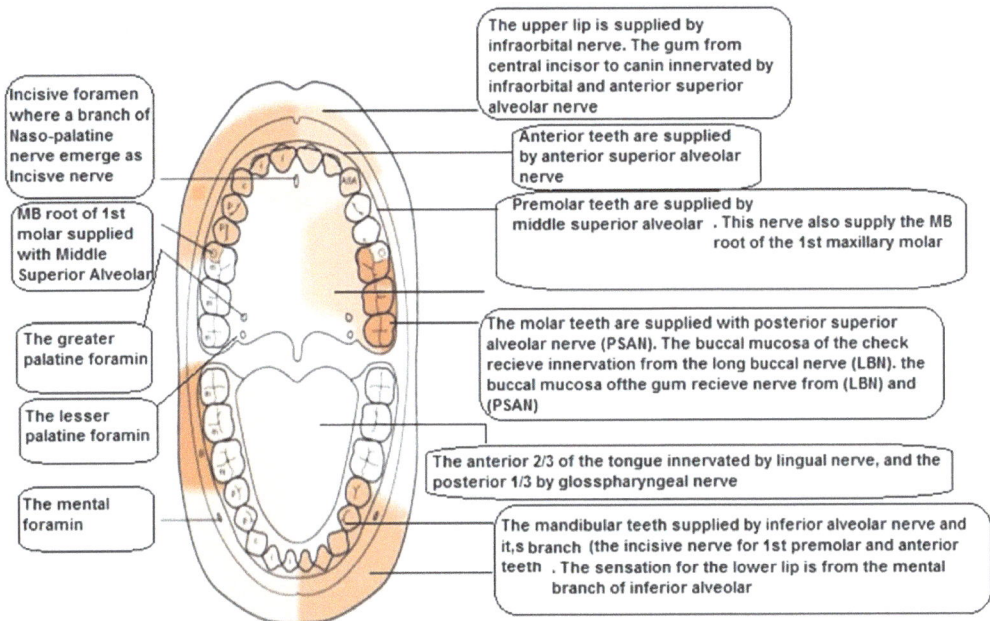

Fig. (1.13). Summary for sensory dental innervations. The middle superior alveolar nerve is present in 28% of anatomically dissected cadavers, in the remaining 72% this nerve can not be recognized and the premolars are mostly supplied by posterior superior alveolar nerve.

BIBLIOGRAPHY

[1]   Sinnatamby CS, Last RJ. Last's anatomy: regional and applied. Edinburgh: Elsevier/Churchill Livingstone 2006.

[2]   Gray H, Clemente CD. Anatomy of the human body. Philadelphia: Lea & Febiger 1985.

[3]   Instant Anatomy. Learn human anatomy online Available at: https://www.instantanatomy.co.uk/

Physiology of Pain

Esam Ahmad Z Omar[*]

Department of Oral & Maxillofacial Surgery, College of Dentistry, Taibah University, Madinah, Saudi Arabia

Abstract: In this chapter, the mechanism of pain, pain pathway from Oro-facial area and the physiological principle of pain have been discussed in detail. In order to understand the mode of action of local anesthesia, it is essential to understand the pain physiology. This chapter contains the essential details of pain physiology that may be needed for an understanding of the mechanism of local anesthesia. The endogenous analgesic system is an important modulator part for pain intensity and a major contributor to pain gate theory, all that has been discussed in a concise and precise way to give the complex information in a simple way to understand and remember.

Keywords: Endogenous pain killer system, Impulse generation, Pain fibers, Pain pathway, Pain physiology, Principle of pharmacology for pain management.

PART 1 - ACTION POTENTIAL

Action Potential

An *impulse* of electrical nature comprising of self-spreading series of depolarization and repolarization, transmitted over the plasma membrane of neurons, as the nerve impulse is transmitted passes over the plasma membrane of the neural and muscular cells when it is contracting.

The Resting Membrane Potential

When the neuron is not actively sending signals, it is referred as being at a state of 'Rest Membrane Potential.' The cell membrane of neurons possesses a pump of protein nature that is known as the sodium-potassium pump (Na+ K+ ATPase). The cell membrane at rest utilizes active transport by using ATP energy to pump three sodium ions out of the neuron (3 Na+) and two potassium ions (2 K+) into the cell (Table **2.1** shows the concentration of different essential ions around the cell membrane of the neuron).

[*] **Corresponding author Esam Ahmad Z Omar:** Department of Oral & Maxillofacial Surgery, College of Dentistry, Taibah University, Madinah, Saudi Arabia; Tel: 0569536708; Fax: 00966148494710; E-mail: esamomar@hotmail.com

Table 2.1. Ions concentration within and outside the excited cell at a state of rest.

Ions	Inside cell/mmol dm^{-3}	Outside cell/mmol dm^{-3}	Ions move down their concentration gradient
Potassium (K+)	150.0	2.5	The buildup of positive charges outside the cell membrane prevents potassium ions from moving out of the neuron down their concentration gradient.
Sodium (Na+)	15.0	145.0	
Chloride (Cl-)	9.0	101.0	The negatively charged protein molecules prevent Cl- ions from the movement of these ions into the cytoplasm.

Graded Potentials

Graded potentials (or receptor potentials) are temporary hyperpolarization or depolarization within a specific area of the plasma membrane that is able to produce changes causing local flow of current in response to stimuli that reduces separation.

The receptor potential's magnitude is an indication of and directly related to the intensity of the stimulus. When the strength of the stimulus is high, it causes greater molecule channels to open and thereby a greater voltage change, whether it is depolarization or hyperpolarization. As a result, the current travels farther (Table **2.2**).

Table 2.2. Comparison of Graded Potentials (GP) with Action Potentials (AP) features.

GP (Graded Potentials)	AP (Action Potentials)
The signals are short-distance.	The signals are long-distance.
Stimulus-dependent magnitude.	Non-Magnitude and dependent on stimulus (magnitude is stable).
Local current flow signal.	Saltatory conduction (myelinated nerve) and local current (not-myelinated nerve). Flow depends on the presence of my-line sheath.
The signal magnitude disappears as it runs away from the stimulus.	The signal magnitude is continued and propagated along the length of the excitatory cell.
Synapses and receptors are the areas of initiation.	The axon hillock is the area of impulse propagation and flow.
Activity is hyperpolarization or depolarization.	Depolarization is the only activity.

Definitions

Threshold is the amount of stimulus at the level of the receptors (Graded potentials or **receptor potentials**) needed to start the action potential.

If the stimulus strength is high enough to cause depolarization crossing a basic critical level then the layer keeps on depolarizing alone, and does not depend on the stimulus. The threshold edge is roughly 20mV less negative as compared to the resting membrane potential. When threshold edge is achieved (-55mV), depolarization occurs automatically.

Depolarization takes place as the membrane potential reaches a less negative figure (the threshold point), shifting towards zero, making the neuron more excitable. It occurs through the activation of the voltage-gated Na^+ channels, allowing the influx of Na^+ ions into the neuron.

Repolarization is the point at which a cell layer's charge comes back to negative after depolarization. This occurs when the Na^+ channel gates become inactive and closed. At the same time, the K^+ channel gates become active and open, causing movement of K^+ outside the neuron.

Hyperpolarization happens when the layering potential turns out to be more negative, moving far from zero, and below the rest membrane potential.

After-hyperpolarization occurs by increasing Potassium (K^+) ion permeability. The neuron's membrane potential is far from the point of threshold causing the cell to undergo a **relative refractory period (RRP)**. The neuron needs an extraordinary stimulus to create an activity (action potential). These activities (depolarization and hyperpolarization signs) are transient. The neuron's membrane potential returns back to its resting state, once the stimulus is removed.

Action Potentials

Electrical signals travelling long distances are called *action potentials* (Fig. **2.1**). These signs move along the entire neuronal membrane. In graded potentials the greatness of the sign disseminates, however, the size of the activity potential is kept up all through the length of the axon. Furthermore, action potentials are not stimulus dependent as the graded potentials. The magnitude of action potentials always remains constant.

Action potentials of similar magnitudes exist. A supra-threshold activator (stimuli), one that is bigger than the expected value and requires depolarizing the plasma membrane essentially to threshold, does not form greater action potentials, rather, it increases recurrence (*frequency*) of action potential production and generation.

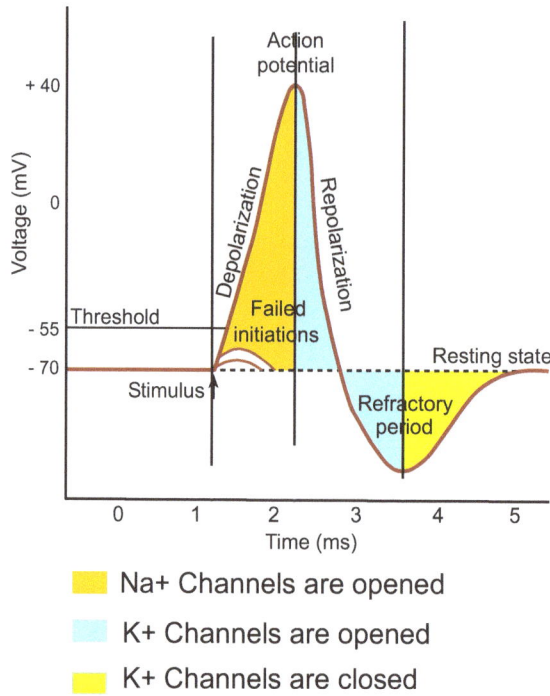

Fig. (2.1). Steps of action potential.

The permeability of K+ ions and Na+ ions through voltage-gated ion channels are the key for the generation of an action potential. However, changes in permeability occur at distinctive times (Fig. **2.2**). Voltage-gated channels direct *open* and *close* because of changes in membrane potential. At first, a boost (stimulus) will bring about membrane depolarization towards a constant specific limit (threshold).

Steps of action potential (Fig. **2.1**):

Depolarization

The Na$^+$ channels, which are voltage gated, begin to open, resulting in entrance of Na$^+$ ions into the cell as a result of both, electrical and concentration gradients. The flood of Na+ ions (influx of Na+ ions) brings about additional depolarization, causing more Na+ channels to open, precipitating the influx of Na+ ions, *etc*. This procedure continues until the membrane is depolarized to the maximum threshold level and soon thereafter a greater part of the Na+ channels allow Na+ ions movement which is fast and plentiful. The penetrability to Na+ particles is around

600 times greater at this point than ordinary. This particle flux results in an upward spike in the activity potential. This period of the activity of the action potential with (+) charges influx causes the cell membrane to reverse polarity. The membrane potential at the top of the activity of action potential is +30mV.

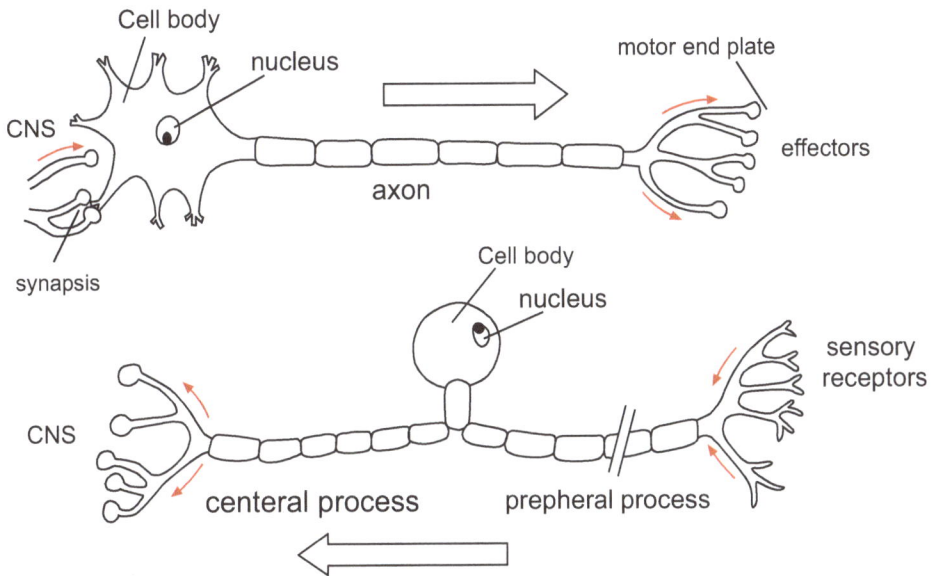

Fig. (2.2). Types of the neurons.

Repolarization

The open Na+ channels are shut approximately after 1msec, in this manner controlling further influx of (+) charge into the cell. In the meantime, K+ channels, which are also voltage-gated, open, causing K+ particles leave the cell down their electrical and concentration gradient. During this period of activity, K^+ ions permeability is around 300 times greater than ordinary. The efflux of (+) charge causes repolarization. Repolarization is a change of the membrane potential towards a resting state.

As Sodium-channels are more voltage sensitive, so it opens more rapidly than K+ channels and small depolarization is adequate to open them. Fortunately, to open K+ channels there is a need for larger changes in membrane potential to further cell excitation as K+ channels are less sensitive to voltage. This explains the reason for the opening of K+ ion channels later to Na+ ion channels.

This is practically important because if both ion channels open simultaneously, an adjustment in membrane potential occurs due to Na+ ion influx countering the K+ ion efflux resulting in no generation of action potential.

Action potential would not be achieved again as Na$^+$ channels cannot reopen until voltage-gated channels resume their resting state. The neuron should be repolarized to -70 mV first from the existing action potential. This duration when all the Na$^+$ channels are open till their inactivation is known as the absolute refractory period characterized as such because no new activity can be created. The period lasts roughly 2-msec, limiting the quantity of activities of action potential and can create upwards of 500 neurons every second.

After-Hyperpolarization

The rise in K+ ions permeability is a long process because the voltage-gated K+ channels close and open gradually. Therefore, K+ particles keep on exiting the cell, causing membrane potential to reach an equilibrium potassium potential. This period is known as after-hyperpolarization. As the membrane potential furthers from the threshold, extraordinary stimulus is required to cause depolarization. At the occurrence of hyperpolarization, it is more difficult but still possible, for the excitatory cell (neuron) to produce another potential activity. This relative refractory period continues after the absolute refractory period until the K+ voltage-gated channels return to their resting state, with the neural membrane at resting potential.

Refractory Period: is necessary to enable the voltage-sensitive glycol-protein (ion channels) to return to their original polarity.

- When a neuron is in the **absolute refractory period:** a second activation or stimuli will **not** cause a new action potential (Na+ channels are recovering or open).
- The **relative refractory period** is a period of relative inactivity as a second action potential would **only** be created if the stimulus activator is extraordinarily greater than normal threshold (Occurs when the K+ channels are opened and the membrane is in a hyperpolarized state (-80mV). Generation action potentials are more difficult during this relative period compared with rest of the membrane potential.

Summary of Action Potential

- Graded potential or (**receptor potential)** initiates action potential by increasing the membrane permeability to Na+ down its concentration gradient. Threshold point is the key for initiation of an action potential if the threshold point of membrane depolarization is achieved.
- Na+ channel is a voltage-sensitive channel, it is opened by changes generated by receptors potential and is closed when the voltage reaches +30. K+ channel is opened at a voltage of +30 and closed when the voltage approaches less than -70

(hyperpolarized point) as it is closed slowly, hyperpolarization is developed.

1. **Depolarization**: Receptor potentials generate a change in membrane potential from -70 mV to -55 mV. The voltage-gated Na+ ion channels are sensitive to these changes, which are enough to open gates for the influx of Na+. The flow (influx) of Na+ causes changes in the polarity of the neuron and the cell becomes more positive. When a positive charge inside the cell approaches +30 mV, the Na+ gate closes and voltage-gated K+ ion channels activate.

2. **Repolarization**: Voltage-gated K+ channels are less sensitive than voltage-gated Na+ channels, this explains the late activation of the K+ channels when a change in the voltage approaches +30 mV, allowing a 0.5ms opening of potassium channels causing K+ ions efflux, for restoring the original polarity of the neuron, this is called repolarization.

3. The 'overshoot' in the K+ ions movement as the polarity restored is called (**hyperpolarization**). The **after-hyperpolarization** is a restoration of the resting potential membrane state by using Na+ ATPase and K+ ATPase (active pump).

Conduction of the Action Potential (Impulse Transmission)

Types of impulse propagation (conduction - transmission):

1. Local current flow (Non-myelinated nerve).
2. Saltatory conduction (Myelinated axons - faster): differs from local current flows as it results in a greater increase of conduction velocity and propagation down the axon, along nerve fibers.

The neuron (Nerve cell) comprises of four integral parts:

1. Axon terminal.
2. Axon.
3. Axon hillock.
4. Cell body.

The cell body of the excitatory cells (neuron) contains a nucleus and organelles that are essential for cell functions and activity, including, synthesis of protein, transportation of materials and production of energy. A neuron additionally has unique parts that permit data and information transmission in the form of impulses. Dendrites are branch-like structures that receive signals. The axon, which frequently looks like a long tail, takes impulse messages away from the cell. The axon closes in a terminal containing connectors called neurotransmitters, which permits the sign to move over the space between the neurons (synaptic cleft) to sends data and information to adjacent neurons. Whenever axons and dendrites of various cells are clustered together, they produce nerve fibers (Fig. **2.2**).

- Sensory neurons: conduct nerve action potential (impulse) from tactile and sensory receptors to the central nervous system (CNS- Brain and Spinal cord).
- Efferent neurons – transmit the impulse towards CNS.
- Relays information (messages) from CNS to the muscles and other organs. The cell body of the neuron is not involved in impulse transmission, and it is just for metabolic purposes.

Motor neurons: to the muscles and organs:

- The cell body is a part of the neuron and included in drive (impulse) transmission.
  Interneurons: interconnected cells in the nervous system, with numerous interconnections.
- Relays message from sensory and motor neurons.
- Makeup the central nervous system (spinal cord and brain).

Dendrites of the cell body, projections expanding surface range, and the cell body are sites responsible for communication with different neurons. These sites receive inputs, which initiate graded potentials that travel a short distance to where axons originate from the cell body known as the axon hillock. Adequate neuronal stimulation results in an action potential at the site of axon hillock. Thereafter, it is necessary that this action potential be regenerated, as well as propagated until it reaches the axon, the third partition of the neuron.

The axon, also known as nerve fiber, is primarily a projection of the cell body that is prolonged for the purpose of transmission of action potentials towards other cells. The terminal part of the neuron is called the axon terminal, whereby neuronal communication occurs with one or multiple cells by a specific method.

The axon hillock area is responsible for generation of action potential. This area of a neuron is especially excitable due to high presentation of Na+ voltage-gated channels. As the axon hillock receives excitatory input and is stimulated, there is a prominent flow (influx) of Na+ particles and the plasma membrane becomes positive within the cell, result in an action potential, while the remaining part of the axon maintains a resting state (rest membrane potential) and is negative from the inside. Similarly, as with reviewed possibilities and graded potentials, local current flow is the method of spread of the signals.

This present stream depolarizes the new nerve region, increasing sodium ions (Na+ ions) permeability of the plasma cell membrane through channels controlled by the voltage. The consequent flood of Na+ ions depolarizes the cell membrane further with the goal of achieving its limit. This results in generation of another action potential. In the meantime, the axon hillock, being the first site of an action potential repolarizes, because of the efflux of potassium ions (K+). This makes the initiation of new action potential impossible sequentially along this part of the axon. Thereby, the impulse helps sustain quality during transmission to the axon terminal.

Some type of neural axon is wrapped around with lipid sheath at regular intervals, which are called Myelin. Schwann cells are producers for nervous myelin; the myelin is not considered as a part of the axon. The myelin (lipid sheath) consists of multiple layers of lipids wrapping the axon of a neuron. This lipid provides greater protection, keeping the development of current over the cell membrane of the neuron.

The Action potential cannot be created (generated) in the region of the axon cover with myelin. Rather, this occurs just at the myelin sheath gaps known as the Nods of Ranvier. These nods are situated around 1 to 2 mm distance. The stream of current (impulse) from a dynamic nod "skips" along the axon to the nearby nod to bring about depolarization and initiate another new activity (potential). This conduction of the action potential (impulse), jumping of impulse between the node of Ranvier known as (Saltatory Conduction).

Factors that affect speed of action potential conduction:

1- Myelinated Axons (Saltatory Conduction):
The Saltatory impulse transmission results in prominent rise in speed of impulse conduction as compared to that of local unmyelinated axon's current flow. The speed of propagation and conduction of the impulse is specifically related to the earnestness of the data passed on by a given neuron. Nerve filaments are conveying less vital data, for example, those controlling low digestive procedures, are unmyelinated. A case of a nerve fiber with myelin is one that is responsible for innervating skeletal muscle, so that developments may take place quickly (Fig. **2.3**).

Another advantage of myelin presence along an axon is that it results in a more energetically efficient impulse transmission. Since action potential happens just at the Nods of Ranvier, less K+ and Na+ ions move all through the cell membrane. In this way, low metabolic vitality is needed for these ions to return to their original rest membrane state.

Node of Ranvier

Area of Relative Refractory Period

Area of absolute Refractory Period

Area of stimulation (Action Potantial)

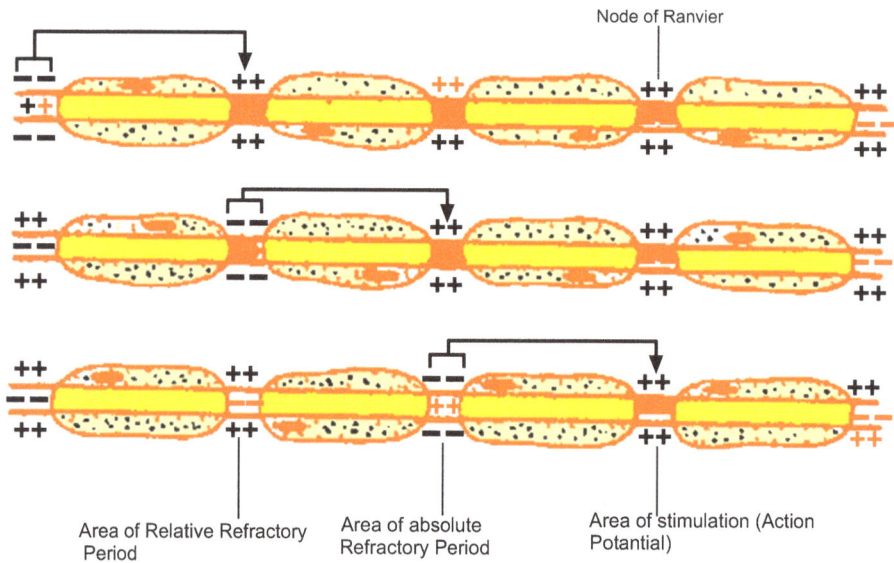

Fig. (2.3). The saltatory conduction takes place in myelinated axons.

2- The Diameter of the Axon:

Axon diameter is an important factor in determining the speed of action potential conduction. The impulse velocity through the axon depends on the diameter of the axon (Table **2.3**). As the diameter increases, resistance to impulse flow decreases along the axon.

The action potential impulse transmission is unidirectional along the axon. Nerve impulses run from the axon hillock and the cell body, moving towards the terminal part of the axon. As the present impulse streams from the initial region of movement to the nearby area, the new area of axon depolarizes and produces an impulse (action potential). Simultaneously, the previous region reaches its ARP (absolute refractory period) because of sodium gate inactivation. The impulse, therefore, travels away from the subsequent active region. The current continues unidirectional and depolarizes the following adjoining area of the axon. During this time, the original site is capable of being re-stimulated after recovery from the refractory period; the activity potential is present at a great distance along the axon to influence this site by a method for neighborhood current stream. This unidirectional conduction guarantees that the sign achieves the axon terminal, a site having impact on the movement of the innervated cell rather than going forward and backward along the axon inadequately.

Table 2.3. Diameter of the Axon and the Velocity of Conduction.

Fiber Type(s)	Name	Subtype	Diameter (mm)	Conduction Velocity (m/s)
Myelinated Somatic Afferent/Efferent				
Cutaneous afferent	A	β	6–12	35–75
		δ	1–5	5–30
Muscle afferent	A	α	12–21	80–120
		β	6–12	35–75
		δ	1–5	5–30
Muscle efferent	A		6–12	35–75
Anterior horn cells (α and γ motor neurons)				
Myelinated Autonomic Efferent				
Preganglionic efferent	B		3	3–15
Unmyelinated Somatic/Autonomic Afferent/Efferent				
Postganglionic efferent	C		0.2–1.5	1–2
Afferent to dorsal root ganglion (pain)	C		0.2–1.5	1–2
Sensory Receptor	Fiber Type			
Hair follicle	Aβ			
Skin follicle	Aβ			
Muscle spindle	Aα			
Joint receptor	Aβ			
Pain, temperature	Aδ, C			

Pain is a defensive functional process that alerts a person to the event of tissue harm (injuries). Activation of pain receptors (nociceptors) modifies permeability of membrane towards ions. The major effect of this is the influx of Na+ particles due to their electrical gradients and concentration slopes. Adequate Na+ particle convergence (influx) causes an impulse (action potential) that travels along the ascending neuron to the central nervous system (CNS) and pain centers where painful perception takes place.

Nearby analgesics, for example, lidocaine and procaine anticipate or calm the view of pain by interfering with the anxious impulse being conducted. These medications tie to a particular site on the Na+ voltage-gated channels and suppresses ion development. Without Na+ ion movement, an activity of action potential cannot be produced in the afferent neurons and the signs neglect to reach the CNS. As a rule, the activity of these medications is confined to the site of use and turns out to be a less endless supply of the medication far from the site of activity in the nerve.

Generally, there are five theories in explanation of the mode of action of local anaesthesia:

- Acetylcholine Theory.
- Ca++ Displacement Theory.
- Surface charging Theory.
- Membrane Expansion Theory.
- Specific Receptor Theory.

1. **Acetylcholine Theory:**
   The action of acetylcholine takes place at the nerve synapses where it acts as a neurotransmitter. It also plays a part in nerve conduction. However, no evidence exists to support this theory.

2. **Calcium Displacement Theory:**
   LA produces its effects by movement of Ca2' from a membranous site regulating Na permeability. Facts establish that LA potency is not affected if Ca2' ion concentration is varied around the nerve.

3. **Surface Charge Theory:**
   According to this theory, the membrane surface undergoes electrical potential alteration as the local anesthetics binds to the membrane of the nerve. Drug molecules of cat-ionic (RNH+) line up at the membrane exchange interface and make neuron's action potential more positive at the membrane surface. As a result, the excitability of the nerve decreases and the threshold potential expands.
   - **Demerits of the Theory:**
     - Rest membrane potential of the nerve is unaltered by local aesthetics.
     - Action of local aesthetics conventionally does not occur at the surface of the cellular membrane, instead it works within membrane channels.
     - This theory is unable to describe what happens to uncharged anesthetic molecules for the purposes of nerve impulse blocking (*e.g.* Lignocaine).

4. **Membrane Expansion Theory:**
   The lipid soluble local anesthetics penetrate the lipid part of the cell membrane thereby, altering the nerve membrane's configuration. As Na channels decrease in diameter, the neural excitation and Na conduction is inhibited. This theory is beneficial as it explains un-ionized drugs like benzocaine and the effect of local anesthetics on them.

5. **Specific Receptor Theory:**
   - The action of local aesthetics occurs as they bind to specific Na+ channel receptors. Such receptors may be present outside or inside the Axoplasmic surface.
   - After aesthetic substances attaches with Na+ receptors, the sodium ion permeability is greatly impacted, and in certain cases are completely

diminished causing interference in nerve conduction.

○ External Receptor sites: naturally occurring Biotoxins - Saxitoxin and Tetrodotoxin act on external receptors thus, blocking influx of Na+ ions.

○ Internal Receptor sites: As Na+ permeability suddenly increases, Ca2' ions are released from sites within the cell membrane. Local anesthetics are in competition for the same receptor with Ca. Thus, Ca2 is displaced by LA; preventing initiation of depolarization.

○ All local anesthetics are amphipathic, *i.e.* they posses both, Lipophilic and Hydrophilic characters.

○ Basic molecular structure of local anesthetic agents: The pKa (pKa = -log pKa), The Acid Dissociation Constant, Ka, is the harmony constant for the response in which a weak acid is in balance with its counterpart base in the fluid arrangement. The balance expression beneath the concentration of water is excluded. This is because water is vastly in excess and changes its amount insignificantly on balance being built up. Ka can be considered as a MAC (modified equilibrium constant). A Molecule's affinity for Hydrogen ions is measured through the dissociation constant, pKa.

○ The smaller the pKa value, the more acidic solution is. Ka is a superior measure of the strength and quality of an acid than pH. This is because as more water is added to the acid solution will not change the constant Ka (the value of the equilibrium constant), however, it will change the H+ particle concentration on which pH depends.

How to calculate drug absorption by pKa?

Percent-Ionized Formula:

$$\frac{100}{1+10^{x\,(pH\,-\,Pka)}}$$

Where x = - 1 if acidic medication or 1 if alkaline medication.

Fundamental Rules:

• pKa is characterized as the pH where medication exists as *half ionized* and half *un-ionized.*
• If pKa - pH = 0, then half is un-ionized and half of medication is ionized.
• Acid in an acid solution will not ionize.
• An acid in an alkaline solution will ionize.
• Alkaline in an alkaline solution will not ionize.
• Alkaline in an acidic solution will ionize.

If pKa - pH = 0.5, then the three courtiers of solution will be ionized (75% ionized) and only one courtier will be in non-ionized form (25% un-ionized), or three courtiers of solution will be non-ionized (75% non-ionized) and only one courtier will be in ionized form (25% ionized).

If pKa - pH > 1 then the arrangement is 99-100% un-ionized or 99-100% ionized.

Charged cat-ions and uncharged base is related to the solution's pH and the compound's PKG. When these two are the same, the drug exists half in base form and the other half in cat-ions. This relationship is related by pH = PKG-log (RNH+-RN). The relative proportion of charged cat-ions and a free base in the LA is largely dependent on the solution's pH and the compound's PKG remains constant.

PART 2 - PHYSIOLOGY OF PAIN

The International Association for the Study of Pain defines *pain* as, *"An unpleasant sensory and emotional experience arising from actual or potential tissue damage"*.

Nociceptors

Nociceptors are free nerve endings; with no adaptation, or continued response to stimuli that repeat or are sustained. It is responsible for awareness of the damaging stimuli. It is branched in the skin, periosteum, dental pulp, meninges, some internal organs and joints.

Nociceptors are divided into three categories:

• Polymodal nociceptors.
• Mechanical nociceptors and
• Thermal nociceptors.

Polymodal nociceptors are stimulated by all three types of damages, including mechanical, chemical, and thermal. They are also activated in the presence of exogenous irritants, possibly penetrating the skin. These receptors may also cause pain by stimulation from endogenous substances, such as:

1. Acids,
2. Bradykinin; histamine; substance P,
3. Potassium released from damaged cells, and
4. Proteolytic enzymes.

These polymodal nociceptors give rise to a feeling of burning and slow pain.

Mechanical nociceptors are activated through mechanical injuries such as, pinching, cutting, tissue distortion, and intensive pressure on the skin (the more destructive the mechanical stimuli, the greater their firing rates).

Extreme temperatures cause stimulation of thermal nociceptors. There are two groups of thermal nociceptors responding to different stimuli. One is activated in the presence of noxious cold (<5°C) and the other in noxious heat (>45°C). At these temperatures tissues begin to damage.

Nociceptors are associated with afferent neurons of two types:

- A-delta fibers (Mylanated - fast impulse transmission), and
- C fibers (Non-mylanated - slow impulse transmission).

A-delta fibers are associated with thermal and mechanical nociceptors. These fibers are characterized as small and myelinated, transmitting with 5 to 30 m/sec impulse rate. Polymodal nociceptors, however, are linked with C fibers. These fibers are unmyelinated and small, transmitting impulses at a range between 0.5 to 2.0 m/sec, with rate usually lower than 1.0 meter/sec.

Pain types:

- Fast (sharp) pain, and
- Slow (dull) pain.

Fast (sharp - prickling) pain: Perception of such pain is fast, usually within 0.1 sec, as it is transmitted through nerve fibers that are rapid in action. Fast pain is conducted by A-delta fibers. It occurs as certain mechanical or thermal nociceptors are stimulated, therefore, it is largely localized.

Slow (throbbing, aching, or dull) pain: This pain is perceived a second after fast sharp pain (usually after 1 sec or more) as it is transmitted through C fibers. This kind of pain lasts longer and causes a sensation that is unpleasant. It also increases over time in certain cases. Polymodal receptors are stimulated by inflammatory chemical mediators directly from damaged cells or activated in damaged tissue's interstitial fluid. Slow pain is also differentiated as being less localized, and can occur in any organ, deep tissue or skin. (Table **2.4**).

Table 2.4. Characteristics of Fast and Slow Pain.

Fast pain	Slow pain
Occurs first.	Occurs second, persists longer.

(Table 2.4) contd.....

Fast pain	Slow pain
Sharp, prickling sensation.	Dull, aching, throbbing sensation; more unpleasant.
A-delta fibers.	C fibers.
Thermal or mechanical nociceptors.	Polymodal nociceptors.
Easily localized.	Poorly localized.

Chemical Activating or Sensitizing Nociceptors

There are endogenous chemical substances, which activate nociceptors, and make it more sensitizing than usual. These are the inflammatory chemical mediators. In case of inflammation, nociceptors become more sensitive (Table **2.5**).

Table 2.5. Endogenous Chemical Activating or Sensitizing Nociceptors.

Chemical	Source	Enzyme involved in synthesis	Effect on first-order sensory neuron	Pharmacological intervention
Potassium	Damaged cells		Activation	
Serotonin	Platelets	Tryptophan hydroxylase	Activation	
Bradykinin	Plasma kininogen	Kallikrein	Activation	
Histamine	Mast cells		Activation	H$_1$ receptor antagonists (*e.g.*, diphenhydramine chloride, Benadryl®)
Prostaglandins	Arachidonic acid/ damaged cells	Cyclooxygenase	Sensitization	Non-steroidal anti-inflammatory drugs (*e.g.* aspirin, ibuprofen)
Leukotrienes	Arachidonic acid/ damaged cells	Lipoxygenase	Sensitization	
Substance P	First order sensory neuron		Sensitization	Opioid receptor agonists (*e.g.*, morphine)

Hyperalgesia

Sensitivity to stimuli increases if it occurs after an area is injured. Even when the given stimulus generally causes no pain, previous injury results in replication of excessive pain. This rise in sensitivity of nociceptors is known as primary hyperalgesia. The sensation of burning is a common hyperalgesia example. If the burned area is touched, even gently, it causes great pain.

Nociceptors are greatly sensitized at the site of inflammation and tissue damage due to release and activation of different chemicals (Table **2.5**). The threshold for nociceptor activation is decreased and sensitization increased.

Bradykinin is one such substance (Inflammatory mediators), producing a greater pain sensation than many others. Stimulation of this substance occurs with the release of damaged tissue enzymes, and it takes a neuro-chemical mechanism resulting in pain sensation.

Mechanisms of Hyperalgesia

1. Activation of C fibers and A-delta occurs directly.
2. Prostaglandin release and synthesis is promoted within nearby tissues and cells. This increases the sensitization of pain receptors of all three kinds, resulting in greater strength of noxious stimulus replication. The nonsteroidal anti-inflammatory drugs (NSAIDs) suppress synthesis of prostaglandins, this is why this group of medication has an analgesic effect. In the case of astringent or sedulous tissue injury.
   - the second-order sensory neurons in the spinal cord's dorsal horn become hyperexcitable due to central mediated hyperalgesia. The way in which this enhanced replication, also known as, "wind-up", occurs is related to the neurotransmitter glutamate's relinquishment from C fibers. The glutamate which is an excitatory neurotransmitter, with mediation from the NMDA (N-methyl-D-aspartate-type) of receptor glutamate, causes calcium gates to open. With the influx of calcium, bio-chemical long-lasting changes occur and the dorsal horn of the spinal cord reaches a state of general hyperexcitability.

Afferent fibers and their nociceptive neurotransmitter.

Fibers involve two neurotransmitters in the trigeminal spinal nucleus for facial sensation and the spinal cord's dorsal horn for the remaining part of the body. Second-order sensory neurons are activated by these neurons which include:

- Substance P, and
- Glutamate.

Mechanisms of These Amino Acids as Neurotransmitters

Glutamate is a basic amino acid neurotransmitter, which the C fibers and A-delta release. This amino acid attaches with glutamate receptor (N-methyl-D-aspartte-type, AMPA-type) of the second-order sensory neuron to cause action potential and thereby, an impulse which perpetuates conduction of the impulse (neural signal) to the higher Central nervous system level (CNS level).

Production and release of substance P occur largely from C nerve fibers. In a state of sedulous pain, this neurotransmitter level greatly increases. Substance P neurotransmitter causes glutamate action to last longer and stimulation in the spinal cords' ascending pathways.

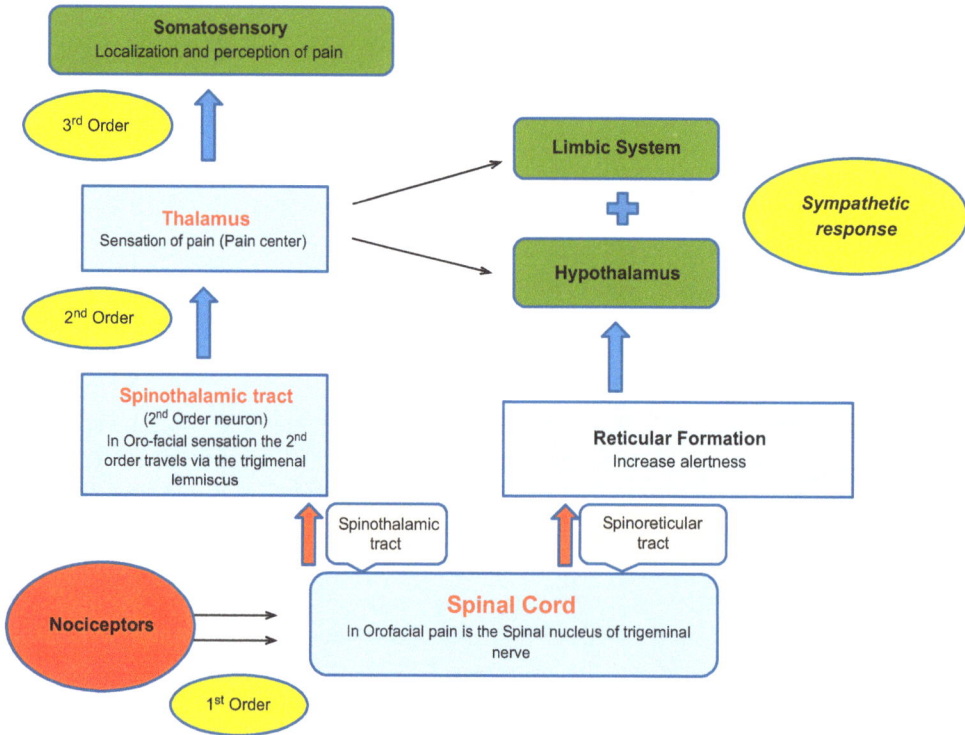

Fig. (2.4). Pain Pathway of the Trigemenal nerve.

Pain pathway (Fig. **2.4**)

1. **First-Order Neurons:**
   The nociceptor stimulation located in the body's periphery produces an action potential associated with first-order neurons. These in turn deliver signals to spinal cord or spinal nucleus of trigeminal nerves in case of oro-facial sensation.

2. **Second-Order Neurons:**
   These neurons are located in the spinal cord's dorsal horn and spinal nucleus in mid-brain (for oro-facial sensation). From these, the signal travels to several brain regions.

The path taken by ascending nociceptive is:

○ The trigeminal limeniscus (for facial sensation) and spinothalamic tract. The Trigeminal lemniscus transmits pain, tactile and temperature impulses and is a part of the CNS. It conveys these impulses from mucous membranes of nasal and oral cavities, the ocular perceiver, and facial skin and from the masticatory and facial muscles, it gathers proprioceptive information. The proprioceptive information is carried by the brainstem's ascending axonal tract to the ventral posterior medial nucleus of the thalamus from the mesencephalic nucleus which is the contralateral principal nucleus of the trigeminal system. Within the spinal cord, axons of the second-order sensory neurons project to the contralateral side and medulla obligate reaching the white matter and terminating in the ventral posterior medial nucleus of the thalamus which is its pain center. (Fig. **2.4**).

The thalamus is the basic nucleus for pain awareness and sensation; however, specific location of the pain source cannot be determined.

The spino-reticular tract is responsible in transmitting impulses to the brainstem's reticular formation. An important part in response to pain is played by the reticular formation, that is:

- The avoidance reflex is activated within the spinal cord at all levels.
- The function of pain arousal is performed. The reticular formation sends impulses stimulating electrical activity at the level of cerebral cortex causing an increase in the alertness.
- It is also responsible in supplying the hypothalamus with neural signals which influence its activity and tasks linked to alertness, including increasing blood pressure and heart rate. The autonomic nervous system, specifically its sympathetic part, mediates these functions.

  The hypothalamus and limbic system receives impulses from the reticular formation and thalamus. Thus they reach the center of autonomic nervous system. All these CNS regions work together to form emotional and behavioral responses to fear, pain and stress. The attention and mood changing influence of pain is accounted to the limbic system.

3. **Third-Order Sensory Neurons:**

   Third-order sensory neurons commence from the thalamus. Transmission of pain impulses to the cortes takes place through these neurons. The somatosensory cortex of the CNS is responsible in perceiving and localizing the painful stimulus and its intensity. The signal is also transmitted to other regions within the cerebral cortex, significant in perception and providing the pain stimulus with meaning.

Endogenous Analgesic System

This system is a part of pain pathway that controls nervous signal (impulses) transmission in the pain pathway. It primarily works by releasing neurotransmitters in the pain pathway-CNS (Fig. **2.5**):

Endorphins

• Dynorphin
• Enkephalins

Endorphins primarily occur in the:

1. Hypothalamus
2. Brainstem
3. Limbic system.

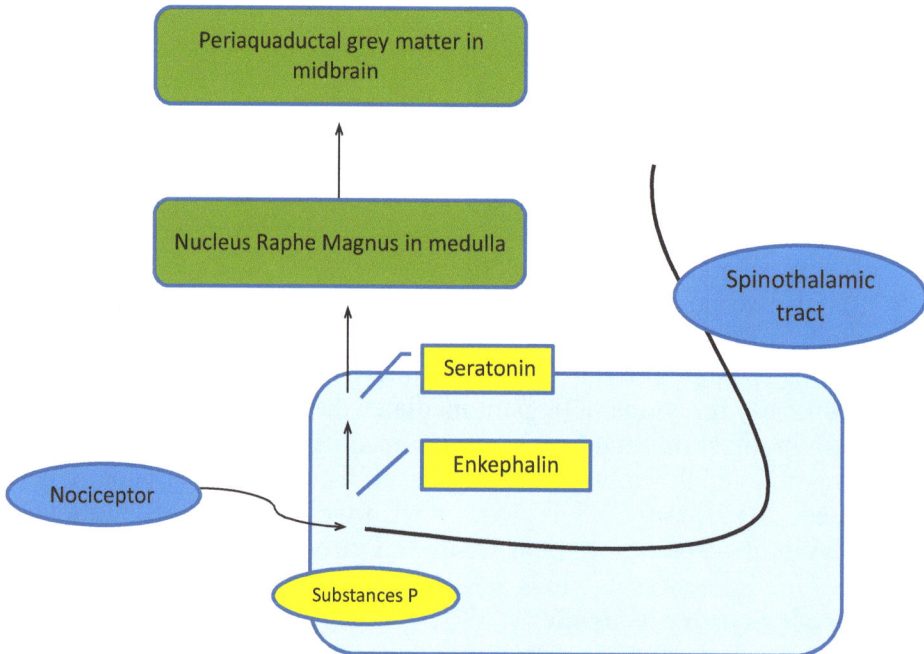

Fig. (2.5). Analgesic system.

Dynorphin and enkephalins are found primarily in a part of midbrain called periaqueductal gray matter (PAG), and in the hypothalamus and the limbic system. These substances of endogenous nature have similar effects as that of opiate drugs in the analgesic system, as well as in the Spinal nucleus for oro-facial sensation and the spinal cord's dorsal horns.

There is a large concentration of opioid receptors in the periaqueductal gray matter (PAG) areas present in the midbrain. Long term analgesic effects result from stimulation of this region, without affecting the consciousness level. As a result, the periaqueductal gray matter area is often called the endogenous analgesic center. The input received comes from a number of brain regions, including hypothalamus, cortex, reticular formation, and the spinothalamic tracts at the spinal cord or trigeminal limeniscus (for facial sensation). This area is associated with the emotion generator of pain, the limbic system.

The endogenous analgesic system consists of three major parts (pathway):

• Periaqueductal gray area (PAG),
• Nucleus raphe magnus (NRM), and
• Pain inhibitory system in the spinal cord's dorsal horns.

The periaqueductal gray matter (PAG) marks the beginning of the endogenous analgesic pathway, which moves forward with neural connections towards the medulla specifically the nucleus raphe magnus (NRM), (Fig. **2.5**). From the nucleus raphe magnus (NRM) the neurons then descend to the spinal cord's dorsal horn forming a synapse with spinal interneurons. These in turn synapse with afferent pain fibers. A number of neurons descending from the periaqueductal gray matter (PAG) area are responsible in secreting enkephalin in the nucleus raphe magnus (NRM from their axon terminals. The neurons descending from the nucleus raphe magnus release serotonin in the spinal nucleus from their axon terminals for oro-facial sensation and the spinal cord for the other part of the body.

The interneurons local cord is stimulated by the serotonin to secrete endogenous analgesic enkephalin. The encephalin, endogenous analgesic, blocks the incoming pain fiber impulse by presynaptic inhibition. As the endogenous analgesic enkephalin attaches to opioid receptors present on these pain fibers, the calcium channels are closed within the terminal axons. The exocytosis of neurotransmitter requires an influx of calcium therefore when the gates are blocked; release of substance P is prevented. This system is responsible for interruption of pain impulses at the spinal cord level and at level of trigeminal limeniscus (for oro-facial sensation).

It remains obscure how the endogenous analgesic system becomes activated because it is normally inactive. Potential factors that cause activation include exercise, acupuncture, stress, and hypnosis.

PART 3 - OUTLINE OF PHARMACOLOGIC TREATMENT OF PAIN

The analgesic medications suppress or eliminate pain, by acting on the nervous system without causing loss of consciousness.

The analgesic should exhibit the following criteria:

- Non-sedative
- Potent
- Minimal adverse effects
- Does not cause tolerance
- Inexpensive
- Effective without changing the state of awareness

Pain medications are branched into three main divisions:

- Non-narcotic analgesics
- Opioid analgesics
- Adjuvant analgesics

Non-Opioid (Non-narcotic) Analgesics:

The nonnarcotic analgesics include paracetamol (acetaminophen) and Non-steroidal Anti-inflammatory (NSAIDs). These act peripherally as well as centrally, blocking pain signals (impulses) from being transmitted. In addition it reduces fever, inflammation, and inhibits synthesis of prostaglandins that are responsible for increases the sensitivity of pain receptors (nociceptors).

The Mechanism of the NSAIDs:

The cyclooxygenase is the enzyme which limits the rate of prostaglandin synthesis. The Non-steroidal Anti-inflammatory (NSAIDs) works by inhibiting the release and the activity of cyclooxygenase. The two main types of cyclooxygenase are: the cyclooxygenase 1 - COX-1; constitutive and cyclooxygenase 2 - COX-2, both of them are induced in inflamed areas. The Non-steroidal Anti-inflammatory (NSAIDs) usually associated with gastric ulcers as a complication for high dose for long time use, to avoid this a more specific medications for COX-2 (Vioxx®, rofecoxib) have been created. These agents work by reducing inflammation, pain and fever and do not have any undesirable side effects (gastric ulcer). The Non-steroidal Anti-inflammatory (NSAIDs) inhibits the blood vessels' sensitivity to bradykinin and histamine, reversing the effects of vasodilation, and suppressing the inflammatory chemical mediators being released from mast cells, granulocytes and basophils.

The Mechanism of Opioid Drugs:

Their effects are exerted *via* opioid receptors, with three major categories: mu (μ), delta (Δ) and kappa (κ). Analgesia seems to involve κ-receptors within the spinal cord while μ-receptors at supraspinal sites. Analgesic effects of Morphine are produced with μ-receptor involvement. Most opioids used on clinical level are μ-receptor selective. Morphine is capable of stimulating spinally *via* μ2-receptors or supraspinally *via* μ1-receptors after systematical provision. However it tends to act largely through μ1-receptors supraspinally. The μ-receptor activation also causes other effects including respiratory system depression; decrease in gastrointestinal motility, with possible constipation; and a feeling of well-being being induced (euphoria).

Morphine can be administered orally, intravenously, or epidurally. Epidural administration is considered the most efficient as it produces the least central depressant depression as compared to other routes of effective analgesia. The action of opioid medication takes the route of first-order sensory neurons and their opioid receptors in the dorsal root ganglia while their axon terminals lie in the dorsal horn. The release of substance P is inhibited as these receptors are stimulated, causing an interruption in the transmission of the signal of pain impulse being send to the pain pathway of the second order neuron.

Adjuvant Analgesics:

Medications like antiseizure and antidepressants are included in adjuvant analgesics. Their success lies in the presence of non-endorphin synapses within the endogenous analgesic pain pathway.

This is clear as when the neurotransmitter serotonin is elevated in the central nervous system by both types of antidepressant (the selective serotonin reuptake inhibitors and Tricyclic antidepressant medications), these hinder serotonin removal through the synapse and control sensation of pain. The antiseizure medications like carbamazepine and phenytoin display certain specific analgesic effects under specific conditions. These medications, for example, control the spontaneous neuronal action potential. It is especially effective after nerve injury for the management of pain.

Certain agents, like the corticosteroids, significantly decrease inflammatory response by different mechanism including reducing of chemical mediator synthesis and release.

BIBLIOGRAPHY

[1]   Kelly L. Essentials of human physiology for pharmacy. Boca Raton, FL: CRC Press 2004.
       [http://dx.doi.org/10.1201/9780203495339]

[2]   Despopoulos A, Silbernagl S. Color atlas of physiology. Stuttgart: G. Thieme 1991.

[3]   Malamed SF. Handbook of local anesthesia. St. Louis, MS: Elsevier/Mosby 2013.

[4]   Goodman LS, Gilman A. The Pharmacological basis of therapeutics. New York: Macmillan 1975.

[5]   Brunton LL, Chabner BA, Knollmann Björn C. Goodman & Gilman's the pharmacological basis of therapeutics. New York: McGraw-Hill 2011.

[6]   Costanzo LS. Physiology: cases and problems. Philadelphia: Lippincott Williams & Wilkins 2006.

[7]   Guyton AC, Hall JE. Textbook of medical physiology. Philadelphia: W.B. Saunders 1996.

[8]   Raff H. Physiology secrets. Philadelphia: Hanley & Belfus 2003.

[9]   Sherwood L. Human physiology: from cells to systems. Australia: Thomson/Brooks/Cole 2007.

[10]   Silverthorn DU, Johnson BR. Human physiology: an integrated approach. San Francisco: Pearson/Benjamin Cummings 2010.

[11]   Purves D. Neuroscience. Sunderland, MA: Sinauer 2008.

[12]   Procacci P, Maresca M. Descartes' physiology of pain. Pain 1994; 58(2): 133.
[http://dx.doi.org/10.1016/0304-3959(94)90193-7] [PMID: 7816481]

[13]   Brodie ME, Richardson M. Physiology of pain. Hatfield: University of Hertfordshire Press 2005.

[14]   Central Pain. Human Studies of Physiology.

[15]   Blackwell RE, Olive DL. Physiology of Pain 1998.
[http://dx.doi.org/10.1007/978-1-4612-1752-7_2]

[16]   Blackwell RE, Olive DL. Physiology of Pain. Chronic Pelvic Pain 1998; pp. 7-18.

[17]   Physiology of Pain Development. Atlas of Injection Therapy in Pain Management. 2012.

[18]   Livingston WK. The Physiology of Pain. Pain Mechanisms 1976; pp. 44-61.

[19]   Smith J. Anatomy and Physiology of Pain Managing Pain in Children. 17-28.
[http://dx.doi.org/10.1002/9781444322743.ch2]

[20]   Zimmermann M. Basic Physiology of Pain Perception. Pathophysiology of Pain Perception 2004; 1-24.
[http://dx.doi.org/10.1007/978-1-4419-9068-6_1]

[21]   Sukiennik AW. Pain Physiology and Neuroblockade. Integrative Pain Management 2016; pp. 119-38.

[22]   Bijlani R. Chapter-127 Pain and Relief from Pain. Understanding Medical Physiology 2011; pp. 597-606.

[23]   Chambers D, Huang C, Matthews G. Pain physiology. Basic Physiology for Anaesthetists. 269-74.
[http://dx.doi.org/10.1017/CBO9781139226394.059]

[24]   Bijlani R. Chapter-127 Pain and Relief from Pain. Understanding Medical Physiology 2011; pp. 597-606.

[25]   Sembulingam K. Chapter-90 Physiology of Pain. Essentials of Physiology for Dental Students. 2011; pp. 555-7.
[http://dx.doi.org/10.5005/jp/books/11397_104]

[26]   Serpell M. Anatomy and physiology of pain. Handbook of Pain Management. 2008; pp. 9-24.
[http://dx.doi.org/10.1007/978-1-908517-12-8_2]

[27]   Chambers D, Huang C, Matthews G. Pain physiology. Basic Physiology for Anaesthetists. 269-74.
[http://dx.doi.org/10.1017/CBO9781139226394.059]

[28]   Flor H, Turk DC. Pain-related cognitions, pain severity, and pain behaviors in chronic pain patients. Pain 1987; 30.

[29]   Hernandez S, Cruz ML, Seguinot II, Torres-Reveron A, Appleyard CB. Impact of Psychological Stress on Pain Perception in an Animal Model of Endometriosis. Reprod Sci 2017; 24(10): 1371-81.
[http://dx.doi.org/10.1177/1933719116687655] [PMID: 28093054]

[30]   Corder G, Tawfik VL, Wang D, *et al.* Loss of μ opioid receptor signaling in nociceptors, but not microglia, abrogates morphine tolerance without disrupting analgesia. Nat Med 2017; 23(2): 164-73.
[http://dx.doi.org/10.1038/nm.4262] [PMID: 28092666]

[31]   Liu RX, Luo Q, Qiao H, *et al.* Clinical significance of the sympathetic nervous system in the development and progression of pulmonary arterial hypertension. Curr Neurovasc Res 2017; 14(2): 190-8.
[http://dx.doi.org/10.2174/1567202614666170112165927] [PMID: 28088894]

[32]   Yvone GM, Zhao-Fleming HH, Udeochu JC, *et al.* Disabled-1 dorsal horn spinal cord neurons co-express Lmx1b and function in nociceptive circuits. Eur J Neurosci 2017; 45(5): 733-47.
[http://dx.doi.org/10.1111/ejn.13520] [PMID: 28083884]

[33]   Hartling L, Ali S, Dryden DM, *et al.* How Safe Are Common Analgesics for the Treatment of Acute Pain for Children? A Systematic Review. Pain Res Manag 2016; 2016: 5346819.
[http://dx.doi.org/10.1155/2016/5346819] [PMID: 28077923]

[34]   Costa YM, Baad-Hansen L, Bonjardim LR, Conti PC, Svensson P. Reliability of the nociceptive blink reflex evoked by electrical stimulation of the trigeminal nerve in humans. Clin Oral Investig 2017; 21(8): 2453-63.
[http://dx.doi.org/10.1007/s00784-016-2042-6] [PMID: 28074292]

[35]   Kim MJ, Park YH, Yang KY, *et al.* Participation of central GABAA receptors in the trigeminal processing of mechanical allodynia in rats. Korean J Physiol Pharmacol 2017; 21(1): 65-74.
[http://dx.doi.org/10.4196/kjpp.2017.21.1.65] [PMID: 28066142]

[36]   Xin Q, Bai B, Liu W. The analgesic effects of oxytocin in the peripheral and central nervous system. Neurochem Int 2017; 103: 57-64.
[http://dx.doi.org/10.1016/j.neuint.2016.12.021] [PMID: 28065792]

[37]   Ozgocer T, Ucar C, Yildiz S. Cortisol awakening response is blunted and pain perception is increased during menses in cyclic women. Psychoneuroendocrinology 2017; 77: 158-64.
[http://dx.doi.org/10.1016/j.psyneuen.2016.12.011] [PMID: 28064085]

[38]   Sperry MM, Ita ME, Kartha S, Zhang S, Yu YH, Winkelstein B. The Interface of Mechanics and Nociception in Joint Pathophysiology: Insights From the Facet and Temporomandibular Joints. J Biomech Eng 2017; 139(2)
[http://dx.doi.org/10.1115/1.4035647] [PMID: 28056123]

[39]   Li X, Hu L. The Role of Stress Regulation on Neural Plasticity in Pain Chronification. Neural Plast 2016; 6402942.
[http://dx.doi.org/10.1155/2016/6402942]

[40]   Kilinc E, Guerrero-Toro C, Zakharov A, *et al.* Serotonergic mechanisms of trigeminal meningeal nociception: Implications for migraine pain. Neuropharmacology 2017; 116: 160-73.
[http://dx.doi.org/10.1016/j.neuropharm.2016.12.024] [PMID: 28025094]

[41]   Lee SJ, Kim DH, Hahn SJ, Waxman SG, Choi JS. Mechanism of inhibition by chlorpromazine of the human pain threshold sodium channel, Nav1.7. Neurosci Lett 2017; 639: 1-7.
[http://dx.doi.org/10.1016/j.neulet.2016.12.051] [PMID: 28017662]

[42]   De Gregori M, Muscoli C, Schatman ME, *et al.* Combining pain therapy with lifestyle: the role of personalized nutrition and nutritional supplements according to the SIMPAR Feed Your Destiny approach. J Pain Res 2016; 9: 1179-89.
[http://dx.doi.org/10.2147/JPR.S115068] [PMID: 27994480]

[43]   Faircloth AC. Anesthesia Involvement in Palliative Care. Annu Rev Nurs Res 2017; 35(1): 135-58.
[http://dx.doi.org/10.1891/0739-6686.35.135] [PMID: 27935778]

[44]   Pometlová M, Yamamotová A, Nohejlová K, Šlamberová R. Can Anxiety Tested in the Elevated Plus-maze Be Related to Nociception Sensitivity in Adult Male Rats? Prague Med Rep 2016; 117(4): 185-97.
[http://dx.doi.org/10.14712/23362936.2016.19] [PMID: 27930896]

[45]   Okine BN, Gaspar JC, Madasu MK, *et al.* Characterisation of peroxisome proliferator-activated receptor signalling in the midbrain periaqueductal grey of rats genetically prone to heightened stress, negative affect and hyperalgesia. Brain Res 2016. pii: S0006-8993(16)30778-8

[46]   Aurora SK, Brin MF. Chronic Migraine: An Update on Physiology, Imaging, and the Mechanism of Action of Two Available Pharmacologic Therapies. Headache 2017; 57(1): 109-25.
[http://dx.doi.org/10.1111/head.12999] [PMID: 27910097]

[47]   Baron R, Maier C, Attal N, *et al.* Peripheral neuropathic pain: a mechanism-related organizing principle based on sensory profiles. Pain 2017; 158(2): 261-72.
[http://dx.doi.org/10.1097/j.pain.0000000000000753] [PMID: 27893485]

[48]   Tayeb BO, Barreiro AE, Bradshaw YS, Chui KK, Carr DB. Durations of Opioid, Nonopioid Drug, and Behavioral Clinical Trials for Chronic Pain: Adequate or Inadequate? Pain Med 2016; 17(11): 2036-46.
[http://dx.doi.org/10.1093/pm/pnw245] [PMID: 27880651]

CHAPTER 3

The Outline of the Local Anesthesia - Pharmacology and Techniques

Fadi Jarab[1,*] and Esam Ahmad Z Omar[2]

[1] *Department of Oral & Maxillofacial Surgery, Jordan University of Science and Technology, Jordan*

[2] *Department of Oral & Maxillofacial Surgery, College of Dentistry, Taibah University, Madinah, Saudi Arabia*

Abstract: The pharmacology of local anesthesia is considered as the gate to dental anesthesia techniques. In the biomedical field, the human should not be injected with any medication unless the practitioner is well oriented about the nature of the medicine, the mechanism of action, the recommended dose, the maximum allowed dose, and possible complications. In this chapter, the techniques of local dental anesthesia have been discussed in detail as well, including the anatomical landmarks and regional nerve anatomy. The possible local and systemic complications have been added with the proper way of management and percussions. The relation of common systemic diseases to possible complications of local anesthesia medication has been discussed with emphasis on some wrong practiner,s opinion regarding using of vasoconstrictors in hypertensive patient (for details about management of medically compromised patients, read chapter 5, page: 131-195).

Keywords: Complications, Controversy regarding vasoconstrictors, Details of techniques, Local and possible systemic complications, Pharmacology of local anesthesia.

PART 1 - PHARMACOLOGY OF LOCAL ANESTHESIA

Definition

The local anesthetic is defined as a therapeutic modality which brings about a reversible loss of conduction from periphery to its interpretation in the central nervous system.

---

[*] **Corresponding author Fadi Jarab:** Department of Oral & Maxillofacial Surgery, Jordan University of Science and Technology, Jordan; Tel: 0096279505 0342; Fax: 00966148494710; E-mail: fsjarab@just.edu.jo

Chemical structure (Fig. **3.1**):

Composed of 3 parts:

1. The Lipophilic Part: is the largest portion,aromatic,derived from benzoic acid or aniline
2. The Hydrophilic Part: is an amino derivative of ethyl alcohol or acetic acid
3. Intermediate Chain: either amide or ester linkage,determines the type of L.A

• Local anesthetics are weak bases, poorly soluble in water and unstable, but they combine readily with acids to form salts which are stable and water soluble. Thus, local anesthetics used for injection are dispensed as salts, most commonly the hydrochloride salts.
• Local anesthetics without a hydrophilic part are not suited for injection but are good for topical application.
• Local anesthesia temporarily blocks the normal generation and conduction action of the nerve impulses.

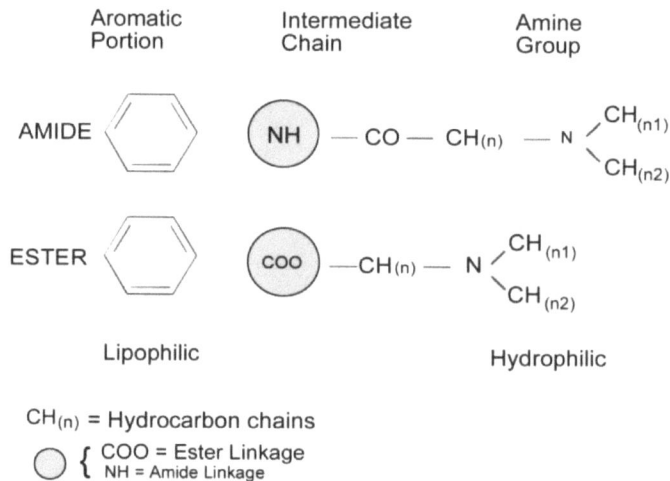

Fig. (3.1). Local anesthetic Chemical structure.

Factors Affecting the Local Anesthetic Action

• pKa
• Lipid Solubility
• Protein Binding
• Tissue Diffusibility
• Vasodilator Activity

The Effect of PH on Local Anesthetic Nerve Blocking Action (for more explanation read page: 35)

- PKa is defined as the PH at which half of the molecules are ionized and half nonionized,it is constant and characteristic for each agent
- most local anesthetic agents without vasoconstrictor have a PH of 5.5-7
- when tissue PH is below an anesthetics PKa, excess H+ is present, and the proportion of RN declines

$$RNH+ \leftrightarrow RN + H+$$

Since RN is the form of diffusion, effectiveness decreases

So,

- Acidification of tissues (as in infection) decreases effectiveness
- The closer the local anesthetic PKa to the tissue PH, the faster the onset of action

Summary

The onset of local anesthesia is strongly correlated with pKa of the various local anesthetics and lipid solubility. The pKa determines ionization and ionization influences diffusion of anesthetics across the neural membrane sheath of the nerve. The uncharged base form diffuses more quickly than the charged cationic form. The closer pKa of the local anesthesia to physiologic pH of the tissues, the more anesthetic exists in the uncharged base form. Lower pKa results in a more rapid onset. It should be remembered that the onset is also reduced by increasing the solution pH.

Classification of Local Anesthetic Agents Based on Chemical Structure

AMIDES	ESTERS
LIDOCAINE	PROCAINE
MEPIVACAINE	PROPOXYCAINE
ARTICAINE	CHLOROPROCAINE
ETIDOCAINE	TETRACAINE
BUPIVACAINE	
PRILOCAINE	

Note: articaine contains both ester and amide linkages in its chemical structure,but is considered as an amide local anesthetic agent.

Relationship of Physical-Chemical Properties to Local Anesthetic Activity

Agent	Relative Potency	App. Lipid Solubility	Duration (min.)	App.P.B.
LOW POTENCY - SHORT DURATION				
Procaine	1	< 1	60-90	5
INTERMEDIATE POTENCY/DURATION				
Mepivacaine	2	1	120-240	75
Prilocaine	2	1.5	100-240	55
Lidocaine	2	4	90-200	65
HIGH POTENCY - LONG DURATION				
Bupivacaine	8	30	180-600	95
Tetracaine	8	80	180-600	85
Etidocaine	6	140	180-600	94

Vascular Effect of Local Anesthetics

Local anesthetics are mostly vasodilators which decrease the duration of action:

• Cocaine: the only vasoconstrictor
• Procaine: most potent vasodilator
• Mepivacaine: least potent vasodilator

Central Nervous System Effects of Local Anesthetics

• Local anesthetic agents readily cross the blood-brain barrier, and toxic levels can produce signs of CNS excitation and depression.
• The initial symptoms of local anesthetic toxicity in man consist of a generalized feeling of lightheadedness and dizziness, followed by auditory and visual disturbances, such as difficulty in focusing and tinnitus. Drowsiness, disorientation, and a temporary lack of consciousness may also occur.
• Slurred speech, shivering, muscle twitching, and tremors of the face and extremities appear to be the immediate precursors of a generalized convulsive state.
• A further increase in the dose of local anesthetic agents during the excitation period results in cessation of convulsive activity, respiratory arrest, and a flattening of the brain wave pattern consistent with generalized central nervous system depression.
• The signs and symptoms of CNS excitation followed by depression are related to an inhibition of cerebral cortical neurons.
• An initial selective blockade of inhibitory cortical neurons or synapses allows

excitatory fibers to function unopposed leading to excitation and convulsions
- Further increases in dosage depress both inhibitory and facilitatory pathways causing a generalized state of central nervous system depression.
- Local anesthetic toxicity is due usually to an inadvertent rapid intravenous injection or extravascular administration of an excessive dose.

Cardiovascular Effect of Local Anesthetics

- HYPOTENSION: Arteriolar dilation is a result of:
- Direct effect (procaine and lidocaine have most effect) *
- *Block of postganglionic sympathetic fiber function
- *CNS depression
- Avoid by adding vasoconstrictor to prep
- Note: cocaine is exception: produces vasoconstriction, blocks NE reuptake
- ARRHYTHMIAS: direct effect (More resistant than CNS)-
- Decrease cardio excitability and contractility
- Decreased conduction rate
- Increased refractory rate (bupivacaine)
- Note: cocaine is exception, it stimulates heart
- ALL can cause arrhythmias if concentration is high enough

Biotransformation and Excretion

- Amide local anesthetics are metabolized by the liver
- Ester local anesthetics are metabolized in plasma *via* pseudocholinesterase
- Procaine is hydrolyzed into PABA and diethylamine alcohol(more allergy) both amide and ester local anaesthetics are excreted *via* kidneys

Pharmacology of Commonly Used Local Anesthetic Agents

Lidocaine

- Lidocaine
- Xylocaine
- AmidePotency 2 (compared to procaine)-
- Toxicity 2 (compared to procaine)
- Metabolized in liver
- Excreted *via* kidneys with around 10% unchanged
- Pka 7.9
- PH without vasoconstrictor 5.5
- PH with vasoconstrictor 3.5-4.5
- Almost no allergy
- Rapid onset of action 2-3 min.

- More profound anesthesia
- Longer duration of action
- pulpal anesthesia 45-60 min.
- soft tissue anesthesia 3-5 hr. less vasodilator properties
- Max. dose without vasoconstrictor 4.4mg/kg
- Max. dose with vasoconstrictor 6mg/kg -
- available in many forms
- 2% +/- vasoconstrictor (1-50000,1-80000, 1-10000,1-200000)
- 4%
- 10% sprays
- 2% gel
- 5% ointment
- 2% means 20 mg per 1 ml, so a cartridge of 1.8 ml contains 36 mg.

Prilocaine

- Amide
- Potency 2(compared to procaine)
- Toxicity 1(same as procaine)
- Metabolized primarily by liver and some by lungs and kidneys
- Excreted by kidneys
- Slower onset of action 4 min Pulpal anesthesia 4% (10min.)
- Pulpal anesthesia 3% + V.C. (60 min.)
- Soft tissue anesthesia 4-5 hrs.
- Max. dose 4% (6mg/kg)
- Available in * plain 4%, 3% + felypressin (0.03 IU/mL)
- Methemoglobinemia as a side effect

Mepivacaine

- Amide
- Potency 2
- Toxicity 1.5-2
- Metabolized in liver
- Excreted *via* kidneys
- The least vasodilator
- Rapid onset of action 2 min
- Available as 3% plain or 2% with 1:80000 adrenaline
- Pulpal anesthesia 30 min
- Soft tissue anesthesia 2-3 hours
- 3% maximum dose is 4.4mg/kg 3%
- mepivacaine is recommended in:- Pediatric patients*, Geriatric patients* and Procedures not requiring long pulpal anesthesia *

Bupivacaine

- Marcaine
- Amide
- Metabolized by liver
- Excreted *via* kidneys
- Potency 4 times more than lidocaine
- Toxicity 4 times less than lidocaine
- Long duration of action(and etidocaine)
- Long onset of action(6-10 min)
- 0.5% is an effective dental concentration…potent
- Available as(0.5% or0.75%)with adrenaline
- Maximum dose 1.3 mg/kg
- Cardiotoxic(ropivacaine significantly less)
- Used in: *Long dental procedures (pulpal anaesthesia 90 min) and *Management of postoperative pain

Procaine

- Ester
- Metabolized in plasma
- Excreted *via* kidneys
- Potency 1
- Toxicity 1
- Effective dental concentration 2%-4%
- Maximum dose 6mg/kg
- Major disadvantages
- Long onset of action 10 min with pKa9.1
- Very short pulpal anaesthesia duration
- Highly allergic
- Indications: As a vasodilator and In patients allergic to amide L.A

Tetracaine

- Ester
- Slow onset
- Longest duration of action among esters
- 10x more toxic and more potent than procaine

Topical Local Anesthesia

Higher concentration than injection local anesthesia
Provides anesthesia up to 2-3mm depth of dry mucous membrane
The onset of action 1-5 minutes

Can induce systemic toxicity
Topical local anesthetic agents
Lidocaine 5%
Benzocaine up to 20%
EMLA 5%, mixture of lidocaine and prilocaine.

Pharmacology of Vasoconstrictors

Vasoconstrictors are highly valuable additions to a local anesthetic solution:

- Decrease blood flow to the site
- Decrease rate of absorption of local anesthetic agent and lower its blood level and toxicity
- Increase the duration of action of the local anesthetic agent
- Decrease bleeding and achieve hemostasis at the site

Types of Vasoconstrictors

1. Catecholamine
   ○ Epinephrine
   ○ Norepinephrine
   ○ Dopamine
2. Non-catecholamine
   ○ Amphetamine
   ○ Ephedrine
3. Felypressin (synthetic analogue)

Dilution of Vasoconstrictors

Concentration

1:1000 = 1 gm / 1000 ml solution, this means 1000 mg/1000ml = 1mg/1ml

1:10000 = 0.1mg/ml

1:100000 = 0.01mg/ml

1:80000 = 0.0125mg/ml

1:200000 = 0.005mg/ml

Adrenergic Receptors

- Epinephrine remains the most effective and most used vasoconstrictor in medicine and dentistry.

- Nor- epinephrine is not recommended, because it produces intense peripheral vasoconstriction with a possible elevation of blood pressure, with nine times higher side effects than epinephrine.
- Adrenaline relaxes the smooth muscle of skeletal muscle arterioles, noradrenaline constricts, noradrenaline thus raises diastolic blood pressure and causes, by the baroreceptors, a slowing of the heart rate or little change whereas adrenaline by its action on the heart and peripheral resistance causes tachycardia. Adrenaline relaxes bronchiole smooth muscle . noradrenaline has no effect.
- Epinephrine as the acid salt is highly soluble in water.
- Slightly acid solutions are relatively stable if they are protected from air.
- Sodium bisulfate is usually added to epinephrine solutions to delay its deterioration (through oxidation). By acidification. So they are quite soluble in water and comparatively stable.
- Epinephrine is available as synthetic and is also obtained from the adrenal medulla of animals (approximately 80% of adrenal medullary secretions being epinephrine). adrenaline stored in chromaffin cells before being released following sympathetic nerve stimulation.
- Epinephrine acts directly on both α- and β- adrenergic receptors ; β effect predominates.

Adrenaline has a number of systemic action; adrenaline affects:

1. The Heart
    - Increase the rate and force of contraction of the heart raising cardiac output.
    - Increase in pulse rate.
    - Rise in systolic (standard dose has little effect).
    - Increase in myocardial oxygen consumption.

These actions lead to an overall decrease in cardiac efficiency.

2. Effect on Blood Vessels
    - Vessels supplying the skin, mucous membrane, and kidneys contain primarily α receptors (epinephrine produces constriction in these vessels).
    - Blood vessels supplying the skeletal muscles contain both β2 and α receptors, with β2 predominating . β2 adrenoreceptor stimulation produces vasodilatation by activation of adenylate cyclase resulting in fall in diastolic pressure.
    - The injection of epinephrine directly into surgical sites leads to high tissue concentrations, a predominant α-receptor stimulation, and hemostasis.
    - As epinephrine tissue levels decrease with time, the primary action on blood vessels will revert to vasodilation, as β2 actions predominate. It is not

uncommon, therefore, for some bleeding to be noted at about 6 hours following surgery.

3. Effect on the Lungs
   ○ β2 adrenoreceptor stimulation in the lungs lead to bronchiolar muscle relaxation ; it is important life-threatening in the case of bronchoconstriction (acute asthma).

- Clinical applications-epinephrine:
  ○ Management of acute allergic reactions
  ○ Management of bronchospasm
  ○ Treatment of cardiac arrest
  ○ As a vasoconstrictor, for hemostasis
  ○ As a vasoconstrictor in local anesthetic, to decrease absorption into the cardiovascular system
  ○ As a vasoconstrictor in local anesthetic, to increase duration of action
  ○ To produce mydriasis.
- The treatment of adrenaline overdose:
  ○ Stop the treatment
  ○ Reduce cerebral blood pressure by sitting the patient upright
  ○ Oxygen administration
- Felypressin (octapressin)
  ○ Non- sympathomimetic amine.
  ○ Pronounced on venous than arteriolar microcirculation
  ○ No effect on adrenergic nerve transmission, so safety given to:
    ▪ Hyperthyroid patient
    ▪ MAO inhibitor, tricyclic antidepressants
    ▪ No clinical evidence.
  ○ Contraindicated for pregnant women; (oxytocic actions on the uterus)
  ○ In high dose, it my produce facial pallor
  ○ Available in 0.03 IU/ml + 3% Prilocaine
  ○ Few contraindications of epinephrine ; instead with use of felypressin
  ○ A Patient with a significant cardio-vascular disease, but there is no evidence that it is any safer.
  ○ A Patient with thyroid dysfunction, diabetes, sulfite, sensitivity
  ○ A patient who is receiving MAO inhibitors, tricyclic antidepressant.

The Armamentarium

1. Syringe
2. Cartridge/carpule
3. Needle

The Needle

Component

1. Hub
2. Shank(body)
3. Bevel(facilitates penetration)
4. Syrinnge penetrating end

Gauge

1. Diameter of internal lumen of a needle
2. As gauge increases, the diameter decreases

Aspiration

Is the application of negative pressure. It Is used before administration of L.A to make sure that the L.A. solution is not injected into the blood vessel, especially important in block anesthesia.

Length

1. From hub to tip
2. Ultra short 12 mm
3. Short 20 mm
4. Long up to 35 mm

Care and Handling

1. Never use a needle for more than one patient.
2. Chang it after 3-4 penetrations
3. Cover with protective sheath when not in use, using scoop technique
4. Dispose of it in sharp container

The Cartridge

• Supplied prefilled by manufacturer for dental use
• Packed in cylindrical containers or blister packs

Component

1. Cylindrical wall
2. Metal cap containing a basal diaphragm which is penetrated by the needle
3. A rubber bung which contacts the syringe plunger

Contents

1. Local anesthetic agent
2. Vasopressor
3. Sodium chloride as a buffering agent
4. Sodium metabisulfite as an antioxidant of adrenaline
5. Methylparben as a preservative
6. Thymol (sometimes added) as a fungicide
7. Distilled water

Handling

1. The contents of a cartridge are used for one patient only
2. The cartridges are not autoclavable
3. Store in original container at room temperature
4. Avoid sunlight to prevent oxidation
5. Don't soak in anything(alcohol or sterilizing agent)
6. Warmer not necessary
7. Check expiry date before use

The Syringe

Types

1. Conventional
    a. Non-aspirating
    b. Aspirating
    c. Self aspirating
2. Specialized
    a. Disposable
    b. Intraligamental
    c. Intraosseous
    d. Safety
    e. Jet

Components of Conventional Syringes

1. Threaded hub
2. Barrel
3. Plunger

Breech Loading, Plastic Cartridge Type Aspirating

Advantages

1. Light weight
2. Visible cartridge
3. Aspiration with one hand
4. Rust resistant
5. Lower cost
6. Long lasting with proper maintenance

Disadvantages

1. Possible infection with improper care
2. Deterioration of plastic with repeated autoclaving
3. Size

Breech Loading, Metallic Cartridge Type Aspirating Advantages

1. Visible cartridge
2. Aspiration with one hand
3. Rust resistant
4. Long lasting with proper maintenance

Disadvantages

1. Weight
2. Size

Disposable Syringe

Advantages

1. Sterile till opened
2. Light
3. Disposable

Disadvantages

1. Does do not accept prefilled cartridges
2. Awkward to first-time users

Safety Syringe

Advantages

1. Sterile till opened
2. Light
3. Disposable

Disadvantages

1. Cost
2. Awkward to first-time users

Jet Injector

Advantages

1. Does do not require a needle
2. Very small amount of L.A delivered
3. Replaces topical anesthesia

Disadvantages

1. Cost
2. Inadequate pulpal or regional block
3. May damage periodontal tissues

Pressure Syringe

Advantages

1. Measure dose
2. Overcome tissue resistance
3. Cartridge protected

Disadvantages

1. Cost
2. Easy to inject too rapidly

Care and Handling of the Syringes

- After each use, wash and rinse then autoclave
- Dismantle and lightly lubricate all threaded joints after 5 autoclaves
- Clean the harpoon with a brush after each use
- Replace piston and harpoon if there is decreased sharpness

Additional Armamentarium

- Topical antiseptic
- Applicator sticks for topical application
- Topical local anesthesia

PART - 2: BASIC INJECTION TECHNIQUES (FIG. 3.2 – 3.23)

Basics of technique (Fig. **3.2-3.23**):

- **Use a Sterilized Sharp Needle**

- **The Flow of Local Anesthetic Solution:** After properly loading the cartridge into the syringe, to ensures a free flow of anesthetic solution when it is injected into the target area a few drops of local anesthetic solution should be ousted from the cartridge. The anesthetic cartridge stoppers are made of a silicone rubber to ensure ease of administration. A few drops of the solution are recommended to be expelled from the needle to determine if a free flow of solution exists.

- **Determine Whether or not to Warm the Anesthetic Cartridge or Syringe**: The cartridge is stored at room temperature (approximately 72°F, 22°C).There is no reason for the warming of the local anesthetic cartridge before its injection into target tissues.

- **The Patient Position:** The patient should be in a physiologically sound position before and during the injection. Common faint (vasodepressor syncope - the most commonly seen medical emergency in dentistry), most often occurs before, during, and, on occasion, immediately after administration of local anesthesia. It is a temporary cerebral ischemia secondary to vaso-vagal over activity, in response to stress. This result in the bowling of the blood in the venous compartment of the circulation, this mean there is insufficient blood return to the heart from the venous system. This lead to insufficient stroke volume and inadequate volume of oxygenated blood supply to the brain.

- **Dry the Tissue:** The site of needle penetration should be dried with A 2x2 inch gauze to remove any gross debris. The lip retraction is necessary for visibility and accessibility to obtain adequate visibility during the injection, it too should be dried to make retraction easier.

- **Apply Topical Disinfectant (Antiseptic - Optional):** A reasonable topical sterile oro-base antiseptic to be can be used, after the tissues had got dried, This decreased the risk of introducing septic materials into the soft tissues, producing either infection or inflammation. Antiseptics include Alcohol-containing antiseptics, Merthiolate (thimerosal) and Betadine (povidone-iodine) can cause soft tissue dryness and burn; these should be avoided.

- **Topical Anesthetic:** After the topical antiseptic application, the topical anesthetic can be applied. Application of excessive amounts of topical anesthetic on large areas of soft tissues, may produce undesirably wide areas of anesthesia, an unpleasant taste, and, perhaps even more importantly, with some topical anesthetics (such as lidocaine), a rapid absorption into the cardiovascular system (CVS), theoretically, may be leading to higher local anesthetic blood levels and an increased risk of overdose.

- **Reassure & Communicate with the Patient:** To place a concrete idea in the patient's mind concerning the upcoming injection and dental procedures.

- **Establish a Firm Hand Rest (A Firm Hand Rest is Necessary):** It is essential to maintain complete control over it at all times of injection procedure. The types of hand rest vary according to the practitioner's physical abilities. Any finger or hand rest that permits the anesthetic syringe to be stabilized without increasing the risk to a patient is acceptable. Two techniques to be avoided are using no syringe stabilization of any kind and placing the arm holding the syringe directly on the patient's arm or shoulder Hand position for injection;
  - a. Palm-down: poor control over the syringe, not recommended.
  - b. Palm-up: better control over the syringe because it is supported by the wrist; recommended.
  - c. Palm up and finger support: greatest stabilization; highly recommended.

- **Make the Tissue Taut:** The tissues at the site of needle penetration should be stretched before insertion of the needle. This can be accomplished in all areas of the mouth except the palate (where the tissues are naturally quite taut). Stretching of the tissues permits the sharp stainless steel needle to cut through the mucous membrane with a minimum of resistance. The loose tissues, on the other hand, are pushed and torn by the needles as it is inserted, producing more discomfort on injection and more postoperative soreness.

- **Keep the Syringe Out of the Patient's Line of Sight:** With the tissue prepared and the patient positioned, the assistant should pass the syringe to the administrator behind the patient's head or across and in front of the patient but below the patient's line of sight (less preferred). A right-handed practitioner administrating a right-side injection can sit facing the patient or, if administering a left-side injection, facing in the same direction as the patient.

- **Insert the Needle into the Mucosa:** With the needle bevel properly oriented (see specific injection technique for bevel orientation; however, as a general rule the bevel of the needle should be oriented toward bone), insert the needle gently into the tissue at the injection site (where the topical anesthetic was placed) to the depth of the bevel. With a steady hand rest and adequate tissue preparation, this potentially traumatic procedure is accomplished without the patient ever being aware of it.

- **Watch and Communicate with the Patient:** During Step 11a, the patient should be watched and communicated with; the patient's face should be observed for evidence of discomfort during needle penetration. Signs such as furrowing of the brow or forehead and blinking of the eyes may indicate discomfort . More frequently, no change will be noticed in the patient's facial expression at this time (showing a painless, or atraumatic, needle insertion).

- **Slowly Advance the Needle Toward the Target:** Steps 12 and 13 are carried out together. The soft tissue in front of the needle may be anesthetized with a few drops of local anesthetic solution. After waiting 2 or 3 seconds for anesthesia to develop, the needle should be advanced into the area and a little more anesthesia deposited. The needle should then be advanced again. These procedures may be repeated until the needle reaches the desired target area.

- **Deposit Several Drops of Local Anesthetic Before Touching the Periosteum:** In techniques of regional block anesthesia in which the needle touches or approaches the periosteum, a few drops of solution should be deposited just before contact. The periosteum is richly innervated, and contact with the needle tip produces pain. Anesthetizing the periosteum permits atraumatic contact. Regional block injection techniques that require this are the inferior alveolar, Gow-Gates mandibular, and infraorbital nerve blocks.

- **Aspirate:** Aspiration always must be carried out before deposing a volume of local anesthetic at any site. Aspiration dramatically minimizes the possibility of an intravascular injection. The goal of aspiration is to determine whether the needle tip lies within a blood vessel. To aspirate, one must create a negative pressure within the dental cartridge. The self-aspirating syringe does this whenever the operator stops applying positive pressure to the thumb ring (plunger). With the more commonly used harpoon-type syringe the administrator must make a conscious effort to create this negative pressure within the cartridge. The thumb ring should be pulled back gently. Movement of only 1 or 2 mm is needed. This produces a negative pressure within the cartridge that then translates to the tip of the needle. Whatever is lying in the soft tissues around the needle tip (*e.g.*, blood, tissue, or air) will be drawn back into the anesthetic cartridge. By observing the needle end lying within the cartridge for signs of blood return, the administrator can determine if a positive aspiration has occurred. Any sign of blood is a positive aspiration, and the local anesthetic solution should not be deposited at that site.

- **Slowly Deposit the Local Anesthetic Solution:** With the needle in position at the target area and aspirations completed and negative, the administrator should begin pressing gently on the plunger to start administering the predetermined (for the technique) volume of anesthetic. Slow injection is vital for two reasons: of utmost significance is the safety factor, slow injection also prevents the solution from tearing the tissue into which it is deposited. Rapid injection results in immediate discomfort (for a few seconds) followed by a prolonged soreness when the action of the local anesthetic is terminated. Slow injection is defined as the deposition of 1 ml of local anesthetic solution in not less than 60 seconds. Therefore, a full 1.8-ml cartridge requires approximately 2 minutes. Through slow deposition, the solution is able to diffuse along normal tissue planes without producing postoperative discomfort.

- **Communicate with the Patient:** The patient should be communicated with during deposition of the local anesthetic. Most patients are accustomed to receiving their local anesthetic injections rapidly. Statements such as, "I'm depositing the solution (or I'm doing this) slowly so it will be more comfortable for you, but you're not receiving any more than is usual" go far to allay a patient's apprehension at this time.

- **Slowly Withdraw the Syringe:** After completion of the injection, the syringe should be slowly removed from the soft tissues and the needle made safe by drawing its protective sheath over it (safety syringe) or by capping it immediately with its plastic sheath *via* the scoop technique.

- **Observe the Patient:** After completion of the injection, the doctor should remain with the patient while the anesthetic begins to take effect (and its blood level increases). Most adverse drug reactions, especially those to interiorly administered local anesthetics, develop either during the injection or within 5 to 10 minutes of completion of the injection.

- **Record the Injection on the Patient's Chart:** An entry must be made of the local anesthetic drug used, vasoconstrictor used (if any), dose (in milligrams) of the solution(s) used, the needle(s) used, the injection(s) given, and the patient's reaction. For example, on the patient's dental progress notes the following might be inscribed: R-IANB, 25-long, 2% lido + 1:100,000 epi, 36 mg. Tolerated procedure well.

Nerves Anesthetized: Terminal branches of the dental nerve
Areas Anesthetized: The entire region innervated by the terminal branches of this nerve, including:
- pulp,
- root area of the tooth,
- buccal periosteum,
- connective tissue,
- related mucous membrane.

Indications:
1. Pulp, root, and related bone need to be anesthetized.
Soft-tissue anesthesia is indicated for surgical procedures in a circumscribed area.

Contraindications:
1. Infection or acute inflammation in the area of injection
2. Dense bone covering the apices of teeth (can be determined only by trial and error. This is most likely over the permanent maxillary first molar in children, its apex lies beneath the zygomatic bone, which is relatively dense).

Precautions: This injection should not be used for larger areas:
- A greater number of tissue penetrations increases the possibility of pain both during and after the injection,
and the larger volume of solution administered increases the possibility of local anesthetic overdose and post injection pain.

Failure of Anesthesia
- Depositing anesthetic solution below the apex of a maxillary tooth results in excellent soft-tissue anesthesia but poor or absent pulpal anesthesia.
- The needle tip lies too far from the bone (solution deposited in the buccal soft tissues).

Advantages:
1. High success rate (>95%)
2. Technically easy injection
3. Usually entirely atraumatic

Disadvantages: Not recommended for large areas, because of the need for multiple needle insertions and the necessity to administer larger total volumes of local anesthetic

- **Landmarks**
- **Mucobuccal fold**
- **Crown of the tooth**
- **Root contour of the tooth**
- **Orientation of the bevel: toward bone with 45 degree angulation to the long axis of the tooth.**

- Procedure
- lift the lip, pulling the tissue taut.
- Hold the syringe parallel to the long axis of the tooth.
- Insert the needle into the height of the mucobuccal fold over the target tooth.
- Advance the needle until its bevel is at or above the apical region of the   tooth. In most instances, the depth of penetration is only a few millimetres. Because the needle is in soft tissue (not touching bone), there should be no resistance to its advancement, nor should there be any patient discomfort with this injection.
- Aspirate. If negative, deposit approximately 0.6 ml (one-third of a cartridge) slowly over 20 seconds. (Do not permit the tissues to balloon.)
- Slowly withdraw the syringe.
- Make the needle safe.
Wait for 3 to 5 minutes.

Fig. (3.2). Local infiltration (paraperiosteal injection).

Areas Anesthetized:
- Pulpal anesthesia of the maxillaryIncisors and Canine
- Buccal attached gingival of these same teeth

Indications:
- When Pulpal anesthesia for operative, endodontic or periodontics are indicated.
- For surgical procedure with other supplement injection

Contraindications:
- Infection or acute inflammation in the area of injection.

Precautions: care should be taken to inject the anesthetic solution at the level of apex of the tooth.

Failure of Anesthesia:
Very rare

- **Landmarks**
- **Buccal area of upper 1st and 2nd Incisors and Canine**
- **The long axis of the tooth**
- **Insertion the needle with 45 degree**

- Procedure (Fig: 3.4)
- Insert the needle into the height of the mucobuccal fold over the target tooth with 45 degree to the long axis of the tooth
- Advance the needle until its bevel is at or above the apical region of the tooth. In most instances, the depth of penetration is only a few millimetres. Because the needle is in soft tissue (not touching bone), there should be no resistance to its advancement, nor should there be any patient discomfort with this injection.
- Aspirate . (not strongly recommended because there is no blood vessels with considerable dimention). If negative, deposit approximately 0.6 ml (one-third of a cartridge) slowly over 20 seconds. (Do not permit the tissues to balloon.)
- Slowly withdraw the syringe.
- Make the needle safe.

Wait for 3 to 5 minutes.

Fig. (3.3). Anterior Superior Alveolar Nerve Infilteration.

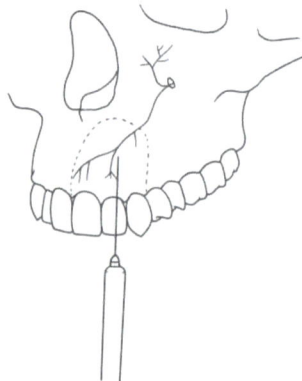

Fig. (3.4). Anterior Superior Alveolar Nerve Infilteration.

Areas Anesthetized:
- Pulpal anesthesia of the maxillary premolars
- Buccal attached gingival of these same teeth
- Attached palatal tissues for the same teeth

Indications:
- When Pulpal anaesthesia for operative, endodontic or periodontics are indicated.
- For surgical procedure with other supplement injection

Contraindications:
- Infection or acute inflammation in the area of injection.

Precautions: care should be taken to inject the anesthetic solution at the level of apex of the tooth.

Failure of Anesthesia:
Very rare

- Landmarks
- Buccal area of upper 1st and 2nd Premolars.
- The long axis of the tooth
- Insertion the needle with 45 degree to the tooth long axis

- Procedure: (Fig: 3.6)
- Insert the needle into the height of the muco-buccal fold over the target tooth with 45 degree to the long axis of the tooth
- Advance the needle until its bevel is at or above the apical region of the tooth. In most instances, the depth of penetration is only a few millimetres. Because the needle is in soft tissue (not touching bone), there should be no resistance to its advancement, nor should there be any patient discomfort with this injection.
- Aspirate (not strongly recommended because there is no blood vessels with considerable dimension). If negative, deposit approximately 0.6 ml (one-third of a cartridge) slowly over 20 seconds. (Do not permit the tissues to balloon.)
- Slowly withdraw the syringe.
- Make the needle safe.

Wait for 3 to 5 minutes.

Fig. (3.5). Middle Superior Alveolar Nerve Infilteration.

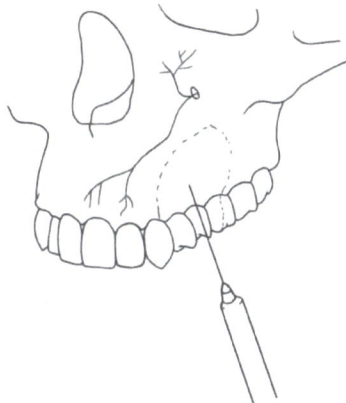

Fig. (3.6). Middle Superior Alveolar Nerve Infilteration.

Areas Anesthetized:

- Pulpal anesthesia of the maxillary Molars

- Buccal free and attached gingival of these same teeth

Indications:
- When Pulpal anesthesia for operative, endodontic or periodontics are indicated.
- For surgical procedure with other supplement injection

Contraindications:
- Infection or acute inflammation in the area of injection.

Precautions: care should be taken to inject the anesthetic solution at the level of apex of the tooth.

Failure of Anesthesia:
Very rare

- Landmarks
- Buccal area of upper 1st, 2nd and 3th Molars.
- The long axis of the tooth
- Insertion the needle with 45 degree to the tooth long axis

- Procedure: (Fig: 3.8)
- Insert the needle into the height of the mucobuccal fold over the target tooth with 45 degree to the long axis of the tooth
- Advance the needle until its bevel is at or above the apical region of the tooth. In most instances, the depth of penetration is only a few millimetres. Because the needle is in soft tissue (not touching bone), there should be no resistance to its advancement, nor should there be any patient discomfort with this injection.
- Aspirate (not strongly recommended because there is no blood vessels with considerable dimention). If negative, deposit approximately 0.6 ml (one-third of a cartridge) slowly over 20 seconds. (Do not permit the tissues to balloon.)
- Slowly withdraw the syringe.
- Make the needle safe.

Wait for 3 to 5 minutes.

Fig. (3.7). Posterior Superior Alveolar Nerve Infilteration.

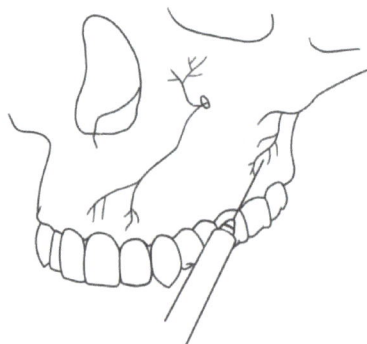

Fig. (3.8). Posterior Superior Alveolar Nerve Infilteration.

Areas Anesthetized:

1. Pulps of the maxillary third, second, and first molars (entire tooth anesthesia can be achieved by using this technique in 72%; the mesiobuccal root of the maxillary first molar is not anesthetized in about 28% of the cases).
2. Buccal periodontium and bone overlay these teeth.

Complications
- Hematoma
- This is commonly produced by inserting the needle too far posteriorly into the pterygoid plexus.

In addition, the maxillary artery may be perforated. Use of a short needle (25 or 27 g) minimizes the risk of pterygoid plexus puncture. A visible intraoral hematoma develops within several minutes, usually noted in the buccal tissues of the mandibular region. There is no easily accessible area to which pressure can be applied to stop the hemorrhage. Bleeding continues until the pressure of the extravascular blood is equal to or greater than that of intravascular blood.

Precaution: The depth of needle penetration should be checked: over-insertion (too deep) increases the risk of hematoma; an insertion that is too shallow might still provide adequate anesthesia.

Examination: Subjective: There is usually none; the patient has difficulty reaching this region to determine the extent of anesthesia, because the mucosa over the gum opposing the maxillary molars are supplied mainly with the long buccal nerve. Objective: absence of pain during therapy

Safety Features: Slow injection, repeated aspirations. There are no anatomical safety features to prevent over-insertion of the needle; therefore, careful observation is necessary.

The goal is to deposit local anesthetic close to the PSA nerves, located posterosuperior and medial to the maxillary tuberosity. It is a highly successful technique (>95%). Nerves Anesthetized: Posterior, superior, alveolar, and branches.

- Landmarks
- Target area: nerves posterior, superior, and medical to the posterior border of the maxilla.
- Mucobuccal fold
- Maxillary tuberosity
- Zygomatic process of the maxilla

- Orientation of the bevel: toward bone during the injection. If bone is accidentally touched, the sensation is less unpleasant.

- Procedure:
- Partially open the patient's mouth, pulling the mandible to the side of injection. Retract the patient's cheek with your finger (for visibility).
- Pull the tissues at the injection site taut.
- Insert the needle into the height of the mucobuccal fold over the second molar.
- Advance the needle slowly in an upward, inward, and backward direction in one movement.
  - a- Upward: superiorly at a 45-degree angle to the occlusal plane
  - b- Inward: medially toward the midline at a 45-degree angle to the occlusal plane
  - c- Backward: posteriorly at a 45-degree angle to the lone axis of the second molars, slowly advance the needle through soft tissue.

Wait for 3 to 5 minutes.

Fig. (3.9). Posterior Superior Alveolar Nerve Block (Tuberosity block, zygomatic block).

Areas Anesthetized:
1. Buccal mucous membrane anterior to the mental foramen, usually from the second premolar to the midline
2. Lower lip and skin of the chin
3. Pulpal nerve fibers to the premolars, canine, and incisors.

Indications:
When the Soft-tissue of anterior part of soft palate anesthesia is indicated for surgical procedures in a circumscribed area.

Contraindications:
1. Infection or acute inflammation in the area of injection

Precautions: it is a traumatic injection, the anesthetic solution should be injected slowly over a long period of time and not more than a quarter of cartridge should be used

Failure of Anesthesia:
Very rare

is a valuable technique for palatal pain control in that, with the administration of a minimum volume of anesthetic solution (maximally, one quarter of a cartridge), a wide area of anterior 2/3 palatal soft-tissue anesthesia is achieved, thereby minimizing the need for multiple palatal injections. Unfortunately, the incisive nerve block has the distinction of being a potentially highly traumatic injection.

- Landmarks
- Incisive foramen
- Incisive papilla located just behind and midway in between the tow upper incisors

Procedure: (Fig: 3.11)
- Slowly advance the needle toward the incisive foramen until bone is gently contacted.
    (1) The depth of penetration is approximately 5 mm.
    (2) Deposit small volumes of anesthetic while advancing the needle. As the tissue is entered, there is increased resistance to the deposition of solution, which is normal with the nasopalatine nerve block.
Technique:
1. A 27-gauge short needle is recommended.
2. Areas of insertion
    a. Labial frenum in the midline between the maxillary central incisors
    b. Interdental papilla between the maxillary central incisors
    c. If needed, palatal soft tissues lateral to the incisive papilla
- Stabilization of the syringe in this second injection is somewhat awkward, but critical. Use of a finger from the other hand to stabilize the needle is recommended. However, the syringe barrel must be held such that it remains within the patient's line of sight, which is potentially disconcerting to some patients.
Wait for 3 to 5 minutes.

Fig. (3.10). Incisive Nerve Block.

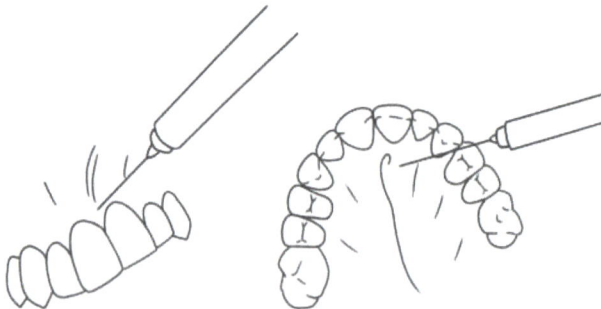

Fig. (3.11). Incisive Nerve Block.

The greater palatine nerve block is useful for dental procedures involving the palatal soft tissues distal to the canine. Minimum volumes of solution (0.45–0.60 ml) provide profound hard- and soft-tissue anesthesia. Although potentially traumatic, the greater palatine nerve block is less so than the nasopalatine nerve block because the tissues surrounding the greater palatine foramen are better able to accommodate the volume of solution deposited.

Contraindications:
1. Infection or acute inflammation in the area of injection

Precautions: This injection should not be used for larger areas:
- A greater number of tissue penetrations increases the possibility of pain both during and after the injection,

and the larger volume of solution administered increases the possibility of local anesthetic overdose and post injection pain.

Failure of Anesthesia
- Depositing anesthetic solution below the apex of a maxillary tooth results in excellent soft-tissue anesthesia but poor or absent pulpal anesthesia.
- The needle tip lies too far from the bone (solution deposited in the buccal soft tissues).

Landmarks:
1. the greater palatine foramen and the junction of the maxillary alveolar process and the palatine bone.
2. The target area is little anterior to foramin:
   - the area between the 6th and 7th molars
   - midway between the occlusal surface of the molars and median palatine raphe.

Nerve Anesthetized: Greater palatine
Areas Anesthetized: The posterior portion of the hard palate and its overlying soft tissues, anteriorly as far as the first premolar and medially to the midline.

Procedure: Assume the correct position .
- For a right greater palatine nerve block, a right-handed administrator should sit facing the patient at the 7 or 8 o'clock position.
- For a left greater palatine nerve block, a right-handed administrator should sit facing in the same direction as the patient at the 11 o'clock position.

Request the patient, who is in a supine position , to do the following:

Open wide., Extend the neck. Turn the head to the left or right (for improved visibility).
- Locate the greater palatine foramen
- Prepare the tissue at the injection site, just 1 to 2 mm anterior to the greater palatine foramen. Pressure is usually indicated since the palatal mucoperiostium is firmly attached by Sharpne,s fibers to the bone of the palate. Note the ischemia (whitening of the soft tissues) at the injection site. If thare is no resistance during injection this is mean you are inject the anesthetic solution at the soft palate.

Fig. (3.12). Greater Palatine Nerve Block.

Nerves Anesthetized:Nasopalatine nerves bilaterally
Areas Anesthetized: Anterior portion of the hard palate (soft and hard tissues) from the mesial of the right first premolar to the mesial of the left first premolar

Local Infiltration of the Palate
Nerves Anesthetized: Terminal branches of the nasopalatine and greater palatine
Areas Anesthetized: Soft tissues in the immediate vicinity of injection
Technique:
1. A 27-gauge needle is recommended, although the 25-gauge short also may be used.
2. Area of insertion: the attached gingival 5 to 10 mm from the free gingival margin

Indications:
When the Soft-tissue of anterior part of soft palate anesthesia is indicated for surgical procedures in a circumscribed area.

Contraindications:
1. Infection or acute inflammation in the area of injection

Precautions: it is a traumatic injection, the anesthetic solution should be injected slowly over a long period of time and not more than a quarter of cartridge should be used

The nasopalatine nerve block is an invaluable technique for palatal pain control in that, with the administration of a minimum volume of anesthetic solution (maximally, one quarter of a cartridge), a wide area of palatal soft-tissue anesthesia is achieved, thereby minimizing the need for multiple palatal injections. Unfortunately, the nasopalatine nerve block has the distinction of being a potentially highly traumatic injection.

- • **Landmarks**
- - **Incisive foramen**
- - **Incisive papilla located just behind and midway in between the tow upper incisors**

Procedure: (Fig: 3.14)
- Slowly advance the needle toward the incisive foramen until bone is gently contacted.
     (1) The depth of penetration is approximately 5 mm.
     (2) Deposit small volumes of anesthetic while advancing the needle. As the tissue is entered, there is increased resistance to the deposition of solution, which is normal with the nasopalatine nerve block.
Technique
- A 27-gauge short needle is recommended.
- Areas of insertion
     a.Labial frenum in the midline between the maxillary central incisors
     b. Interdental papilla between the maxillary central incisors
     c. If needed, palatal soft tissues lateral to the incisive papilla
- Stabilization of the syringe in this second injection is somewhat awkward, but critical. Use of a finger from the other hand to stabilize the needle is recommended. However, the syringe barrel must be held such that it remains within the patient's line of sight, which is potentially disconcerting to some patients.

Fig. (3.13). Nasopalatine Nerve Block.

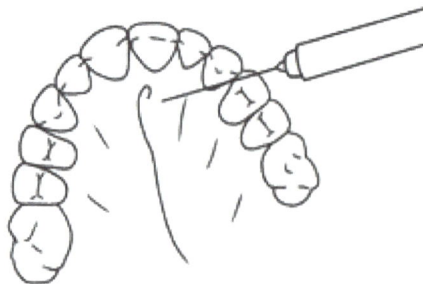

Fig. (3.14). Nasopalatine Nerve Block.

Nerves Anesthetized:
1. Inferior alveolar, a branch of the posterior division of the mandibular
2. Incisive
3. Mental
4. Lingual (commonly)

Areas Anesthetized:
Mandibular teeth to the midline
, Body of the mandible, inferior portion of the ramus , Buccal mucoperiosteum, mucous membrane anterior to the mandibular first molar (mental nerve) , Anterior two thirds of the tongue and floor of the oral cavity (lingual nerve), Lingual soft tissues and periosteum (lingual nerve)

Indications:
When the Soft-tissue of Buccsal mucosa, anterior 2/3 of the tongue floof of the mouth and the posterior teeth from 1st remolar to third molar is indicated for surgical procedures

Landmarks
- Pterygomandibular rapha
- Anterior border of the ramus
- Coronoid notch
- Lingula
- Posterior border of the ramus
- Occlusal plane,
- Contralateral premolars

Contraindications:
1. Infection or acute inflammation in the area of injection

Precautions: it is a traumatic injection, the anesthetic solution should be injected slowly over a long period of time.

Failure of Anesthesia:
Is not uncommon

Procedure: (Fig: 3.16)
- Insert the needle into the tissues lateral to the pterygomandibular rapha. The needle insertion point lies three fourths of the anteroposterior distance from the coronoid notch back to the deepest part of the pterygo-mandibular raphe.
- The average depth of penetration to bony contact will be 20 to 25 mm, approximately two thirds to three fourths the length of a long dental needle.
- If bone is contacted too soon (less than half the length of a long dental needle), the needle tip is usually located too far anteriorly (laterally) on the ramus .
If bone is not contacted, the needle tip is usually located too far posterior.
- Aspirate . If negative, deposit approximately 1.5 ml slowly.
- Slowly withdraw the syringe for 10 mm and deposit few drops of solution(for lingual nerve)
- Slowly withdraw the syringe.
- Make the needle safe.
- Wait 3 to 5 minutes before commencing the dental procedure

Wait for 3 to 5 minutes.

Fig. (3.15). Inferior Alveolar Nerve Block (IANB).

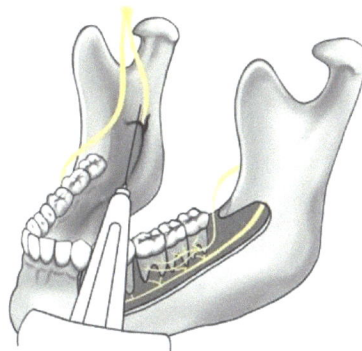

Fig. (3.16). Inferior Alveolar Nerve Block (IANB).

Nerves Anesthetized:
Buccal Nerve

Indications:
When the Soft-tissue of Buccsal mucosa,
is indicated for surgical procedures

Contraindications:
1. Infection or acute inflammation in the area
   of injection

Precautions: it is a traumatic injection, the
anesthetic solution should be injected slowly
over a long period of time.

Failure of Anesthesia:
Is not uncommon

Area Anesthetized:
Soft tissues and periosteum buccal to the mandibular
molar teeth (distal to the mental foramen)
For a right buccal nerve block, a right-handed
administrator should sit at the 8 o'clock position directly
facing the patient .
For a left buccal nerve block, a right-handed
administrator should sit at 10 o'clock facing in the same
direction as the patient

Landmarks
- Pterygomandibular rapha
- Anterior border of the ramus
- Coronoid notch
- Lingula
- Posterior border of the ramus

- Occlusal plane,
- Contralateral premolars

Procedure:
Direct the syringe(long needle) toward the injection site
with the bevel facing down toward bone and the syringe
aligned parallel with the occlusal plane on the side of
injection but buccal to the teeth .
Penetrate mucous membrane at the injection site, distal and
buccal to the last molar

Wait for 3 to 5 minutes.

Fig. (3.17). Buccal Nerve Block.

Nerves Anesthetized:
1. Inferior alveolar, a branch of the posterior division of the mandibular
2. Incisive
3. Mental
4. Lingual (commonly)

Indications:
When the Soft-tissue of Buccsal mucosa, is indicated for surgical procedures

Contraindications:
1. Infection or acute inflammation in the area of injection

Precautions: it is a traumatic injection, the anesthetic solution should be injected slowly over a long period of time.

Failure of Anesthesia:
It is not uncommon
Greater success rate than IAN block with slower time of onset and less aspiration percentage.

Areas Anesthetized:
1. Mandibular teeth to midline
2. Buccal mucoperiosteum and mucous membranes on the side of injection
3. Anterior two thirds of the tongue and floor of the oral cavity , Lingual soft tissues and periosteum
5. Body of the mandible, inferior portion of the ramus
6. Skin over the zygoma, posterior portion of the cheek, and temporal regions

Landmarks
- Pterygomandibular rapha
- Anterior border of the ramus
- Coronoid notch
- Lingula
- Posterior border of the ramus
- Occlusal plane,
- Contralateral premolars

Procedure: (Fig: 3.19)
Target area: Lateral side of the condylar neck, just below the insertion of the lateral pterygoid muscle with 25-30 mm depth of penetration.
Landmarks:

a. Extraoral
- Lower border of the tragus (intertragic notch); the correct landmark is the center of the external auditory meatus, which is concealed by the tragus; therefore its lower border is adopted as a visual aid
- Corner of the mouth

b. Intraoral
- Height of injection established by placement of the needle tip just below the mesiolingual (mesiopalatal) cusp of the maxillary second molar
- Penetration of soft tissues just distal to the maxillary second molar at the height established in the preceding step
- These are the same positions used for a right and a left IAN.
- Position the patient .
- Align the needle with the plane extending from the corner of the mouth to the intertragic notch on the side of injection. It should be parallel with the angle between the ear and the face .
- The syringe barrel lies in the corner of the mouth over the premolars, but its position may vary from molars to incisors, depending on the divergence of the ramus as assessed by the angle of the ear to the side of the face

Wait for 3 to 5 minutes.

Fig. (3.18). Gow Gates Technique.

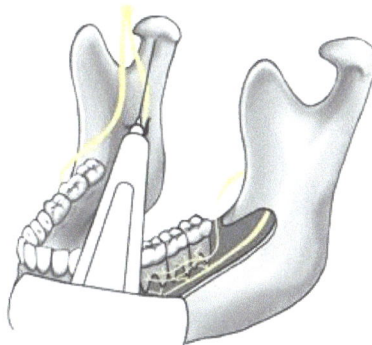

Fig. (3.19). Gow Gates Technique.

Nerves Anesthetized:
1. Inferior alveolar, a branch of the posterior division of the mandibular
2. Incisive
3. Mental
4. Lingual (commonly)

Indications:
When the Soft-tissue of Buccsal mucosa, anterior 2/3 of the tongue floof of the mouth and the posterior teeth from 1st remolar to third molar is indicated for surgical procedures

Contraindications:
1. Infection or acute inflammation in the area of injection

Precautions: it is a traumatic injection, the anesthetic solution should be injected slowly over a long period of time.

Failure of Anesthesia:
It is not uncommon

Areas Anesthetized:
1. Mandibular teeth to the midline
2. Body of the mandible and inferior portion of the ramus
3. Buccal mucoperiosteum and musous membrane in front of the mental foramen
4. Anterior two thirds of the tongue and floor of the oral cavity (Lingual nerve)
5. Lingual soft tissues and periosteum (lingual nerve)

Landmarks
- Pterygomandibular rapha
- Anterior border of the ramus
- Coronoid notch
- Lingula
- Posterior border of the ramus
- Occlusal plane,
- Contralateral premolars

Procedure: (Fig: 3.21)
- Area of insertion: soft tissue overlying the medial (lingual) border of the mandibular ramus directly adjacent to the maxillary tuberosity at the height of the mucogingival junction adjacent to the maxillary third molar .
- The barrel of the syringe is held parallel with the maxillary occlusal plane, the needle at the level of the muco-gingival junction of the maxillary third (or second) molar .
- Orient the bevel away from the mandibular ramus; thus as the needle advances through tissues, needle deflection occurs toward the ramus and the needle remains in close proximity to the inferior alveolar nerve .
Advance the needle 25 mm into tissue (for an average-sized adult). This distance is measured from the maxillary tuberosity. The tip of the needle should lie in the midportion of the pterygomandibular space, close to the branches of mandibular nerve.

Wait for 3 to 5 minutes.

Fig. (3.20). Vazirani-Akinosi Closed-Mouth Mandibular Block.

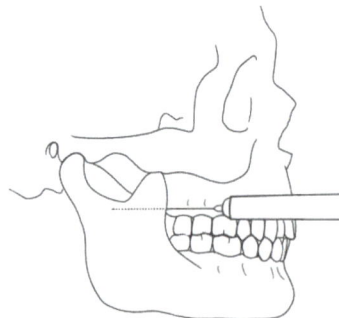

Fig. (3.21). Vazirani-Akinosi Closed-Mouth Mandibular Block.

Nerves Anesthetized:
Mental Nerve

Indications:
When the Pulp, root, and related bone of the incisors, canine and premolars need to be anesthetized.
When the lower lip of the same side of injection need to be anesthetized for both skin and mucosa and associated strectutes

Contraindications:
1. Infection or acute inflammation in the area of injection

Failure of Anesthesia:
It is rare

Areas Anesthetized: Buccal mucous membranes anterior to the mental foramen (around the second premolar) to the midline and skin of the lower lip and chin.

Landmarks
– Mucobuccal fold
– Crown of the tooth
– Root contour of the tooth
– Orientation of the bevel: toward bone with 45 degree angulation to the long axis of the tooth.
– Target area is the area between the 1st and 2nd premolars where the mental foramen is located

Procedure:
If radiograph are available, the mental foramen may be located easily .
- Penetrate the mucous membrane at the injection site, at the canine or first premolar, directing the syringe toward the mental foramen .

- In mental nerve block or incisisve nerve block , the lingual plate and soft tissues are not anasthetized,so to obtain lingual anesthesia

- Buccal approach.Because the buccal soft tissue are already anesthetized, the penetration is atraumatic. Local anesthetic solution should be deposited as the needle is advanced through the tissue toward the lingual .
- Another method of obtaining lingual anesthesia after the incisive nerve block is to   administer a partial lingual nerve block (do IANB from the beginning).

Wait for 3 to 5 minutes.

Fig. (3.22). Mental Nerve Block.

Areas Anesthetized: Bone, soft tissue, and apical and pulpal tissues in the area of injection

Advantages
1. Negligible soft tissue anesthesia
2. Minimum dose
3. No aspiration
4. Rapid onset 30 seconds
5. Overcome failed conventional techniques
6. Used in patients with bleeding diathesis

Disadvantages
1. Damage to the periodontal tissues
2. Damage to the pulp:complete cessation of pulpal flow for 20 minutes
3. Damage to unerupted teeth:cyttotoxic to the cells of the enamel organ
4. Lower success rate in endodontic treatment

Precautions: it is a traumatic injection, the anesthetic solution should be injected slowly over a long period of time and not more than a quarter of cartridge should be used

Intrapulpal Injection
-may be used on any tooth when difficulty in providing pain control exist(during endodontics or surgical tooth division of lower molars most commonly).
-It is used once the pulp chamber is exposed.
-may need to bend the needle and insert the needle in the exposure until it fits snugly then deposit 0.2-0.3ml of solution.
-anesthesia achieved by pressure causing ischemia.
-it is painful.

Failure of Anesthesia:
Very rare

Indications:
1. Pulpal anesthesia of one or two teeth in a quadrant Sed
2. Patients for whom residual soft-tissue anesthesia is undesirable
3. Situations in which regional block anesthesia is contraindicated
4. As a possible aid in diagnosis of pulpal discomfort
5. As an adjunctive technique after nerve block anesthesia if partial anesthesia is present

Procedure: :
- Area of insertion:30 degrees to the long axis of the tooth to be treated on its mesial or distal of the root (one-rooted tooth) or on the mesial and distal roots (of multirooted tooth) interproximally
- Target area: depth of the gingival sulcus
Landmarks
      a. Root(s) of the tooth
      b. Periodontal tissues
- a volume of 0.2 ml of local anesthetic solution is injected under strong pressure
- the needle should remain in position for at least 5 seconds following injection(to prevent the loss of the solution *via* the needle tract into the mouth)
Presence of vasoconstrictor is a must special syringes to be used(even conventional syringes can be used effectively)
- Intraseptal Injection :
Same technique as intraosseouss techniqe but after we feel bony contact we introduce the needle under pressure in order to introduce 1-2 mm in the bone then we deposit around0 .2-0.4 ml(so there is no hole created by a perforator or a bur) and lesser volume of local anesthetic solution

Wait for 3 to 5 minutes.

- May associated with high risk of septicemia

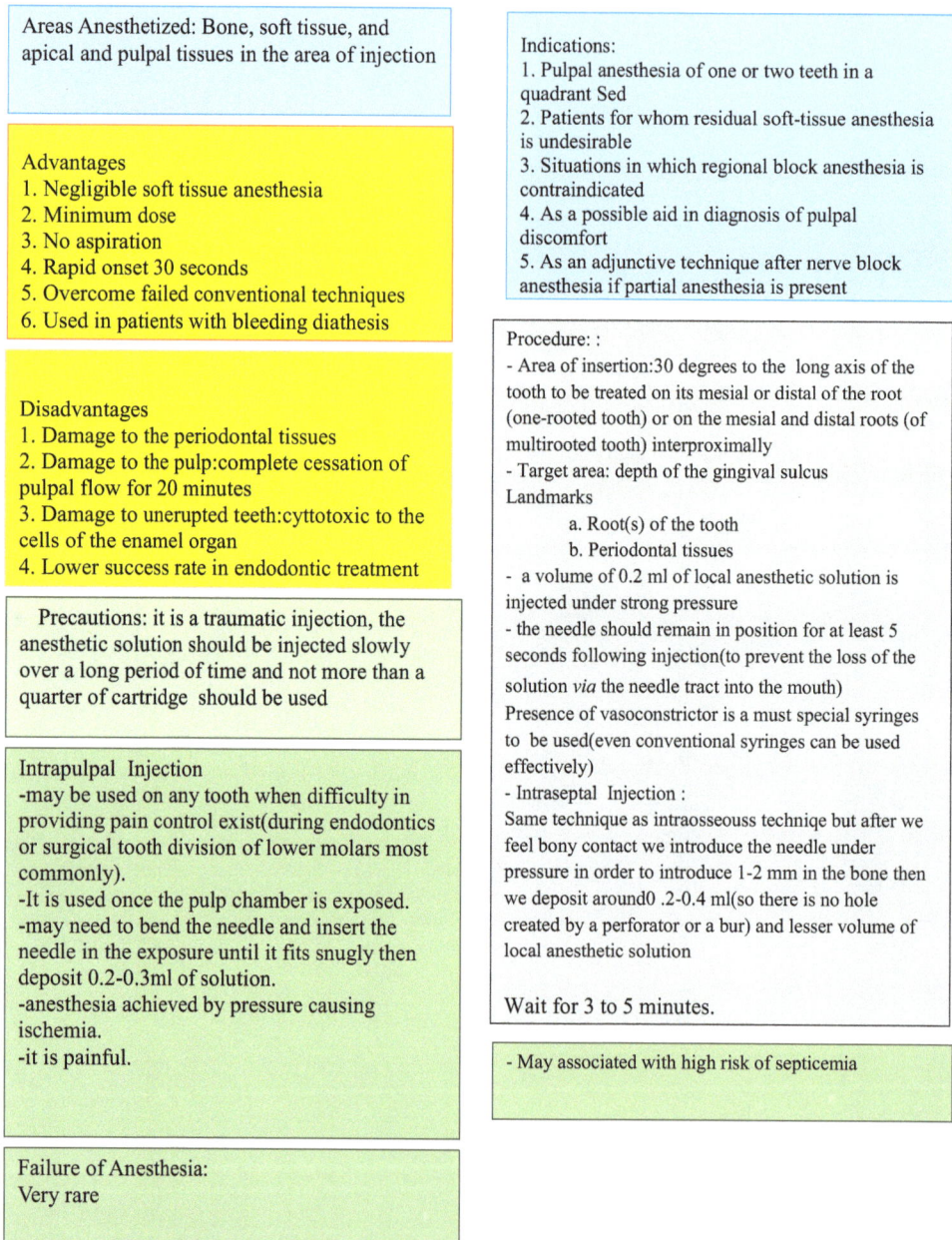

Fig. (3.23). Intraligamentary anesthesia.

PART - 3: OUTLINE OF LOCAL ANESTHESIA COMPLICATIONS

Part - 1: The Systemic Complications of Local Anaesthesia

Systemic Complications can be Calcified as the Following:

1. Psychological reactions induced by anxiety, (not uncommon)
2. Toxic effect as a result of high levels of the anaesthetic drug in the patient's body blood (common)
3. The presence of systemic diseases apart from these (very common)
4. Allergies. (this is extremely rare since the LA is thought to be a hypoallergenic)

- Around 80.3 percent reported some modicum of anxiety or nervousness before the dental anaesthesia, and the procedure itself.
- 61.2 percent said they had no anxiety or nervousness about any procedures they may need in the future, once the dental anaesthesia and procedure had been administered.
- From the sample, the quantity of patients that were satisfied with the procedure rested at 94.3 percent.
- up 94.7 percent of Patients would recommend anaesthesia to others.

What impact does the patient's general condition take on when they are given local anaesthesia?

Evidence From Cardiovascular Diseases

What follows is a very severely rare problem that is caused by local anaesthesia. It only presents itself when the dose administered is too high, and is done so intravenously. This is not typically a practical in dentistry:

- Local anaesthesia can have an impact on the cardiovascular system. This is more so true when the doses are at a higher level. Such manifestations are typically characterised by bradycardia and are seen to be depressants. They also can consist of cardiovascular collapse, and hypotension and the combination of all these factors could lead to cardiac arrest. At doses that are lower, while it can act as a stimulant, the manifestations are not this emphasised.
- The first signs and side effects of compromised cardiovascular system usually come about because of vasovagal responses are fainting and dizziness. This is especially true if the patient assumes an upright pose abruptly (postural hypotension).
- Such diseases can often hinder the use of vasoconstrictors and local anaesthesia. They are discussed many times in terms of their contraindications. However, no absolute contraindications exist for patients that suffer from cardiovascular

problems.

If the patient is not stable then any form of dental care would be postponed till their condition stabilized; if emergency dental treatment is needed, it must be done with close contact, under the care and recommendation of patient's physicians.

Hypertension (High Blood Pressure)

About more than 50 million individuals in the United States have hypertension or are taking antihypertensive prescriptions and around 70% of these patients got dental anaesthesia at least one time in their life.

- One of the common concerns in hypertensive and other cardiovascular compromised patients is the decision regarding giving a local anaesthetic agent with a vasoconstrictor during dental treatment.
- The proper way of approaching this issue is to analyse the patho-physiological impact and mode of action of vasoconstrictors. The main impact here includes:
  ○ A delay of the process of absorbing of the solution into the systemic circulation lead to:
    ▪ increase in the duration,
    ▪ increase the depth of anaesthesia,
    ▪ and also may result in the decrease in the risk of toxicity.

The administration of LA, along with the help of a vasoconstrictor, typically leads to augmented effectiveness of the anaesthesia. It may helps in reducing the likelihood of blood pressure rising beyond the normal margin, due to anxiety and pain.

Can the standard dose of local anesthesia (e.g. 1.8mL of 2% lidocaine with 1:100,000 epinephrine - 18 μ.g of epinephrine) be given to cardiovascular patients during dental treatment?

The answer is yes.

The AHA and ADA (The American Heart Association and the American Dental Association) in 1964, in their joint conference, recommend the following "the concentrations of vasoconstrictors in local dental anaesthesia are not contraindicated for the patients of cardiovascular disease since preliminary aspiration is done, and the local anaesthesia is injected slowly over enough period of time, along with this the smallest amount of this is used, that is recommended to be effective. These recommendations are important if hypertension is to be managed in the patients that suffer from it and require treatment as well. The recommended dose needs to be restricted to 0.04mg of adrenaline for patients that are suffering from cardiovascular risk. This would amount to around two 1:100000 cartridges of epinephrine.

- The Felypressin is approximately 1/5 (one-fifth) as effective adrenalin (epinephrine- vasoconstrictor) and is accordingly utilized as a part of a 1:20,000 concentration. This concentration is five-fold higher than the usual concentration of adrenalin vasoconstrictor in the local anaesthetic agent.
- Levonordefrin is considered to convey the same clinical risk as 1:100,000 adrenaline (epinephrine).
- The results of a number of studies indicate that the use of one to two of 1.8 ml cartridges of local anesthesia with 1:100,000 of the vasoconstrictor (epinephrine) in the local dental anesthesia is of minimal clinical significance for most of the patients with cardiovascular diseases including hypertensive patients.
- However, using more than two local dental anaesthetic cartridges with a vasoconstrictor (epinephrine) should be considered as a relative contraindication rather than an absolute.
- Additional vasoconstrictor-containing local anaesthetic (or local anaesthetic without epinephrine) can be administered, if necessary, only if the administration of the previous two cartridges of vasoconstrictor-containing local anaesthetic exhibits no signs or symptoms of cardiac alteration, (it should always be remembered to administer the local anaesthesia slowly and with preliminary aspiration.
- Some clinician prefers to start the anaesthesia through the use of an agent that contains non-vasoconstrictors like 4% prilocaine plain or 3% mepivacaine. Inadequate anaesthesia is them supplemented with small amounts of local anaesthetics with adrenaline. For patients that have extreme uncontrollable hypertension, this can be a useful path to take. The treatment for such patients should be postponed till the point that their blood pressure is brought back into control. A sedative like valium (diazepam) can also be used so that the use of the LA with a vasoconstrictor can be limited to two or one cartridges.
- The dentist needs to keep the likelihood of an adverse interaction between anti-hypertensive medicines being taken by the patient, along with the LA agents that they are looking to administer. This applies in particular in the case of adrenergic blocking agents. The danger of a reverse response is reduced through the use of cardioselective beta blockers such as Tenormin or Lopressor. Both classes can develop higher than usual serum levels of LA solutions because of the competitive fall of hepatic clearance that occurs within the liver.
- There is medication for hypertension that can lead to adrenergic receptors to become sensitive to sympathomimetics. This can lead to an amplified systemic response to the vasoconstrictor that contains the anaesthetic liquid.

- Then again, as much as the agent is restricted to one or two cartridges, the medicines will not have a considerable risk.
- Several studies have investigated the systemic effect of administration of vasoconstrictor (catecholamines) with dental local anesthesia. Five min after injection of conventional routine dose (1.8mL of 2% lidocaine with 1:100,000 epinephrine - 18 µ.g of epinephrine), Tolas and coworkers 17 found plasma adrenaline level to be 240 (mean) ± 69 (SD) pg/mL compared to a baseline consentration of 98 ± 38 pg/mL. When lidocaine without catecholamines was used, plasma adrenalin did not differ significantly from baseline level. They reported that in the healthy subjects, heart rate, mean arterial pressure, and rate pressure were not significantly altered from baseline after adrenalin (epinephrine) injection [60].
- Cioffi *et al.*, in a study of plasma catecholamine and changes in hemodynamic in amalgam restoration of a single tooth with usual dose local anesthetic solution (1.8 mL of 2% lidocaine with 1: 100,000 epinephrine), found plasma epinephrine to increase from a baseline of 28 (mean) ± 8 (SE) pg/mL to 105 ± 28 pg/mL five minutes after administration. In parallel with the plasma adrenaline level, the heart rates were affected, but mean arterial blood pressure was unaltered [61].
- Chernow *et al.*, reported a transient change in heart rate for 2 min after inferior alveolar nerve block with epinephrine-containing local anesthetic (the heart rate was increased transiently). Eight min after injection, plasma adrenaline concentration was 3.5 times greater than pre-injection control without significant hemodynamic changes [62].
- Two studies in which 54 µ.g of adrenaline was injected demonstrated significant hemodynamic changes (cardiovascular system responses). In these studies, it has been used (5.4 mL of 2% lidocaine with 1: 100,000 epinephrine for unilateral maxillary and mandibular third molar extractions) resulted in plasma adrenaline (epinephrine) titers 5 minutes after injection that were approximately five times greater than the baseline. Both heart rate and systolic blood pressure were significantly increased. Plasma adrenaline level, heart rate and blood pressure were not significantly increased when 2% lidocaine without epinephrine was used for third molar extractions on the opposite sides [63, 64].
- Knoll-Kohler *et al.*, in a study of hemodynamic (cardiovascular) and plasma catecholamine changes to third molar removal with dental local anesthesia, found that an increase in plasma epinephrine level to more than six times the previously reported threshold for blood pressure increase23 did not cause significant cardiovascular changes [65].
- The conclusion that may be obtained from these studies is that, the administration of the conventional dose of adrenaline (epinephrine) found in one standard cartridge of 2% lidocaine with 1: 100,000 epinephrine results in a very

quickly increase in plasma adrenaline level (epinephrine) two times greater than baseline. This increase is not associated with any biologically significant hemodynamic (cardiovascular) change. Administration of three standard cartridges of the same local anesthetic/vasoconstrictor combination is resulted in a fivefold increase in serum (plasma) adrenaline level; significant hemodynamic (cardiovascular system) changes may occur, but are not consistently related and associated with this dose. The changes of epinephrine level in these studies may be related to anxiety associated with dental treatment rather to standard dose of vasoconstrictor in local anesthetic solution, as all the studies have been mentioned, did not investigate the anxiety level in candidates involved in those studies. It can be concluded as well that the limitation to two standard local anesthetic cartridges is safe even in cardiovascular patients according to American association of cardiovascular diseases. As it has been reported that the threshold serum adrenaline (epinephrine) concentration required for increase in blood pressure is +50 to +100 pg/ ml, the concentration required for an increase in systolic blood pressure is +75 to +125 pg/ml, and the concentration required for a decreased diastolic blood pressure is +150 to +200 pg/ml.23 However, the study from which these concentration values were determined used only six healthy subjects. As mentioned, the mean maximum circulating adrenaline level after administration of 18 μ,g of epinephrine were from 105 to 240 pg/ml, and the maximum serum (plasma) epinephrine reported after 54 μ,g of epinephrine was 302 (mean) ± 142 (SD) pg/ml.2 1 The cardiovascular changes that should have occurred based upon concentration values did not occur with 18 μ,g of adrenaline, but were seen when 54 μ g was administered [66].

- As the vasoconstrictor retard local anesthetic absorption into the systemic circulation, indeed, not all studies have demonstrated delayed local anesthetic absorption. Goebel *et al.*, studied peak plasma level of local anesthetics after maxillary supraperiosteal infiltration of 1.8 mL of 2% lidocaine with 1: 100,000 epinephrine or the same volume of 2% lidocaine without vasoconstrictor. These investigators found that addition of 1: 100,000 epinephrine did not contribute significantly to changes in the peak plasma concentration of lidocaine. Even if local anesthetic absorption is retarded, it is not absolutely provide an additional margin of safety. The vasoconstrictor is also absorbed into the systemic circulation, and its presence could conceivably lower the threshold of the central nervous system or cardiovascular system to the local anesthetic agent [67, 68].

It is important to keep in mind that these agents should always be injected very slowly to ensure that even the slightest possibility of ischemia on the site of the injection is avoided. Implementation of proper aspiration and slowly injection is likely minimizing the possible local and systemic complication of the epinephrine.

Over Dosage and Toxicity

Toxicity from Local anesthesia in dental practice is rare. A toxic reaction can occur:

- When the concentration of local anaesthetic in circulation increases too rapidly.
- When injecting into a highly vascular area there is a risk of an intravascular injection.
- When not follow the recommended dose of local anaesthesia.

Determent factors for overdose and toxicity:

1. Patient's factors:
    - Age
    - Weight
    - Sex
    - Other drug
    - Presence of other systemic diseases
    - Mental attitude and environmental factors
    - Genetics
2. Drug factors:
    - Route of administration
    - Rate of injections
    - Vasoactivity
    - Concentration
    - Dose
    - Vascularity of injection site
    - Absence of vasoconstrictor

The toxicity of local anesthesia is primarily effected the central nervous system and cardiovascular system. Typical symptoms are:

- Talkativeness,
- Apprehension,
- Lethargy,
- Restlessness,
- Convulsion,
- and Loss of consciousness.

More severe symptoms include:

- Increase in blood pressure and heart rate
- Coma,

- Respiratory arrest,
- and Even vascular collapse and cardiac arrest.

Toxic signs and symptoms appear usually within five to ten minutes after injection, but if local anesthetic is injected intravenously, responses may be immediate.

Toxicity can also be produced by vasoconstrictors, such as adrenaline, the possible symptoms are:

- Increase in fear and anxiety,
- Tremors,
- Headache and palpitations.

Special caution should be exercised when a patient suffers from hyperthyroidism or hypertension.

Prevention

- Dentist should keep in mind the maximum recommended doses of anaesthetics. In elderly patients and children the safe doses of anaesthetics are lower than healthy adult. For example, a maximum safe dose of lidocaine hydrochloride 20 mg/ml with adrenaline 12.5 mg/ml for healthy adults is 10 ml which means 5.5 cartridges. For children the maximum dose is 4.4 mg/kg, which means in a child of 20 kg less than 2.5 cartridges of anaesthetic. Maximum doses of some injectable local anaesthetic are listed in Table **3.1** (18).

Table 3.1. Maximum doses of some injectable local anaesthetic.

Effective agent	Maximum dosage
Lidocaine HCL 20 mg/ml + adrenaline 12.5 g/ml (1 : 80 000)	For adults 10 ml (5.5 cartridges).For children 4.4 mg/kg (20 kg; less than 2.5 cartridges)
Articaine hydrochloride 40 mg/ml + adrenaline 5 g/ml (1: 200 000)	For adults 12.5 ml (7 cartridges).For children 5.0 mg/kg (20kg; less than 1.5 cartridges)
Articaine hydrochloride 40 mg/ml + adrenaline 10 g/ml	For adults 12.5 ml. For children 0.175 ml/kg
Prilocaine hydrochloride30 mg/ml + felypressin 0.54 g/ml	For adults 10 ml (5.5 cartridges).For children 6.0 mg/kg (20 kg; 2 cartridges)

In Old Patient

- The systemic catabolic increased
- The metabolism deceased
- The situation is the same in patients complaining of a liver insufficiency.
  - The dosage of the local anaesthetic for these patients should be reduced.

- ○ The aspirating technique should be used before injection to avoid the intravenous injection and possible associated toxicity.
- ○ It is important to monitor the patient for possible side effects during injection.
- ○ Anaesthetics should be injected slowly. The slow injection helps to maintain the aesthetic in the target area.

Failure of Local Anesthesia (Lack of Effect)

In spite of implementation of a proper technique, the patient still feels pain during treatment. The failures of dental local anesthesia can be classified as:

- Anatomical,
- Pathological,
- Psychological,
- and Poor injection technique.

Anatomical causes include:

- Presence of accessory nerve supply,
    - ○ Maxillary molar teeth may have pulpal supply from the greater palatine nerve,
    - ○ Maxillary anterior teeth may receive innervation from the naso-palatine nerve.
    - ○ In the mandible, a long buccal or lingual nerve can sometimes provide innervation to molar pulps.
- Variation in foramen location,
- Abnormal course of the nerves,
- Bifid alveolar nerve or mandibular canal.

Pathological causes for failure of local anesthesia include:

- Trismus,
- Inflammation,
- Infection (the low tissue pH),
- Previous surgery or trauma. When mouth opening is limited.

Psychological Factors

Anxiety and fear can cause failure in local anesthesia, to enable successful anesthesia, relaxation and following the stress reduction protocol are needed. The use of a sedative like benzo-diazepines may become indicated in some cases.

Poor Technique

The most common reason for failure of anesthesia is poor technique. In inferior alveolar block the common mistake is:

- Injection of anaesthesia in the ascending ramus as the needle point touches the lingual cortical bone anterior to the lingula.
- Injection of anaesthesia inferior to the mandibular foramen.
- Injection of anaesthesia too forcefully and rapidly.

Precausion

- Be careful
- The key factor in patient management is the medical history of the patient (be well oriented to diseases, medications, precaution and proper management)
- Be well known to the anatomy and possible variation
- Use the proper instruments
- Follow the right technique and
  - ○ bone contact
  - ○ aspirate
  - ○ do not inject forcefully against hard pressure
  - ○ inject slowly
- Use the minimum necessary doses of anesthetic
- Follow the stress reduction protocol and use sedatives if necessary

Postoperative paresthesia or neuralgia:

The trigeminal nerve permanent altered sensation is extremely rare (about 4:100 000). The Inferior alveolar nerve block is the second most common cause for permanent neurological changes; the most common cause is third molar surgical extraction.

Paresthesia can for example result from:

- Nerve injury: the nerve is usually deflected by the needle during needle insertion or withdrawal, when the deflection does not occur a nerve injury may be developed by direct nerve trauma when the needle is penetrating the nerve or when the tip of the needle scratches the nerve. Trauma for the nerve feels like an "electric shock" throughout the distribution of the involved nerve, and the patient may suddenly jerk his/her head or jaw. If this occurs, the Injection must be ceased immediately, and the needle must be replaced in a slightly different location.
- Haematoma: It is reported that haematoma after local anaesthetic administration may cause change in sensation. If one of the small intraneural blood vessels is

injured, a neurotoxic intraneural haematoma may develop. The hemosiderin granules (iron complex from Red Blood Cells – RBCs) and free radicals from the haematoma are very toxic and may affect the nerve (it may induce a sever neuro-toxic and mayo-toxic effect).

The lingual nerve seems to be most commonly affected. When the mouth is wide open, the lingual nerve is held tightly in the tissues and is unable to be deflected by the needle. Inferior alveolar, mental and buccal nerves can also be affected due to local anaesthesia.

- The total or partial anaesthesia altered sensation may present as:
  - deep, burning pain
  - or flushing over the associated cheek.
  - if chorda tympani are involved there may be alteration in taste sensation.

Paresthesia is usually transient, but may be permanent if anesthetic solution is injected directly into the nerve. This is very rare and difficult because the nerve located in tight epineurium Therefore, injection against pressure must be avoided with exception of greater palatine and nasopalatine nerves block. Instead of that, when the needle is withdrawn through the nerve, a little amount of anesthetic into the lumen and onto the needle can cause a chemical damage when the needle has transfixed the nerve after injection (the lingual nerve is the nerve mostly effected).

Temporary blindness and diplopia has been reported following posterior superior alveolar nerve block, this probably is due to a spread of anaesthetic near the nerves innervating muscles of the eye, and/or even into contact with the optic nerve, and therefore disturbs the function of the nerve temporarily.

Angina Pectoris and Post-Myocardial Infarction

- Dental anaesthetics have a smaller chance of adversely affecting patients that have no history of infarction, and have stable angina as opposed to their opposites.
- *Anxiety and stress reduction protocol* has a significant part to play in terms of managing such patients. Ensuring that the pain control is of the best possible quality is imperative during the dental procedure. Using LA which contains a vasoconstrictor has been seen to play a positive role in terms of stress reduction in such patients because of the proper pain control,
- The elective treatment should be avoided in those patients with:
  - myocardial infarctions that occurred within the last 6 months,
  - unstable anginas,
  - or patients have had recently had coronary bypass (around three months prior to procedure).

Emergency treatment can be done only with consultation with the cardiologist

If dental treatment can not be delayed:

- **Stress reduction protocol should be followed**
- **and appropriate sedation may be needed**
- **Anything that goes beyond one or two cartridges of local anesthesia needs to be carefully monitored.**

Cardiac Dysrhythmia

- It is essential to identify patients that have an existing cardiac dysrhythmia condition (also known as arrhythmias), the condition can prove to be a big problem and as such physicians need to ensure the current status of the patient before proceeding with their procedure.

Patients that can be prone to Cardiac Dysrhythmia:

Patients that are suffering from:

- Ischemic heart disease,
- Thyrotoxicosis,
- Congestive heart failure,
- and Coronary atherosclerotic heart disease,
- The above patients are prone to cardiac arrhythmias resulting from stress.

- It is crucial to keep an eye on anxiety, the stress reduction protocol should be followed. LA agents that have vasoconstrictors can be used to maintain pain during the procedure, as such, they are an appropriate course of action to take.
- Patients that have refractory or severe arrhythmias should not be put through elective dentistry till their condition is brought under control by the physician.

Cerebrovascular Accident

Patients with the hypertensive vascular disease, atherosclerosis, along with cardiac pathoses including atrial fibrillation and myocardial infarction, have a higher chance of suffering from a stroke. Patients that have already suffered a stroke are at greater risk of having another one as opposed to a patient that has never had a stroke.

- For such patients, it is advised that their treatment is postponed by at least six months. This is important since someone who has suffered one stroke could suffer another during the procedure.
- Once six months have passed, the procedure may go ahead as planned. However, vasoconstrictors with LA must be used to control the pain and minimize the anxiety.

Pulmonary Disease

The dental officer is most frequently witness to chronic obstructive pulmonary disease and asthma.

Asthma

- It is the objective of dental management to ensure that an acute attack does not occur. Stress can be a contributing factor for asthma patients, and stress needs to be managed. The Food and Drug Administration has also pointed out that medication containing sulphites can also lead to allergic reactions in people that are prone to attacks.
- However, the data on the subject is limited. More than 96% of people that suffer from asthma are not sensitive to sulphites. People that are found to be sensitive to this are typically those with severe conditions. They are generally dependent on steroids.
- Awe *et al.* reported that LA with vasoconstrictors could be implemented in patients that suffered from asthma but were not dependent on steroids. Nevertheless, till we find out more about this sensitivity, it is recommended to avoid using this in asthma patients that are dependent on corticosteroids.
- Another hallmark of metabolism of ester LAs is that their hydrolysis leads to the formation of para-aminobenzoic acid (PABA). PABA and its derivatives carry a small risk potential for allergic reactions. A history of an allergic reaction to a LA should immediately suggest that a current reaction is due to the presence of PABA derived from an ester LA. However, although exceedingly rare, allergic reactions can also develop from the use of multiple-dose vials of amide LAs that contain PABA as a preservative [70].

Chronic Obstructive Pulmonary Disease

- Chronic bronchitis and emphysema are the most common types of chronic obstructive pulmonary disease. They are mapped through irreversible obstruction of ventilation in the lungs.
- No actual guidelines exist for this type of a problem. Despite the lack of recommended guidelines, those suffering from hypertension and/or coronary heart disease need to be managed as per the guidelines meted out for those diseases.

Renal Disease

- Dental LA at times are not metabolised and do not exit the blood stream with the same speed as they would when the patient has some form of renal disease. The dosage being administered may need to be recalculated for such patients. In most cases, it needs to be reduced, and the intervals between doses may need to be increased.

Hepatic Disease

- The status of the liver in terms of how it's functioning and whether it is diseased is also going to be important. The main reason for this is that anaesthetics are typically metabolised in the liver.
- As the metabolisms of local anesthetic depend on the type of local anesthesia, the esters are metabolized in the plasme and the amides are metabolized in the liver.

Ester LAs are metabolized in plasma by pseudocholinesterase. The rate of hydrolysis of ester LAs depends on the location and type of the substitution in the aromatic ring. For example, chloroprocaine is metabolized about four times faster than procaine, and procaine is metabolized about four times faster than tetracaine. However, the rate of hydrolysis of all ester LAs is prominently decreased in patients with abnormal plasma pseudocholinesterase.

Amide LAs are metabolized in the liver by a dealkalization reaction in which an ethyl group is cleaved from the tertiary amine.

The determinants of the hepatic clearance of these anesthetics include:

- The hepatic blood flow
- And liver function.

Factors that decrease hepatic blood flow or hepatic drug extraction both result in an increased elimination half-life. Renal clearance of unchanged LAs is a minor route of elimination, accounting for only 3% to 5% of the total drug administered [70].

- Patients that have a chronic active hepatitis need to be examined for impaired function. The same is true for hepatitis antigen carriers.
- LA can be used for such people. However, the dose should be kept as low as possible.
- Those suffering from advanced forms of cirrhotic disease the breakdown of LA in the liver is slowed down by a considerable amount. This can result in hiked levels of plasma and higher risks of toxic reactions. The dosage needs to be adjusted based on this scenario. The time intervals may need to be extended while the amount of the drug being administered may be reduced.
- For such cases, the first injection could be lidocaine or mepivacaine because of their rapid onset. This could be subsequently followed with a long-acting agent like bupivacaine or etidocaine.

Diabetes

- Patients are suffering from Type I or Type II diabetes can be given anaesthesia, however, some precautions may be needed for safe local anesthesia administration.
- The consultation and discussion with the patient's doctor about the status and condition of his/her diabetes is important for evaluation the suitability of the patient for surgery. A discussion with the patient is also important, this can help in understanding the patient's needs in terms of diabetes.
- Extra caution and care are required for those that have Type I diabetes and are consuming larger amounts of insulin. Such patients can go from one extreme to another *i.e.* hypoglycaemia and hyperglycaemia. The use of vasoconstrictors needs to be reduced because they can enhance hypoglycaemia.

Adrenal Insufficiency

- No changes need to be made to any dosage for patients that are suffering from this issue. The only important precaution that may be necessary for these patients is to take a supplementary corticosteroid. Such a patient needs to be given 24mg hydrocortisone intravenously. The possible risk of post-operative infection should be considered as well.

Hyperthyroidism

- For such a condition it is advisable to avoid using epinephrine or any other vasoconstrictors. The dosage should at the very least be minimised to one or two shots for patients that have poorly controlled or untreated hyperthyroid issues.[26]
- It is common for such patients to have arrhythmias, hypertension, and cardiac abnormalities. Despite this, a patient that is managing this condition well will not present any issues and can be administered proper doses of vasoconstrictors.

Hypothyroidism

- Patients that are exhibiting mild symptoms are generally not thought to be in any actual danger when they are being put through a dental care procedure. Nevertheless, such patients can have a reaction to the LA agents they are given. The reaction could be mild or severe based on how the depressants impact the central nervous system. The dose needs to be kept low for such patients, and in the event that the patient is suffering from severe hypothyroidism then the procedure or care itself should be delayed.

Malignant Hyperthermia

- This is a potentially fatal complication. It is mostly caused by amide LAs.

Nevertheless, no special precautions have been outlined for this muscle disease by any authorities or organizations.

Malignant hyperthermia (MH) is a life-threatening clinical syndrome of hypermetabolism involving the skeletal muscle. It is triggered in susceptible individuals primarily by the volatile inhalational anesthetic agents and the muscle relaxant succinylcholine, though other drugs have also been implicated as potential triggers [69].

Malignant hyperthermia (MH) is an existence undermining disorder of hypermetabolism, because of subclinical myopathy that permits extensive amounts of calcium to be discharged from the sarcoplasmic reticulum (SR) of skeletal muscle and cause a hypermetabolic state after exposure to an activating agent (triggering agents). It is activated in susceptible people fundamentally by anesthetic agents and the muscle relaxant, however different medications have additionally been implicated as potential triggers. MH is not a hypersensitive disorder (allergy) but rather an inherited disorder that can be discovered both in swine and people.

In people susceptible to MH, the skeletal muscle,s ryanodine receptor is defective, and this defect interferes with the normal regulation of calcium in the muscle. An irregular ryanodine receptor that controls calcium discharge causes a development of calcium in skeletal muscle, bringing about a massive metabolic response.

This hypermetabolism causes:

- Expanded carbon dioxide generation,
- Metabolic and respiratory acidosis,
- Accelerated oxygen utilization,
- Heat creation,
- Initiation of the sympathetic system,
- Hyperkalemia,
- Disseminated intravascular coagulation (DIC),
- and Numerous organ dysfunction, which commonly result in organ failure. Early clinical indications of MH incorporate an expansion in end-tidal carbon dioxide (even with expanding minute ventilation), tachycardia,tachypnea, muscle rigidity and hyperkalemia. Later signs incorporate myoglobinuriafever, fever and organ failure.

Sickle Cell Anemia

- The use of the given anaesthetics is safe so long as the dose that is being administered is limited to a single cartridge or just one more.

- Methemoglobinemia:
  This is basically oxidised haemoglobin that is no longer capable of transporting and binding oxygen. The increase in any levels of this can be a result of the anaesthesia that is being administered. This is particularly the case for prilocaine (Citanest).
- Some drugs that are commonly used that can lead to this interaction include Nardil, Macrobid, Bactrim, Dapsone, *etc.* [32].
- The use of prilocaine needs to be avoided and the dose itself should be minimised when it comes to the anaesthesia.

Drug Interactions

Antipsychotic Drugs (Phenothiazines)

- This has no known contraindications when put into context with local anaesthetics, for patients taking lithium to treat bipolar disorder. This is true irrespective of whether vasoconstrictors are being used or not.
- For bipolar disorder, phenothiazine drugs like Thorazine or Risperdal can lead to blood pressure fluctuations. LAs with vasoconstrictors, when employed in average amounts, will generally lead to no negative reaction [33].
- It is always recommended, nevertheless, that the physician is treating the patient be consulted before treatment begins. The hypotensive episodes are not uncommon in these patients; the blood pressure should be closely monitored.

Tricyclic Antidepressants

- While the use of such drugs *i.e.* Tofranil or Elavil has gone down over the course of time, they are often still given to many patients. The number is significant enough for this to be considered here. The dose is safe to use as long as it doesn't cross one or two cartridges in terms of quantity. Nevertheless, such patients need to be carefully monitored for any signs that they may break into hypertension because of the augmented sympathomimetic impact.

Monoamine Oxidase Inhibitors

- Studies conducted on both animals and humans have failed to show any evidence that the fear of severe hypertension due to the interaction between MAO and agents is well founded.

Antianxiety Drugs

- Diazepam (Valium) is a depressant that has a potent impact on the central nervous system. LA agents need to be kept at the minimum possible doses.

Allergy

- It is possible for adrenal insufficiency to be misdiagnosed as an allergic reaction.
- The most common complication, which accounts for 99 percent of the occurrences, is overdose itself. A clinical manifestation is rare, in most cases, it presents itself in subclinical ways (Johnson: JOURNAL OF Anesth. Angle. 49:173-183).
- Only one case of anaphylaxis was reported during the 1940-1993 time frame in all the publications that exist during this time period.
- LA is a safe thing to implement when it comes to dentistry in general.

Summary

- LAs are safe to give to most patients, even the ones that have complex medical histories and conditions. This is true irrespective of whether vasoconstrictors are being used. The simple safety guidelines need to be observed properly before any patient is given anaesthesia.
- To ensure that the risk of unintentional intravascular injection is reduced, aspirate beforehand.
- The injection should be administered slowly. At most the speed should be a minute per cartridge. This is wide recommended. The patient needs to be observed carefully before and after administration.
- Use the smallest possible amount of solution needed to implement the anaesthesia. The main aim is to keep the patient comfortable.

Never forget that dentists help supply an effective and safe anaesthesia service.

Part 2: Local Complications

LA used for dental procedures are thought to be extremely safe and mostly incur a low rate of adverse reactions.

Prolonged Anesthesia or Paresthesia

- Paresthesia is the prolonged sensation of the tongue or lip; that extend beyond the expected time frame of an LA application.
- This complication is temporary and can include a tingling sensation or burning sensation, dysesthesia or hyperesthesia may also develop.

What Causes These Complications?

1. The needle can at times cause direct trauma. The nerve sheath may experience haemorrhaging which can result in an intraneural hematoma.
2. At times this is the result of an LA being administered through a cartridge that

has been spoiled by sterilising solution or alcohol
3. It can also be a result of scar formation
4. LA can also lead to neurotoxicity
    ○ A study conducted recently has found that of every 785,000 injections, there is one irreversible paresthesia. The study also found that some drugs had a higher probability of being linked with paresthesia.
    ○ Prilocaine (Citanest) and articaine (found in Canada and some European regions under Ultracaine) have been associated with this issue. At present, no known guaranteed method exists when it comes to dealing with the issue. Most of the time this issue is transient and goes away on its own in eight weeks. During the time it presents itself there is no way actually to help a patient. The patient's condition needs to be monitored and recorded if any changes are seen in how the symptoms manifest than it can be considered as a good sign since it could leave to the neuropathy getting resolved. This can mean that the nerve may recover normal function.

Trismus

- Trismus or limited jaw opening is a common problem that results from the administration of LA. Mastication muscles spasm can lead to this issue.
- Causes:
    1. Piercing of the muscle due to needle insertion
    2. The formation of Hematoma
    3. Injecting LA directly into the mass of the muscle can lead to a slight myotoxic response, which can further result in necrosis
    4. Injection that was administered too rapidly.

Management of Trismus

- The site needs to be cared for with a moist, hot towel, for 20 minutes after every hour.
- Analgesics should be used as and when required.
- The patient will be told to close and open their mouth slowly as a form of physiotherapy.

Hematoma

Hematomas are most commonly linked with pterygoid plexus of veins, inferior alveolar vessels, posterior superior alveolar, and mental vessels:

- It must be noted that aspiration results are not always linked to hematoma, it can exist despite a negative aspiration. This is because the needle may poke a blood vessel on its way in or out.

- Aspiration results only highlight what the needle tip contains, at the time it was aspirating. A positive result is also the same.

Hematoma Prevention

- The basic principles of traumatic injection technique need to be followed.
- Ensure that the lowest possible number of needle penetrations take place.
- The posterior superior alveolar nerve block requires a short needle.

Hematoma Management

- Apply pressure directly if visible right after the injection is administered
- Discharge patient after bleeding has ceased. Inform them that they need to apply ice on the affected area for the initial 6 hours. Tell them to avoid applying heat during these hours as well. Tell them how and when to use analgesics. Inform them that some discoloration may occur.

Injection Leading to Pain

At times, an injection that is meant to administer the anaesthetic can cause simultaneous burning sensation or pain.

What is the cause?

1. When te needle is passed through a sensitive structure like a tendon or muscle, it can result in pain.
2. This can happen when the solution is being injected too quickly and ends up listening to the tissue.
3. LA solutions that are too warm or cold can also lead to discomfort.
4. Short term burning sensation can be caused by solutions that are acidic, *i.e.* those with vasoconstrictors.

Prevention of Pain

- The injection should be administered slowly. The length of time that it should take varies, but a minute at least is recommended per cartridge.
- The cartridges should not be stored in the fridge and should not be heated, it should be stored at a temperature of the room.
- It is advisable to avoid storing them in any kind of disinfecting solution.

Management of Pain

- Any kind of pain or painful sensation is generally dealt with by the anaesthesia itself.

Needle Breakage

It is very rare for a needle to break. However, the problem can present itself at times. If the patient moves suddenly or unexpectedly, then such a breakage can occur. There is a higher chance for smaller diameter needles to break as compared to larger ones.

Prevention of Needle Breakage

- A portion of the tissue always needs to be left exposed; it's never advisable to insert a middle all the up to the hub of the tissue
- If a depth longer than 18mm is required then make sure that a longer needle is used
- 25 gauge needles are ideal because of their larger diameters
- Ensure that the needle is not subjected to excessive force when it's being pushed into the tissue
- Withdraw entirely before redirecting the needle, when required. Ensure that no needle is bent more than once

Management of Needle Breakage

- If the needle breaks, the first thing to do is to stay calm
- Tell the patient that they need to be still and ensure that their mouth remains open by keeping your hand where it is
- If the needle is visible, try to remove it through help of a hemostat or any other tool like it
- If you cannot see the needle then tell the patient
- Make an entry about the issue in the patient's chart
- The patient should be referred to an oral surgeon as an emergency case, if the broken needle cannot be retrieved.

Surgical removal needs to be left to someone that has proper experience with performing surgeries of the given region under care. It should also be done after radiographs have been developed to locate the needle.

Injury of the Soft Tissue

- A patient can end up biting their tongue or lip because of the loss of sensation that results from a successful block. Pain and swelling present themselves once the anaesthesia is offset.
- Patients that are mentally incapacitated, demented or suffering from Alzheimer's, along with children, will suffer from this issue more commonly as opposed to other patients.
- The caregiver or parent of the patient needs to be given careful guidelines on

how to take care of the patient during the time of recovery.

Soft Tissue Injury Prevention

- To prevent the issue for patients that are susceptible to injuries, the LA should be administered for only an appropriate time frame
- Warn the caregiver about the manner in which they need to watch over the patient they are taking care of, and inform them about the soft-tissue damage that can result from the anaesthesia administration
- In terms of children specifically, a cotton roll can be placed along the affected area so that they may not hurt themselves
- Expand on the risks of injury to patients that are suffering from bleeding anomalies.

Managing Soft Tissue Injury

- Make use of analgesics as and when required
- Rinses and applications should be administered with dilute solutions of baking soda and salt, at lukewarm temperature
- Considering using petroleum jelly for lip lesions that present themselves

Paralysis of Facial Nerves

- Issues of paralysis may occur if the parotid gland capsule ends up getting penetrated by the needle. If LA ends up being administered therein, it can cause problems.
- If this nerve is administered LA, then the result would be a temporary unilateral paralysis of the upper lip, lower lip, cheek, chin and eye muscles.
- Corneal injuries can result from this. The risk is present because there is a chance that the protective reflex to shut the eyelid can be lost, loss of eye tears and eye dryness.
- Other nerves can also be affected by the face. Cranial nerves III, IV or VI, along with the optic nerve can be affected because of temporary paralysis.

Preventing Facial Nerve Paralysis

- The atraumatic injection technique needs to be implemented
- Ensure that the needle is not over inserted
- In the context of the inferior alveolar nerve block, do not administer the injection until the bone has been contacted at the right depth

Managing the Paralysis

- Ensure that the patient feels reassured about the transient nature of the paralysis.
- Explain to the patient the need for an eye patch, at least till the point their motor

functions come back.
- Contact lenses cannot be used during this period.
- All details of the issue need to be recorded in the patient's chart.

Infection

- Infections are no longer the complications that they used to be thinks to the introduction of sterile disposable needles. An infection is a rare complication when it comes to administering LA to a patient.
- The flora of the oral cavity itself is not seen as a problem since it does not typically result in infections for patients that are not suffering from extreme immunity issues. The situation is different for those that are immunocompromised.
- The fact is that every needle insertion allows bacteria to enter the body through the tissue. However, a person's typical immune system will prevent a clinical infection from taking root. However, patients that suffer from immune problems require an antiseptic rinse or a topical antiseptic application. Chlorhexidine can be used before the needle is used as well.
- If an infection does happen despite these precautions, the likelihood is that it will present itself first through trismus and pain after a day. If the symptoms do not go away for three days and continue to get worse then the likelihood that there is an infection needs to be taken seriously. The patient at this point needs to look analysed to see what other symptoms pointing to an infection are present. Examples of said symptoms include fever, lymphadenopathy, and swelling.
- Needles should not be inserted into an active site of infection. This would include situations like when there is an abscess. Such a problem has the potential for allowing the infection to spread further, which is why it should be avoided.

Preventing Infections

- Ensure that the needles being used are disposable and sterile
- Avoid contamination of the needle by ensuring that there is no contact with nonsterile surfaces
- For patients with severe immunocompromised systems, use some form of antiseptic before giving the injection

Managing the Infection

- An appropriate dose of antibiotics like penicillin can be prescribed for an appropriate duration
- Details should be recorded in the patient's chart, and progress should be followed up

Mucosal Lesions

- The intraoral mucosa can exhibit evidence of ulceration or sloughing, at times.
- Prolong use of a topical option can lead to desquamation of the epithelial layer.
- Tissue necrosis may be borne from high concentrations of vasoconstrictor *i.e.* 1:50000. This is not common, but there is a chance it may occur.

Preventing Mucosal Lesion

- In terms of mucosa, avoid leaving on topical anaesthetic for prolonged periods of time.

Mucosal Lesion Management

- Advise the patient of the possible duration of two or one weeks. Make sure to reassure them so that they are not worried about their condition.
- Rinses can be implemented with lukewarm dilute solutions made from baking soda or salt until the symptoms have subsided.

Summary

- Localised complications stemming from LA administration can be reduced if the basic principles of the LA injection technique are followed. The suggestions that were shared beforehand can also help but it does not grantee the complications prevention. Despite this, even if proper technique and protocols are followed there is always a chance that there may be a problem. Most issues, however, can still be resolved without any permanent long term problem. Appropriate management can help the patient recover from any complications.

BIBLIOGRAPHY

[1]   Barash PG, Cullen BF, Stoelting RK. Clinical anesthesia. Philadelphia: Lippincott Williams & Wilkins 2006.

[2]   Malamed SF. Handbook of local anesthesia. St. Louis, MO: Elsevier/Mosby 2004.

[3]   AP C Manual of local anesthesia in dentistry. New Delhi: Jaypee Brothers Medical Publishers 2010.

[4]   Logothetis DD. Local anesthesia for the dental hygienist. St. Louis, MO: Elsevier/Mosby 2012.

[5]   Bassett KB, DiMarco AC, Naughton DK. Local anesthesia for dental professionals. Boston: Pearson 2010.

[6]   Jastak JT, Yagiela JA, Donaldson D, Jastak JT. Local anesthesia of the oral cavity. Philadelphia: Saunders 1995.

[7]   Evers H, Haegerstam G. Buckhöj Poul Introduction to dental local anaesthesia. Fribourg: Mediglobe 1990.

[8]   Local anesthesia in dentistry. Book On Demand Ltd 2013.

[9]   Kelly L. Essentials of human physiology for pharmacy. Boca Raton, FL: CRC Press 2004.

[10]   Despopoulos A, Silbernagl S. Color atlas of physiology. Stuttgart: G. Thieme 1991.

[11]   Malamed SF. Handbook of local anesthesia. St. Louis, MS: Elsevier/Mosby 2013.

[12]   Goodman LS, Gilman A. The Pharmacological basis of therapeutics. New York: Macmillan 1975.

[13]   Brunton LL, Chabner BA, Knollmann Björn C. Goodman & Gilman's the pharmacological basis of therapeutics. New York: McGraw-Hill 2011.

[14]   Costanzo LS. Physiology: cases and problems. Philadelphia: Lippincott Williams & Wilkins 2006.

[15]   Guyton AC, Hall JE. Textbook of medical physiology. Philadelphia: W.B. Saunders 1996.

[16]   Raff H. Physiology secrets. Philadelphia: Hanley & Belfus 2003.

[17]   Sherwood L. Human physiology: from cells to systems. Australia: Thomson/Brooks/Cole 2007.

[18]   Silverthorn DU, Johnson BR. Human physiology: an integrated approach. San Francisco: Pearson/Benjamin Cummings 2010.

[19]   Purves D. Neuroscience. Sunderland, MA: Sinauer 2008.

[20]   Procacci P, Maresca M. Descartes' physiology of pain. Pain 1994; 58(2): 133.
[http://dx.doi.org/10.1016/0304-3959(94)90193-7] [PMID: 7816481]

[21]   Brodie ME, Richardson M. Physiology of pain. Hatfield: University of Hertfordshire Press 2005.

[22]   Central Pain, Human Studies of Physiology.

[23]   Blackwell RE, Olive DL. Physiology of Pain. 1998; pp. 7-18.
[http://dx.doi.org/10.1007/978-1-4612-1752-7_2]

[24]   Blackwell RE, Olive DL. Physiology of Pain. Chronic Pelvic Pain 1998; pp. 7-18.

[25]   Physiology of Pain Development. Atlas of Injection Therapy in Pain Management. 2012.

[26]   Monheim LM, Bennett CR. Monheim's Local anesthesia and pain control in dental practice. St. Louis: Mosby 1984.

[27]   Reader A, Nusstein J, Drum M. Successful local anesthesia for restorative dentistry and endodontics. Chicago: Quintessence Pub. Co. 2011.

[28]   Watson DS, Kaempf G. Monitoring the patient receiving local anesthesia. Denver, CO: Association of Operating Room Nurses 1991.

[29]   Livingston WK. The Physiology of Pain. Pain Mechanisms 1976; pp. 44-61.

[30]   Smith J. Anatomy and Physiology of Pain. 17-28.
[http://dx.doi.org/10.1002/9781444322743.ch2]

[31]   Zimmermann M. Basic Physiology of Pain Perception. 2004; pp. 1-24.

[32]   Sukiennik AW. Pain Physiology and Neuroblockade. Integrative Pain Management 2016; pp. 119-38.

[33]   Bijlani R. Chapter-127 Pain and Relief from Pain. Understanding Medical Physiology 2011; pp. 597-606.

[34]   Chambers D, Huang C, Matthews G. Pain physiology Basic Physiology for Anaesthetists. 269-74.
[http://dx.doi.org/10.1017/CBO9781139226394.059]

[35]   Bijlani R. Chapter-127 Pain and Relief from Pain. Understanding Medical Physiology 2011; pp. 597-606.

[36]   Sembulingam K. Chapter-90 Physiology of Pain Essentials of Physiology for Dental Students. 2011; pp. 555-7.
[http://dx.doi.org/10.5005/jp/books/11397_104]

[37]   Serpell M. Anatomy and physiology of pain Handbook of Pain Management. 2008; pp. 9-24.

[38]　Chambers D, Huang C, Matthews G. Pain physiology Basic Physiology for Anaesthetists. 269-74.
[http://dx.doi.org/10.1017/CBO9781139226394.059]

[39]　Flor H, Turk DC. Pain-related cognitions, pain severity, and pain behaviors in chronic pain patients. Pain 1987; 30.

[40]　Hernandez S, Cruz ML, Seguinot II, Torres-Reveron A, Appleyard CB. Impact of Psychological Stress on Pain Perception in an Animal Model of Endometriosis. Reprod Sci 2017; 24(10): 1371-81.

[41]　Corder G, Tawfik VL, Wang D, *et al.* Loss of μ opioid receptor signaling in nociceptors, but not microglia, abrogates morphine tolerance without disrupting analgesia. Nat Med 2017; 23(2): 164-73.
[http://dx.doi.org/10.1038/nm.4262] [PMID: 28092666]

[42]　Liu RX, Luo Q, Qiao H, *et al.* Clinical significance of the sympathetic nervous system in the development and progression of pulmonary arterial hypertension. Curr Neurovasc Res 2017; 14(2): 190-8.
[http://dx.doi.org/10.2174/1567202614666170112165927] [PMID: 28088894]

[43]　Yvone GM, Zhao-Fleming HH, Udeochu JC, *et al.* Disabled-1 dorsal horn spinal cord neurons co-express Lmx1b and function in nociceptive circuits. Eur J Neurosci 2017; 45(5): 733-47.

[44]　Hartling L, Ali S, Dryden DM, *et al.* How Safe Are Common Analgesics for the Treatment of Acute Pain for Children? A Systematic Review. Pain Res Manag 2016; 2016: 5346819.
[http://dx.doi.org/10.1155/2016/5346819] [PMID: 28077923]

[45]　Costa YM, Baad-Hansen L, Bonjardim LR, Conti PC, Svensson P. Reliability of the nociceptive blink reflex evoked by electrical stimulation of the trigeminal nerve in humans. Clin Oral Investig 2017; 21(8): 2453-63.
[http://dx.doi.org/10.1007/s00784-016-2042-6] [PMID: 28074292]

[46]　Kim MJ, Park YH, Yang KY, *et al.* Participation of central GABAA receptors in the trigeminal processing of mechanical allodynia in rats. Korean J Physiol Pharmacol 2017; 21(1): 65-74.

[47]　Xin Q, Bai B, Liu W. The analgesic effects of oxytocin in the peripheral and central nervous system. Neurochem Int 2017; 103: 57-64.
[http://dx.doi.org/10.1016/j.neuint.2016.12.021] [PMID: 28065792]

[48]　Ozgocer T, Ucar C, Yildiz S. Cortisol awakening response is blunted and pain perception is increased during menses in cyclic women. Psychoneuroendocrinology 2017; 77: 158-64.
[http://dx.doi.org/10.1016/j.psyneuen.2016.12.011] [PMID: 28064085]

[49]　Sperry MM, Ita ME, Kartha S, Zhang S, Yu YH, Winkelstein B. The Interface of Mechanics and Nociception in Joint Pathophysiology: Insights From the Facet and Temporomandibular Joints. J Biomech Eng 2017; 139(2)
[http://dx.doi.org/10.1115/1.4035647] [PMID: 28056123]

[50]　Li X, Hu L. The Role of Stress Regulation on Neural Plasticity in Pain Chronification. Neural Plast 2016; 6402942.

[51]　Kilinc E, Guerrero-Toro C, Zakharov A, *et al.* Serotonergic mechanisms of trigeminal meningeal nociception: Implications for migraine pain. Neuropharmacology 2017; 116: 160-73.
[http://dx.doi.org/10.1016/j.neuropharm.2016.12.024] [PMID: 28025094]

[52]　Lee SJ, Kim DH, Hahn SJ, Waxman SG, Choi JS. Mechanism of inhibition by chlorpromazine of the human pain threshold sodium channel, Nav1.7. Neurosci Lett 2017; 639: 1-7.

[53]　De Gregori M, Muscoli C, Schatman ME, *et al.* Combining pain therapy with lifestyle: the role of personalized nutrition and nutritional supplements according to the SIMPAR Feed Your Destiny approach. J Pain Res 2016; 9: 1179-89.
[http://dx.doi.org/10.2147/JPR.S115068] [PMID: 27994480]

[54]　Faircloth AC. Anesthesia Involvement in Palliative Care. Annu Rev Nurs Res 2017; 35(1): 135-58.

[55]   Pometlová M, Yamamotová A, Nohejlová K, Šlamberová R. Can Anxiety Tested in the Elevated Plus-maze Be Related to Nociception Sensitivity in Adult Male Rats? Prague Med Rep 2016; 117(4): 185-97.

[56]   Okine BN, Gaspar JC, Madasu MK, *et al.* Characterisation of peroxisome proliferator-activated receptor signalling in the midbrain periaqueductal grey of rats genetically prone to heightened stress, negative affect and hyperalgesia. Brain Res 2016. pii: S0006-8993(16)30778-8.

[57]   Aurora SK, Brin MF. Chronic Migraine: An Update on Physiology, Imaging, and the Mechanism of Action of Two Available Pharmacologic Therapies. Headache 2017; 57(1): 109-25.

[58]   Baron R, Maier C, Attal N, *et al.* Peripheral neuropathic pain: a mechanism-related organizing principle based on sensory profiles. Pain 2017; 158(2): 261-72.
[http://dx.doi.org/10.1097/j.pain.0000000000000753] [PMID: 27893485]

[59]   Tayeb BO, Barreiro AE, Bradshaw YS, Chui KK, Carr DB. Durations of Opioid, Nonopioid Drug, and Behavioral Clinical Trials for Chronic Pain: Adequate or Inadequate? Pain Med 2016; 17(11): 2036-46.
[http://dx.doi.org/10.1093/pm/pnw245] [PMID: 27880651]

[60]   Tolas AG, Pflug AE, Halter JB. Arterial plasma epinephrine concentrations and hemodynamic responses after dental injection of local anesthetic with epinephrine. J Am Dent Assoc 1982; 104(1): 41-3.

[61]   Cioffi GA, Chernow B, Glahn RP, Terezhalmy GT, Lake CR. The hemodynamic and plasma catecholamine responses to routine restorative dental care. J Am Dent Assoc 1985; 111(1): 67-70.

[62]   Chernow B, Balestrieri F, Ferguson CD, Terezhalmy GT, Fletcher JR, Lake CR. Local dental anesthesia with epinephrine. Minimal effects on the sympathetic nervous system or on hemodynamic variables. Arch Intern Med 1983; 143(11): 2141-3.
[http://dx.doi.org/10.1001/archinte.1983.00350110127026] [PMID: 6639234]

[63]   Goldstein DS, Dionne R, Sweet J, *et al.* Circulatory, plasma catecholamine, cortisol, lipid, and psychological responses to a real-life stress (third molar extractions): effects of diazepam sedation and of inclusion of epinephrine with the local anesthetic. Psychosom Med 1982; 44(3): 259-72.
[http://dx.doi.org/10.1097/00006842-198207000-00004] [PMID: 7134364]

[64]   Dionne RA, Goldstein DS, Wirdzek PR. Effects of diazepam premedication and epinephrine-containing local anesthetic on cardiovascular and plasma catecholamine responses to oral surgery. Anesth Analg 1984; 63(7): 640-6.

[65]   Knoll-Köhler E, Knöller M, Brandt K, Becker J. Cardiohemodynamic and serum catecholamine response to surgical removal of impacted mandibular third molars under local anesthesia: a randomized double-blind parallel group and crossover study. J Oral Maxillofac Surg 1991; 49(9): 957-62.

[66]   Clutter WE, Bier DM, Shah SD, Cryer PE. Epinephrine plasma metabolic clearance rates and physiologic thresholds for metabolic and hemodynamic actions in man. J Clin Invest 1980; 66(1): 94-101.
[http://dx.doi.org/10.1172/JCI109840] [PMID: 6995479]

[67]   Braid DP, Scott DB. The systemic absorption of local analgesic drugs. Br J Anaesth 1965; 37: 394-404.

[68]   Goebel WM, Allen G, Randall F. The effect of commercial vasoconstrictor preparations on the circulating venous serum level of mepivacaine and lidocaine. J Oral Med 1980; 35(4): 91-6.

[69]   Hopkins PM. Malignant hyperthermia: pharmacology of triggering. Br J Anaesth 2011; 107(1): 48-56.
[http://dx.doi.org/10.1093/bja/aer132] [PMID: 21624965]

[70]   NYSORA, Inc (The New York School of Regional Anesthesia) 2753 Broadway, Suite 183 New York, NY 10025. http://www.nysora.com/

CHAPTER 4

Simple Extraction

Fadi Jarab[1,*] and **Esam Ahmad Z Omar[2]**

[1] *Department of Oral & Maxillofacial Surgery, Jordan University of Science and Technology, Jordan*

[2] *Department of Oral & Maxillofacial Surgery, College of Dentistry, Taibah University, Madinah, Saudi Arabia*

        Abstract: Understanding of the basic principles of exodontia is the essential part for understanding of this subject of dentistry. This introductory chapter discusses the indications, the instrumentation, the definitions and basic steps of simple extraction.

Keywords: Contraindications, Indications, Instrumentations, Introduction, Principles, Steps of exodontia.

PART 1: INTRODUCTION AND INSTRUMENTATIONS

Exdontias (Dental Extraction)

Exodontia is a painless removal of a tooth or tooth root from its socket with minimal injury to the bone and surrounding structure so that postoperative healing is uneventful.

Instrumentations of Dental extractions: The most commonly used instruments in dental extraction: (Fig. **4.1-4.18**)

Patient Position (Fig. 4.16)

1. To ensure adequate visualization and comfort during the various manipulations required for the tooth extraction,
2. The dental chair must always be positioned correctly. For the extraction of a maxillary tooth, the patient's mouth must be at the same height as the dentist's shoulder and the angle between the dental chair and the horizontal (floor) must be approximately 120°.

---

* **Corresponding author Fadi Jarab:** Department of Oral & Maxillofacial Surgery, Jordan University of Science and Technology, Jordan; Tel: 0096279505 0342; Fax: 00966148494710; E-mail: fsjarab@just.edu.jo

3. The occlusal surface of the maxillary teeth must be at a 45° angle compared to horizontal when the mouth is open.
4. During mandibular extractions, the chair is positioned lower, so that the angle between the chair and the horizontal is about 110°
5. The occlusal surface of the mandibular teeth must be parallel to the horizontal when the patient's mouth is open.
6. The position of right-handed dentists during extraction using forceps is in front of and to the right of the patient; left-handed dentists should be in front of and to the left of the patient.
7. For the extraction of anterior mandibular teeth right-handed dentists should be positioned in front of the patient, or behind them and to their right; left-handed dentists should be in front of them or behind them and to their left.

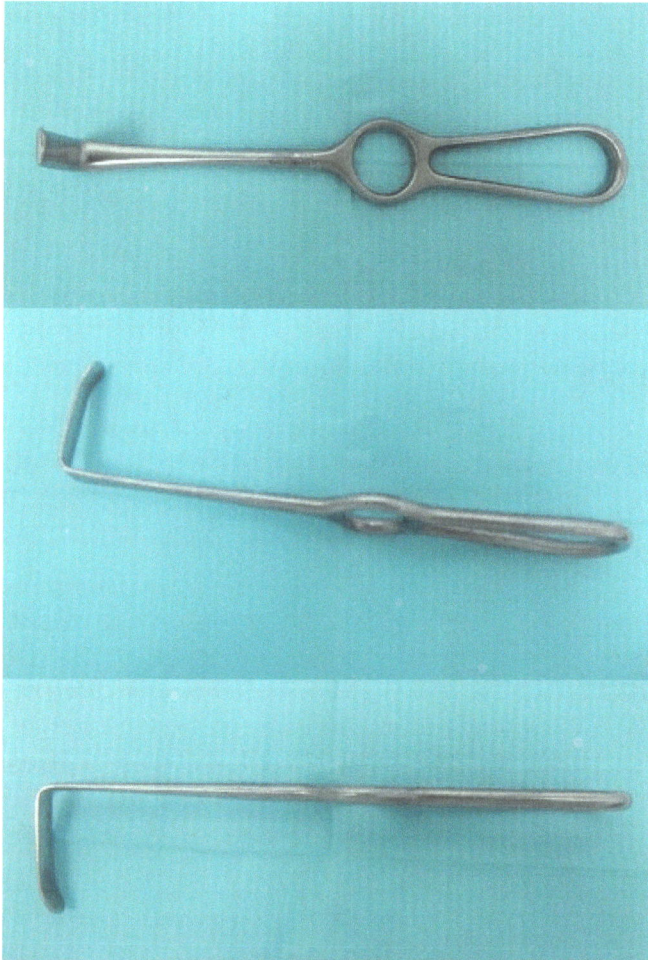

Fig. (4.1). Kocher–Langenbeck retractors, used in the same way as Farabeuf retractors.

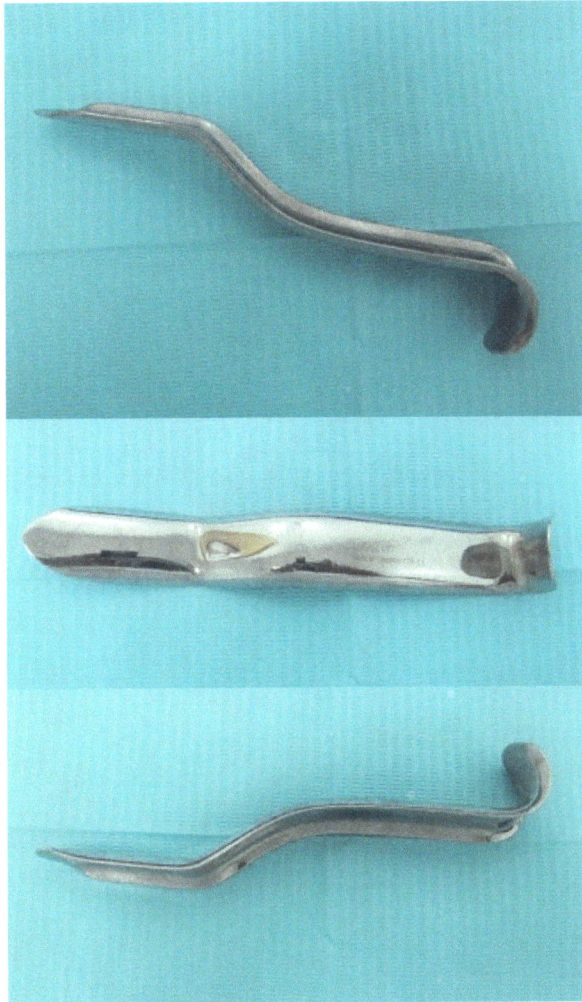

Fig. (4.2). Minnesota retractors for retraction of the cheek and tongue.

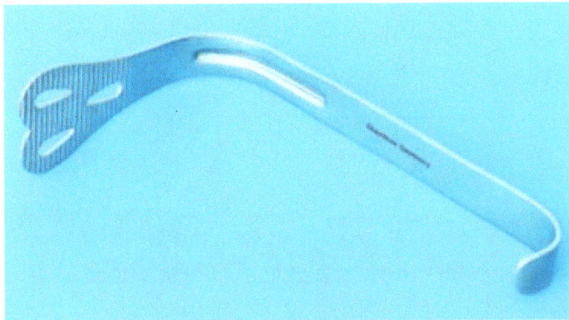

Fig. (4.3). Weider retractor for retraction of tongue to the side during surgical procedure.

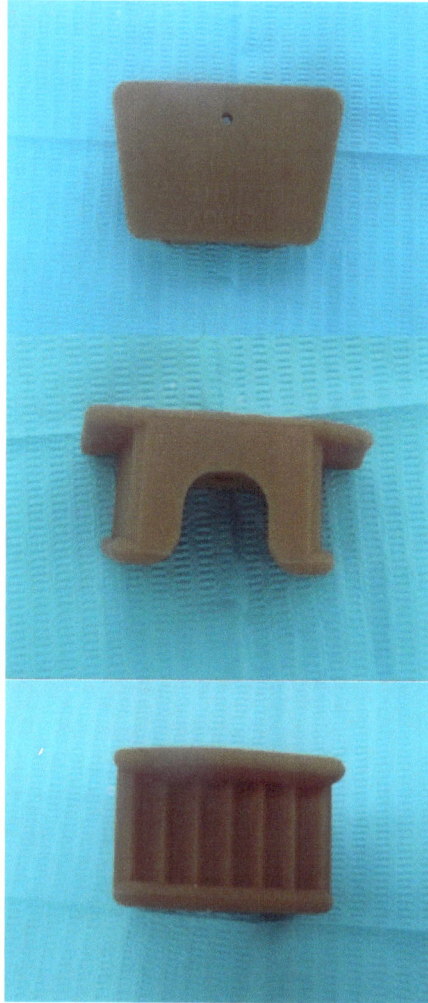

Fig. (4.4). Rubber bite blocks for adults.

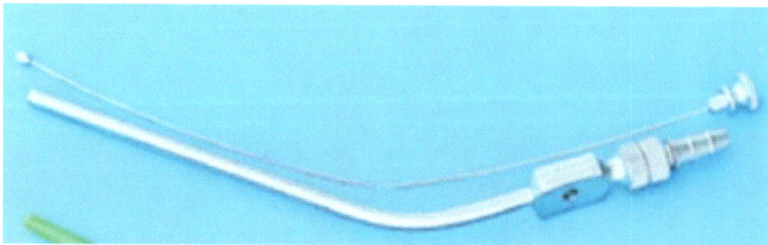

Fig. (4.5). a. Fergusson suction tip with wire stylet used as a cleaning instrument. **b.** Disposable suction tip.

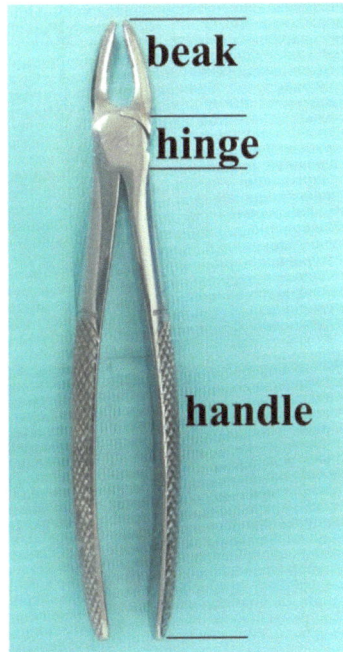

Fig. (4.6). The parts of the forceps.

Maxillary extraction forceps used for the six anterior teeth of the maxilla Beaks that are found on the same level as the handles characterize these forceps, and the beaks are concave and not pointed.

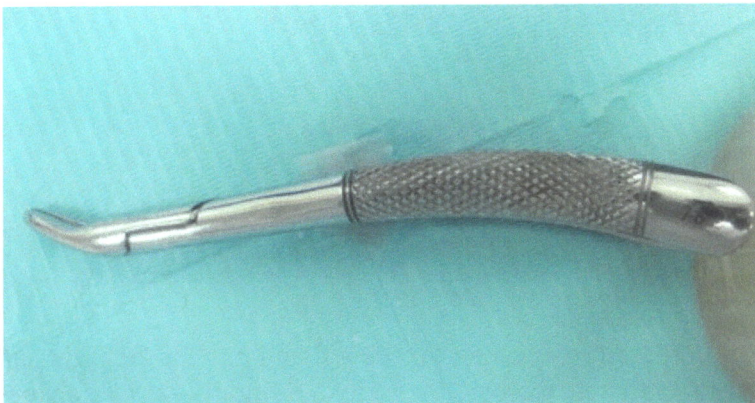

Fig. (4.7). The forceps used for premolars have a slightly curved shape and look like an "S." Holding the forceps in the hand, the concave part of the curved part of the handle faces the palm,while the concave part of the beaks is turned upwards. The ends of the beaks of the forceps are concave and are not pointed.

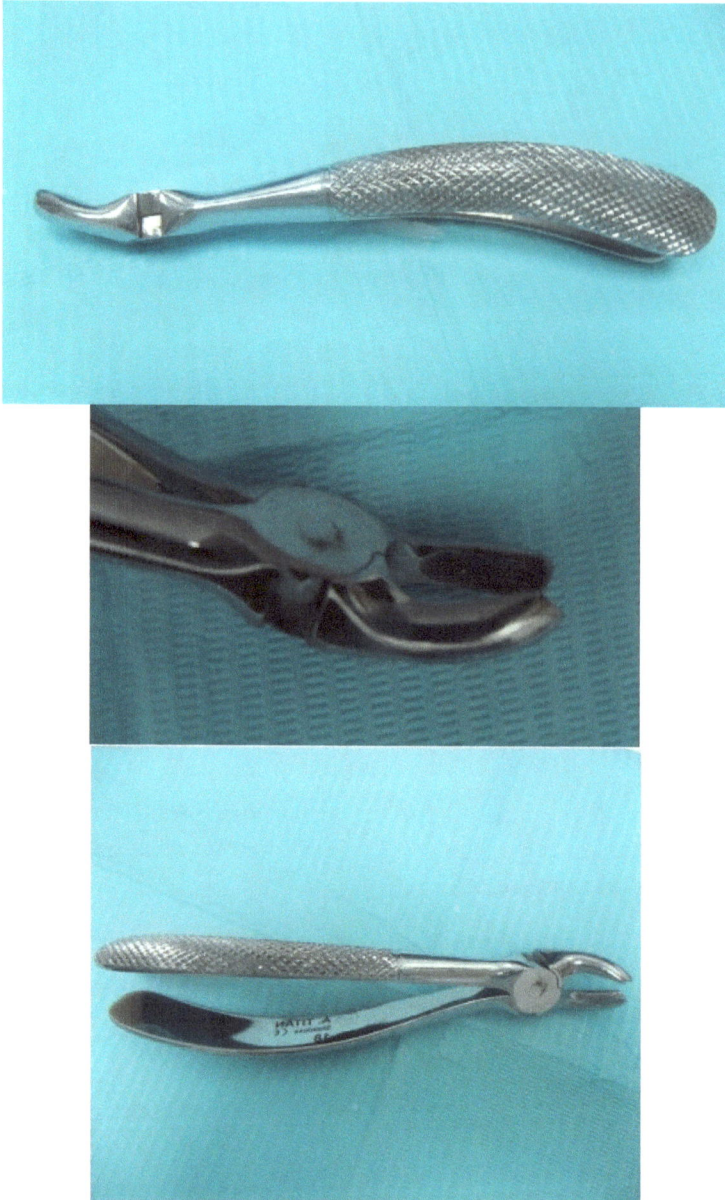

Fig. (4.8). Maxillary left molar forceps, for the first and second upper molars of the left side.

There are two of these forceps: one for the left and one for the right side. Just like the previously mentioned forceps, they have a slightly curved shape that looks like an "S". The buccal beak of each forceps has a pointed design, which fits into the buccal bifurcation of the two buccal roots, while the palatal beak is concave and fits into the convex surface of the palatal root.

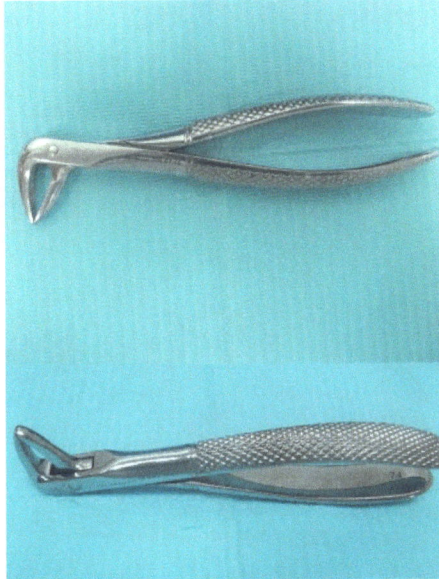

Fig. (4.9). Mandibular molar forceps (English style). **Vertical Hinge Forceps.** These English-style forceps differ from the aforementioned forceps in that their hinges have a vertical direction. Their use is limited, because large amounts of force can be generated during extraction with this type of forceps, so that if the bone is not elastic, there is increased risk of fracture of the alveolar bone.

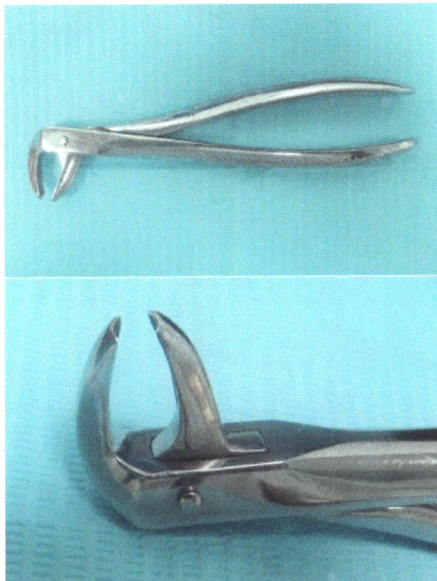

Fig. (4.10). Mandibular molar forceps These forceps are used for both sides of the jaw and have straight handles while the beaks are curved at approximately a right angle compared to the handles. Both beaks of the forceps have pointed ends, which fit into the bifurcation of the roots buccally and lingually .These forceps are used for the removal of both the first and second molar of the right and left side of the lower jaw.

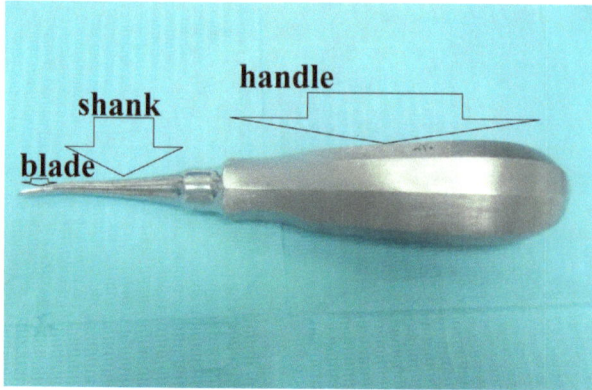

Fig. (4.11). The parts of elevator. Straight Bein elevator.

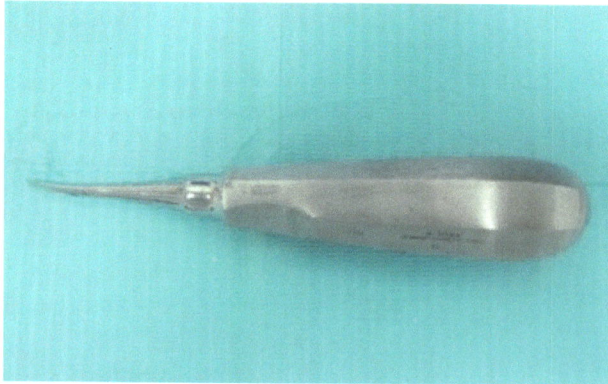

Fig. (4.12). StraightWhite elevator with slightly curved blade, suitable for extracting posterior maxillary teeth.

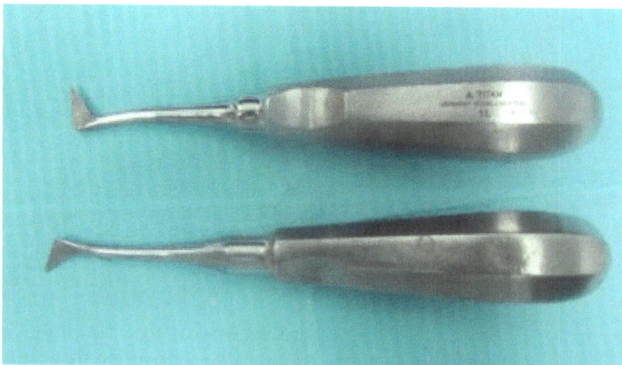

Fig. (4.13). Pair of angled Seldin elevators suitable for extracting roots in the mandible.

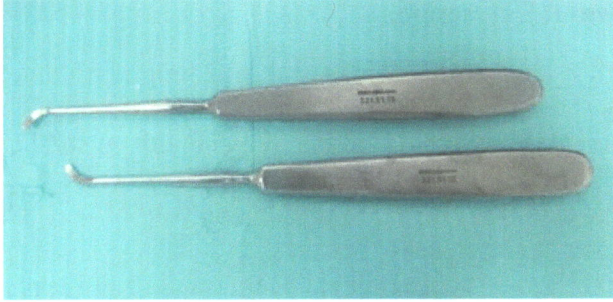

Fig. (4.14). Warwiq James elevators.

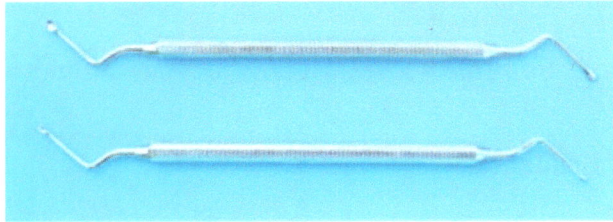

Fig. (4.15). Periapical curettes with ends of different sizes.

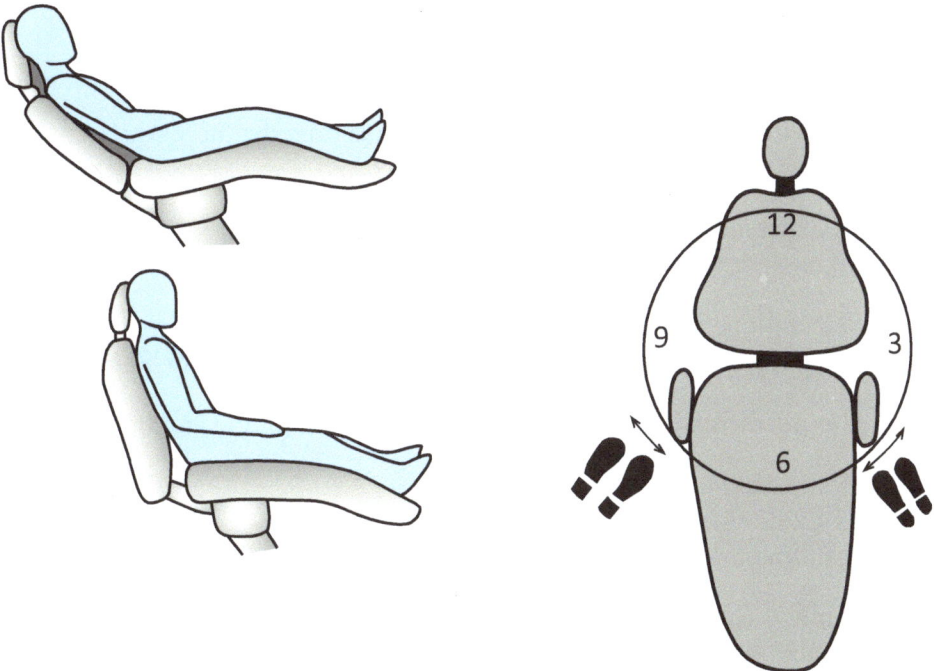

Fig. (4.16). Patient Position.

Basic Steps in Dental Extraction

1. Reflects the soft tissues of the cheeks, lips, and tongue, so that there is adequate visualization of the surgical field.
2. Supports the alveolar process of the maxilla and aids in stabilizing the patient's head.
3. Controls the expansion of the alveolar bone by way of feel, as well as luxation of the tooth during the various maneuvers.
4. Supports and stabilizes the mandible, counteracting the forces applied by the extraction forceps, which, when very great, may injure the temporomandibular joint.
5. Separated the tooth from the soft tissues surrounding it using a desmotome or elevator.
6. Elevate the tooth from the socket using forceps or an elevator (Luxation & Extraction).

Classification of Exodontias

The most common classification is either:

Based on the:

a. The technique used in exodontias or
b. The difficulty of the exodontias

According to the technique used in exodontias the dental extraction can be classified as:

1. The closed technique (Non-Surgical) or
2. The open technique (Surgical also call Trans-Alveolar).

The closed technique is also known as the simple technique or forceps technique, while the open technique is also known as a surgical extraction or flap technique.

According to the difficulty in exodontias the dental extraction can be classified as:

1. Simple Extraction
2. Complex Extraction
3. Surgical Extraction

Difficulty in any Surgical procedures mean presence of factors that may create possible Challenges intra-Operatively, or/and may result in development of possible complications post-Operatively.

The basic requirements for a successful tooth extraction are as follows:

1. Taking of good Medical and Dental History.
2. Informing and reassuring the patient, so that stress and fear levels are minimized, and so to ensure desirable cooperation during the procedure.
3. Knowing tooth anatomy well, which can be variable.
4. Detailed clinical and radiographic examinations, since these provide important information pertaining to procedure planning and selecting the appropriate technique.

The most important step in dental extraction procedure is the ability to assess the systemic and local factors (difficulty) that may contribute to the procedure and the ability to determine the possible difficulties and challenges that may develop in a certain extraction procedure.

Proper way for Holding of the instruments:

Holding of the Forceps

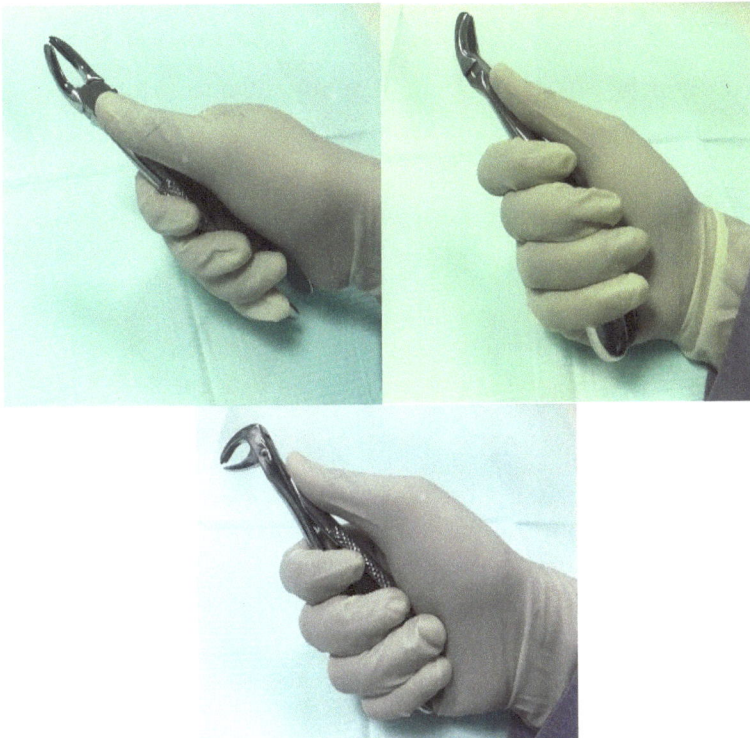

Fig. (4.17). The extraction forceps are held in the dominant hand, while the thumb is simultaneously placed between the handles directly behind the hinge, so that pressure applied to the tooth is controlled.

Holding of the Elevators

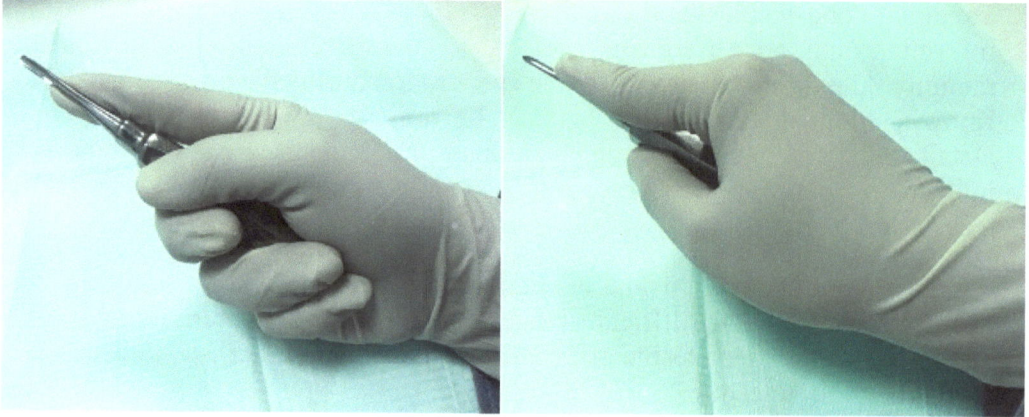

Fig. (4.18). The straight elevator must be held in the dominant hand and the index finger placed along the blade, leaving its anterior end exposed, which is used to luxate the tooth or root.

Indications for Dental Extractions

The main indication is:

If the tooth cannot be saved by Dental treatment due to one of the following reasons:

Technical reasons ...   and/or

Local reasons ...   and/or

Systemic reasons ...   and/or

Psychological reasons ...   and/or

Financial reasons.

In general the following indications can be considered:

1. Fractured teeth with pulp exposure
2. Non-vital teeth which can not be treated endodontically
3. Complete bifurcation exposure (Grade III)
4. Periodontal disease with loss of >50% bone
5. Periodontal Disease with secondary endodontic disease
6. Untreatable tooth Mobility >1mm
7. Retained deciduous teeth
8. Orthodontics consideration
9. Supernumerary teeth, if causing problem such as Dentigerous Cyst
10. Malpositioned teeth causing trauma
11. Retained roots if associated with inflammation or drainage

12. Prosthodontic considerations
13. Impacted tooth especially those associated with pathology or may cause malocclusion and/or when there is orthodontic recommendation
14. Cases that client is unwilling to treat (patient advices should be considered).

Contraindications for Dental Extractions

There is no absolute contraindication for dental extraction. All the contraindications are relative and may present due to a certain systemic or local conditions. Almost in all cases these relative contraindications can be solved which make the extraction possible sometime with special precautions.

BIBLIOGRAPHY

[1]   Archer WH. Oral and maxillofacial surgery. Philadelphia: Saunders 1975.

[2]   Gans BJ. Atlas of oral surgery. Saint Louis: C.V. Mosby Co. 1972.

[3]   Fragiskos FD. Oral surgery. Berlin: Springer 2007.
      [http://dx.doi.org/10.1007/978-3-540-49975-6]

[4]   Hooley JR, Whitacre RJ. A Self-instructional guide to oral surgery in general dentistry. Seattle, Wa.: Stoma Press 1979.

[5]   Howe GL. Minor oral surgery. 3rd ed., Oxford: Wright 1997.

[6]   Dimitroulis G. A synopsis of minor oral surgery. Oxford: Wright 1996.

[7]   Kruger GO. Textbook of oral and maxillofacial surgery. St. Louis: Mosby 1984.

[8]   Laskin DM. Oral and maxillofacial surgery. St. Louis: C.V. Mosby 1992.

[9]   Laskin DM, Abubaker AO. Decision making in oral and maxillofacial surgery. Chicago: Quintessence Pub. Co. 2007.

[10]   Kwon PH, Laskin DM. Clinician's manual of oral and maxillofacial surgery. Chicago: Quintessence Pub. Co. 1991.

[11]   Rounds CE, Rounds FW. Principles and technique of exodontia. St. Louis: Mosby 1962.

[12]   Peterson LJ. Contemporary oral and maxillofacial surgery. St. Louis: Mosby 1998.

[13]   Contemporary H. Oral and Maxillofacial Surgery. Elsevier 2014.

[14]   Sailer HF, Pajarola GF. Oral surgery for the general dentist. Stuttgart: Thieme 1998.

[15]   Dym H, Ogle OE. Oral surgery for the general dentist. Philadelphia: Saunders 2012.

[16]   Waite DE. Textbook of practical oral and maxillofacial surgery. Philadelphia: Lea & Febiger 1987.

PART 2: THE SIMPLE EXODONTIAS IN SIMPLE STEPS

Extraction of Upper Central Incisor: Fig. (4.19)

Relevant Anatomy

- Single, straight, conical root.
- Thinner labial alveolar bone than the palatal one.
- In relation with nasal floor.

Steps of Extraction

1. Give the patient local anesthesia (buccal and palatal infiltration), and make sure adequate anesthesia obtained.
2. Detach the gingiva (by periosteal elevator).
3. Try to luxate the tooth by straight elevator.
4. Choose the correct forcep.
5. Apply the forcep correctly to the tooth as apical as possible (apical to CEJ), with the long axis of the blades being along the long axis of the tooth.
6. Use the opposite hand to reflect the lip and support the labial and palatal alveolar bone.
7. With a firm grip, apply apical force then combination of both labio-palatal (more labial movement) and rotational movements, with increasing range of movement every cycle until the tooth is extracted.
8. Inspect both of the tooth and the socket.
9. Squeeze the socket.
10. Ensure adequate hemostasis obtained.
11. Apply pressure gauze.
12. Give the patient postoperative instructions.

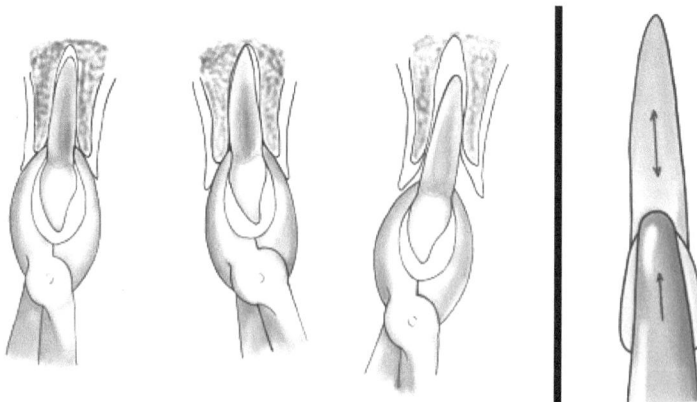

Fig. (4.19). Extraction of Upper Central Incisor.

Extraction of Upper Leteral Incisor: Fig. (4.20)

Relevant Anatomy

- Single, more palatally located, palatally curved apical 3rd.
- Thicker labial alveolar compared to central incisor.
- In relation with nasal floor.

Steps of Extraction

1. Give the patient local anesthesia (buccal and palatal infiltration), and make sure adequate anesthesia obtained.
2. Detach the gingiva (by periosteal elevator).
3. Try to luxate the tooth by straight elevator.
4. Choose the correct forcep.
5. Apply the forcep correctly to the tooth as apical as possible (apical to CEJ), with the long axis of the blades being along the long axis of the tooth.
6. Use the opposite hand to reflect the lip and support the labial and palatal alveolar bone.
7. With a firm grip, apply apical force then palatal force then labio-palatal movement with increasing range of movement every cycle until the tooth is extracted (rotation should be avoid as in usual anatomy the apical one third of the root is inclined palatal), ant rotation movement may result in fracture of this part. The main movement is labially.
8. Inspect both of the tooth and the socket.
9. Squeeze the socket.
10. Ensure adequate hemostasis obtained.
11. Apply pressure gauze.
12. Give the patient postoperative instructions.

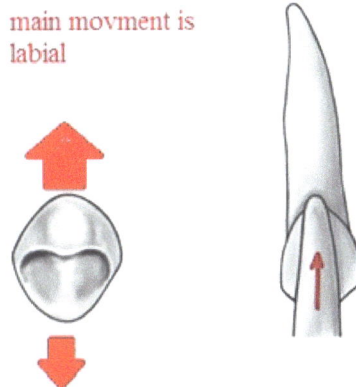

main movment is labial

Fig. (4.20). Extraction of Upper Leteral Incisor.

Extraction of Upper Canine: Fig. (4.21)

Relevant Anatomy

- Single, longest, strongest root.
- Thinner labial alveolar bone than the palatal one.
- Relation: neutral between nasal cavity and maxillary sinus.

Steps of Extraction

1. Give the patient local anesthesia (buccal and palatal infiltration), and make sure adequate anesthesia obtained.
2. Detach the gingiva (by periosteal elevator).
3. Try to luxate the tooth by straight elevator.
4. Choose the correct forcep.
5. Apply the forcep correctly to the tooth as apical as possible (apical to CEJ), with the long axis of the blades being along the long axis of the tooth.
6. Use the opposite hand to reflect the lip and support the labial and palatal alveolar bone.
7. With a firm grip, apply apical force then labio-palatal (more labial) movement, with increasing range of movement every cycle until the tooth is extracted. Rotation can be used after initial luxation of the tooth.
8. Inspect both of the tooth and the socket.
9. Squeeze the socket.
10. Ensure adequate hemostasis obtained.
11. Apply pressure gauze.
12. Give the patient postoperative instructions.

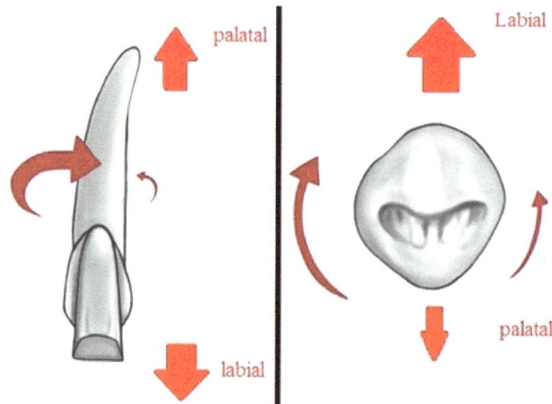

Fig. (4.21). Extraction of Upper Canine.

Extraction of Upper First Premolar: Fig. (4.22)

Relevant Anatomy

- More than 50% have two roots with thin tortuous apical 3rd.
- Thinner buccal alveolar bone than the palatal one.
- In relation with maxillary sinus.

Steps of Extraction

1. Give the patient local anesthesia(buccal and palatal infiltration), and make sure adequate anesthesia obtained.
2. Detach the gingiva (by periosteal elevator).
3. Try to luxate the tooth by straight elevator.
4. Choose the correct forcep.
5. Apply the forcep correctly to the tooth as apical as possible (apical to CEJ), with the long axis of the blades being along the long axis of the tooth.
6. Use the opposite hand to reflect the lip and support the labial and palatal alveolar bone.
7. With a firm grip, apply apical force then bucco-palatal (more buccal) movement, with increasing range of movement every cycle, with extreme caution because of risk of fracture is high since the apical one third is divided into two separated roots, rotation should be avoided.
8. Inspect both of the tooth and the socket.
9. Squeeze the socket.
10. Ensure adequate hemostasis obtained.
11. Apply pressure gauze.
12. Give the patient postoperative instructions.

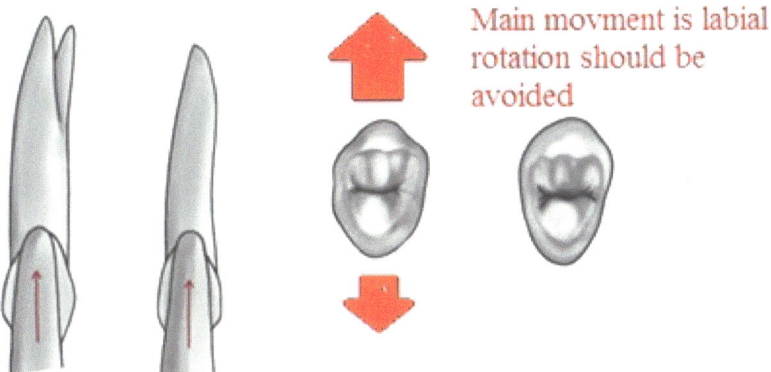

Main movment is labial rotation should be avoided

Fig. (4.22). Extraction of Upper First Premolar.

Extraction of Upper Second Premolar: Fig. (4.23)

Relevant Anatomy

- Mostly single rooted.
- Thinner buccal alveolar bone than the palatal one.
- In relation with maxillary sinus.

Steps of Extraction

1. Give the patient local anesthesia (buccal and palatal infiltration), and make sure adequate anesthesia obtained.
2. Detach the gingiva (by periosteal elevator).
3. Try to luxate the tooth by straight elevator.
4. Choose the correct forcep.
5. Apply the forcep correctly to the tooth as apical as possible (apical to CEJ), with the long axis of the blades being along the long axis of the tooth.
6. Use the opposite hand to reflect the lip and support the labial and palatal alveolar bone.
7. With a firm grip, apply apical force then bucco-palatal (more buccal) movement, with increasing range of movement every cycle, rotation (mainly mesially with less distal rotation) can be used after luxation of the tooth.
8. Inspect both of the tooth and the socket.
9. Squeeze the socket.
10. Ensure adequate hemostasis obtained.
11. Apply pressure gauze.
12. Give the patient postoperative instructions.

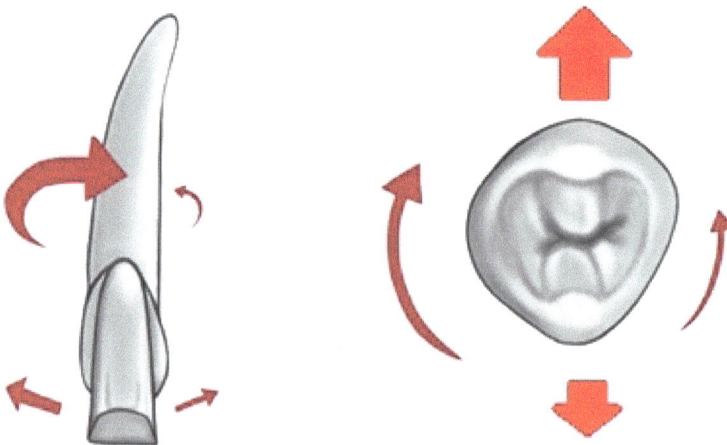

Fig. (4.23). Extraction of Upper Second Premolar.

Extraction of Upper First Molar: Fig. (4.24)

Relevant Anatomy

- Three roots; two buccal and one palatal. which are divergent (more than the second molar).
- Thinner buccal alveolar bone than the palatal one.
- In relation with maxillary sinus especially the palatal root.

Steps of Extraction

1. Give the patient local anesthesia (buccal and palatal infiltration), and make sure adequate anesthesia obtained.
2. Detach the gingiva (by periosteal elevator).
3. Try to luxate the tooth by straight elevator.
4. Choose the correct forcep.
5. Apply the forcep correctly to the tooth as apical as possible (apical to CEJ), with engagement of buccal beak into buccal furcation area, with the long axis of the blades being along the long axis of the tooth.
6. Use the opposite hand to reflect the lip and support the labial and palatal alveolar bone.
7. With a firm grip, apply apical force then bucco-palatal (more buccal) movement, with increasing range of movement every cycle, with distobuccal traction until the tooth is extracted.
8. Inspect both of the tooth and the socket.
9. Squeeze the socket.
10. Ensure adequate hemostasis obtained.
11. Apply pressure gauze.
12. Give the patient postoperative instructions.

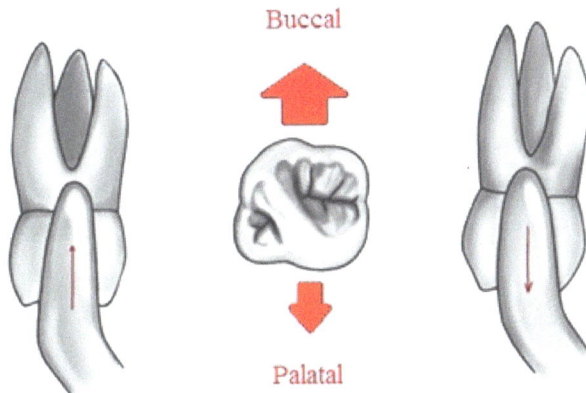

Fig. (4.24). Extraction of Upper First Molar.

Extraction of Upper Second Molar: Fig. (4.25)

Relevant Anatomy

- Three roots; two buccal and one palatal. which are divergent (less than the first molar)
- Thinner buccal alveolar bone than the palatal one.
- In relation with maxillary sinus.

Steps of Extraction

1. Give the patient local anesthesia (buccal and palatal infiltration), and make sure adequate anesthesia obtained.
2. Detach the gingiva (by periosteal elevator).
3. Try to luxate the tooth by straight elevator.
4. Choose the correct forcep.
5. Apply the forcep correctly to the tooth as apical as possible (apical to CEJ), with engagement of buccal beak into buccal furcation area, with the long axis of the blades being along the long axis of the tooth.
6. Use the opposite hand to reflect the lip and support the labial and palatal alveolar bone.
7. With a firm grip, apply apical force then bucco-palatal (more buccal) movement, with increasing range of movement every cycle, with distobuccal traction until the tooth is extracted.
8. Inspect both of the tooth and the socket.
9. Squeeze the socket.
10. Ensure adequate hemostasis obtained.
11. Apply pressure gauze.
12. Give the patient postoperative instructions.

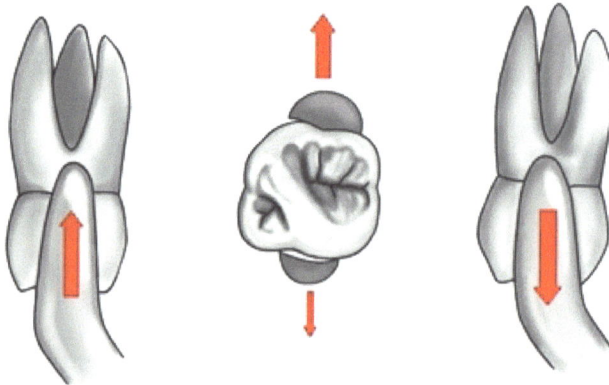

Fig. (4.25). Extraction of Upper Second Molar.

Extraction of Lower Central Incisor: Fig. (4.26)

Relevant Anatomy

- Single, straight root.
- Thin labial alveolar bone.

Steps of Extraction

1. Give the patient local anesthesia (inferior alveolar nerve block+/- infiltration), and make sure adequate anesthesia obtained.
2. Detach the gingiva (by periosteal elevator).
3. Try to luxate the tooth by straight elevator.
4. Choose the correct forcep.
5. Apply the forcep correctly to the tooth as apical as possible (apical to CEJ), with the long axis of the blades being along the long axis of the tooth.
6. Use the opposite hand to reflect the lip and support the labial and lingual alveolar bone and the mandible.
7. With a firm grip, apply apical force then labio-lingual (more labial) movement, with increasing range of movement every cycle until the tooth is extracted.
8. Inspect both of the tooth and the socket.
9. Squeeze the socket.
10. Ensure adequate hemostasis obtained.
11. Apply pressure gauze.
12. Give the patient postoperative instructions.

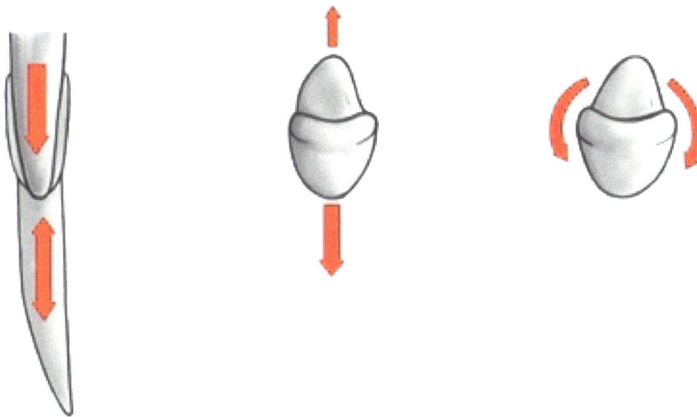

Fig. (4.26). Extraction of Lower Central Incisor.

Extraction of Lower Lateral Incisor: Fig. (4.27)

Relevant Anatomy

- Single, straight root.
- Thin labial alveolar bone .

Steps of Extraction

1. Give the patient local anesthesia (inferior alveolar nerve block+/- infiltration), and make sure adequate anesthesia obtained.
2. Detach the gingiva (by periosteal elevator).
3. Try to luxate the tooth by straight elevator.
4. Choose the correct forcep.
5. Apply the forcep correctly to the tooth as apical as possible (apical to CEJ), with the long axis of the blades being along the long axis of the tooth.
6. Use the opposite hand to reflect the lip and support the labial and lingual alveolar bone and the mandible.
7. With a firm grip, apply apical force then labio-lingual movement, with increasing range of movement every cycle until the tooth is extracted.
8. Inspect both of the tooth and the socket.
9. Squeeze the socket.
10. Ensure adequate hemostasis obtained.
11. Apply pressure gauze.
12. Give the patient postoperative instructions.

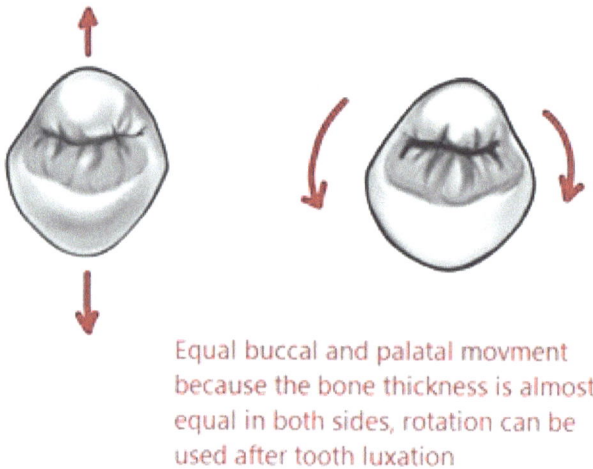

Equal buccal and palatal movment because the bone thickness is almost equal in both sides, rotation can be used after tooth luxation

Fig. (4.27). Extraction of Lower Lateral Incisor.

Extraction of Lower Canine: Fig. (4.28)

Relevant Anatomy

- Single, straight root which is shorter and weaker than the maxillary counterpart.
- Thin labial alveolar bone.

Steps of Extraction

1. Give the patient local anesthesia (inferior alveolar nerve block+/- infiltration), and make sure adequate anesthesia obtained.
2. Detach the gingiva (by periosteal elevator).
3. Try to luxate the tooth by straight elevator.
4. Choose the correct forcep.
5. Apply the forcep correctly to the tooth as apical as possible (apical to CEJ), with the long axis of the blades being along the long axis of the tooth.
6. Use the opposite hand to reflect the lip and support the labial and lingual alveolar bone and the mandible.
7. With a firm grip, apply apical force then labio-lingual movement, with increasing range of movement every cycle until the tooth is extracted.
8. Inspect both of the tooth and the socket.
9. Squeeze the socket.
10. Ensure adequate hemostasis obtained.
11. Apply pressure gauze.
12. Give the patient postoperative instructions.

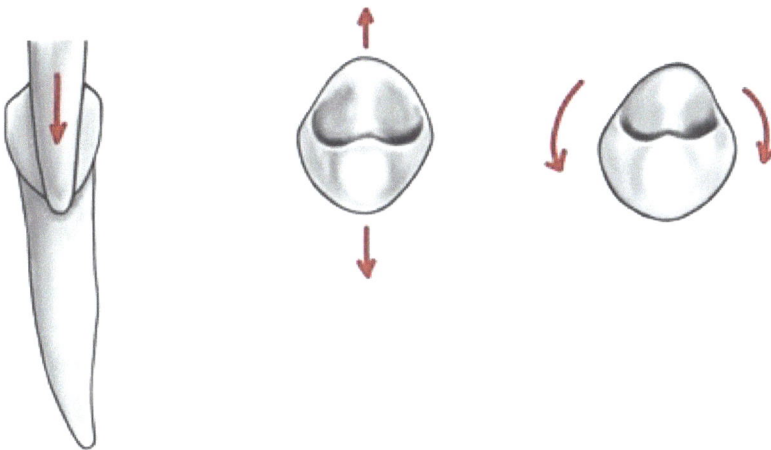

Fig. (4.28). Extraction of Lower Canine.

Extraction of Lower First Premolar: Fig. (4.29)

Relevant Anatomy

- Single, straight, conical root, furcation is possible.
- Thin labial alveolar bone
- In relation with mental foramen.

Steps of Extraction

1. Give the patient local anesthesia (inferior alveolar nerve block), and make sure adequate anesthesia obtained.
2. Detach the gingiva (by periosteal elevator).
3. Try to luxate the tooth by straight elevator.
4. Choose the correct forcep.
5. Apply the forcep correctly to the tooth as apical as possible (apical to CEJ), with the long axis of the blades being along the long axis of the tooth.
6. Use the opposite hand to reflect the lip and support the labial and lingual alveolar bone and the mandible.
7. With a firm grip, apply apical force then combination of both bucco-lingual movement (more ligually because the bone has less thickness ligually) and rotational movements, with increasing range of movement every cycle until the tooth is extracted.
8. Inspect both of the tooth and the socket.
9. Squeeze the socket.
10. Ensure adequate hemostasis obtained.
11. Apply pressure gauze .
12. Give the patient postoperative instructions.

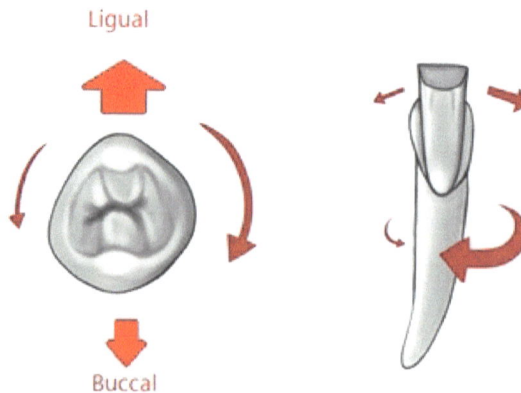

Fig. (4.29). Extraction of Lower First Premolar.

Extraction of Lower Second Premolar: Fig. (4.30)

Relevant Anatomy

- Single, straight, conical root, furcation is possible.
- Thin labial and lingual alveolar bone
- In relation with mental foramen.

Steps of Extraction

1. Give the patient local anesthesia (inferior alveolar nerve block), and make sure adequate anesthesia obtained.
2. Detach the gingiva (by periosteal elevator).
3. Try to luxate the tooth by straight elevator.
4. Choose the correct forcep.
5. Apply the forcep correctly to the tooth as apical as possible (apical to CEJ), with the long axis of the blades being along the long axis of the tooth.
6. Use the opposite hand to reflect the lip and support the labial and lingual alveolar bone and the mandible.
7. With a firm grip, apply apical force then combination of both bucco-lingual (more ligually because the bone has less thickness ligually) and rotational movements, with increasing range of movement every cycle until the tooth is extracted.
8. Inspect both of the tooth and the socket.
9. Squeeze the socket.
10. Ensure adequate hemostasis obtained.
11. Apply pressure gauze.
12. Give the patient postoperative instructions.

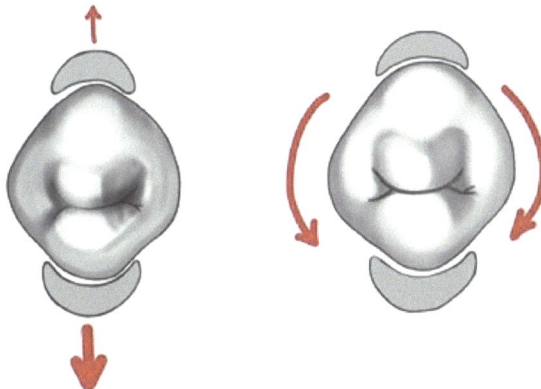

Fig. (4.30). Extraction of Lower Second Premolar.

Extraction of Lower First Molar: Fig. (4.31)

Relevant Anatomy

- Two roots, one mesial and one distal.
- Thick buccal bone and thinner lingual alveolar bone.

Steps of Extraction

1. Give the patient local anesthesia (inferior alveolar nerve block and long buccal nerve block), and make sure adequate anesthesia obtained.
2. Detach the gingiva (by periosteal elevator).
3. Try to luxate the tooth by straight elevator.
4. Choose the correct forcep.
5. Apply the forcep correctly to the tooth as apical as possible (apical to CEJ), with engagement of the beaks into the buccal an lingual furcation areas, with the long axis of the blades being along the long axis of the tooth.
6. Use the opposite hand to reflect the lip and support the labial and lingual alveolar bone and the mandible.
7. With a firm grip, apply apical force then bucco-lingual movement (more ligually because the bone has less thickness ligually) , with increasing range of movement every cycle until the tooth is extracted.
8. Inspect both of the tooth and the socket.
9. Squeeze the socket.
10. Ensure adequate hemostasis obtained.
11. Apply pressure gauze.
12. Give the patient postoperative instructions.

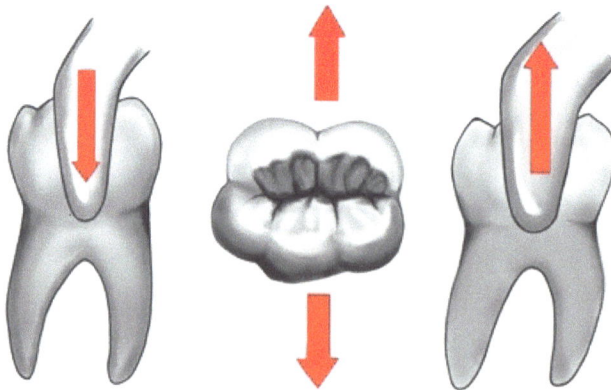

Fig. (4.31). Extraction of Lower First Molar.

Extraction of Lower Second Molar

Relevant Anatomy

- Two roots, one mesial and one distal.
- Much more thicker buccal bone and thinner lingual alveolar bone.

Steps of Extraction

1. Give the patient local anesthesia (inferior alveolar nerve block and long buccal nerve block), and make sure adequate anesthesia obtained.
2. Detach the gingiva (by periosteal elevator).
3. Try to luxate the tooth by straight elevator.
4. Choose the correct forcep.
5. Apply the forcep correctly to the tooth as apical as possible (apical to CEJ), with engagement of the beaks into the buccal an lingual furcation areas, with the long axis of the blades being along the long axis of the tooth.
6. Use the opposite hand to reflect the lip and support the labial and lingual alveolar bone and the mandible.
7. With a firm grip, apply apical force then linguo-buccal movement (more ligually because the bone has less thickness ligually) , with increasing range of movement every cycle until the tooth is extracted.
8. Inspect both of the tooth and the socket.
9. Squeeze the socket.
10. Ensure adequate hemostasis obtained.
11. Apply pressure gauze.
12. Give the patient postoperative instructions.

BIBLIOGRAPHY

[1]　Archer WH. Oral and maxillofacial surgery. Philadelphia: Saunders 1975.

[2]　Gans BJ. Atlas of oral surgery. Saint Louis: C.V. Mosby Co. 1972.

[3]　Fragiskos FD. Oral surgery. Berlin: Springer 2007.
[http://dx.doi.org/10.1007/978-3-540-49975-6]

[4]　Hooley JR, Whitacre RJ. A Self-instructional guide to oral surgery in general dentistry. Seattle, Wa.: Stoma Press 1979.

[5]　Howe GL. Minor oral surgery. 3rd ed., Oxford: Wright 1997.

[6]　Dimitroulis G. A synopsis of minor oral surgery. Oxford: Wright 1996.

[7]　Kruger GO. Textbook of oral and maxillofacial surgery. St. Louis: Mosby 1984.

[8]　Laskin DM. Oral and maxillofacial surgery. St. Louis: C.V. Mosby 1992.

[9]　Laskin DM, Abubaker AO. Decision making in oral and maxillofacial surgery. Chicago: Quintessence Pub. Co. 2007.

[10]   Kwon PH, Laskin DM. Clinician's manual of oral and maxillofacial surgery. Chicago: Quintessence Pub. Co. 1991.

[11]   Rounds CE, Rounds FW. Principles and technique of exodontia. St. Louis: Mosby 1962.

[12]   Peterson LJ. Contemporary oral and maxillofacial surgery. St. Louis: Mosby 1998.

[13]   Contemporary H. Oral and Maxillofacial Surgery. Elsevier 2014.

[14]   Sailer HF, Pajarola GF. Oral surgery for the general dentist. Stuttgart: Thieme 1998.

[15]   Dym H, Ogle OE. Oral surgery for the general dentist. Philadelphia: Saunders 2012.

CHAPTER 5

Complex Exodontia and Guidelines in Management of Medically Compromised Patients in Dental Chair

Esam Ahmad Z Omar*

Department of Oral & Maxillofacial Surgery, College of Dentistry, Taibah University, Madinah, Saudi Arabia

Abstract: Many dental practitioners do not differentiate between the complex extraction and the surgical (trans-alveolar) extraction. By definition, the surgical extraction is one of complex extraction procedures, but the complex extraction is not limited to surgical extraction. In this chapter, the complex extraction has been defined. The pre-operative, intra-operative and post-operative factors that may contribute to the complexity of dental extraction have been discussed. This chapter contains a separated part about the management of medically compromised patients, as those patients can be considered under the definition of complex extraction. This chapter also contains a separated part about physics of elevator's uses.

Keywords: The Complex Exodontia, guidelines in management of medically compromised patients in dental chair, Principles of Elevators, Complications of Exodontia.

PART 1: SYSTEMIC FACTORS CONTRIBUTE TO COMPLEXITY OF DENTAL EXTRACTIONS

A complex extraction is a tooth or root removal that may be associated with possible challenges intra-operatively or may carry a risk of complications postoperatively.

Assessment of the patient in dental extraction starts from the entrance of the patient into the dental clinic by looking at the patient during his or her entrance into the clinic until he or she sits in the dental chair. The following can be observed:

---

* **Corresponding author Esam Ahmad Z Omar:** Department of Oral & Maxillofacial Surgery, College of Dentistry, Taibah University, Madinah, Saudi Arabia; Tel: 0569536708; Fax: 00966148494710; E-mail: esamomar@hotmail.com

1. The built of the patient.
2. The patient's manner of walking.
3. The patient's dress.
4. The patient's age range.
5. Verify the sex of the patient by comparing personal data with appearance.

Unfortunately, patient assessment is started before the entrance of the patient into the dental clinic by reading the patient's personal information. The following may be obtained from the patient's personal file:

1. Age
2. Sex

Age: As patients' become older, the alveolar bone becomes more sclerotic, losing its resiliency, and becomes harder and more prone to fracture of the alveolar process during the extraction procedure.

Sex: It is well known that dental fear and stress is more common in female patients than males. Dental fear is one of the challenges that may create difficulties during the extraction procedure. Built: In overweight patients, dental extraction is more difficult because of the following:

• Limitation of mouth opening.
• Short neck.
• Broad shoulders.
• Presence of other systemic variables (factors) that may add to extraction difficulty.

The Way of Walking: there are five ways of abnormal walking, with different causes, but in general, most of these causes are neurological in origin. There are some orthopedic causes as well. How a patient walks hints at the general condition of their well-being and helps in formulating questions during history taking.

Some causes of the abnormal way of walking:

Neurological Causes

• Cerebrovascular accident (stroke)
• Cerebral palsy
• Long-term brain injury due to alcoholism
• Neuropathy (as with diabetes)
• Head trauma Musculoskeletal causes:

- Spinal cord trauma
- Hepatic Failure
- Cervical spondylosis associated with myelopathy
- Spinal cord tumor
- Congenital hip dysplasia
- Multiple sclerosis
- Muscular dystrophy
- Syphilitic meningomyelitis
- Spinal muscle atrophy Others:
- Syringomyelia
- Pernicious anemia Medications:
- Alcohol intoxication
- Using of Dilantin and other seizure medications

The dressing of the patient gives a lot of information about:

- The patient's attitude
- The patient's financial situation
- The patient's psychology
- The patient's cultural background

When the patient sits on the dental chair and before clinical examination, taking a patient's medical history is crucial. Past medical history available in the patient's record should be rechecked and retaken verbally from the patient themselves, in their own words.

Medical history is key for the management of any medical emergency that may develop in the dental chair because once a patient becomes unconscious; it becomes difficult to understand the cause and to manage the patient properly.

Medical history is significant in the expectation of a possible intra-operative and post-operative local and systemic complication that may develop in a patient at risk. It is a cornerstone in patient assessment and an important part of patient management.

Factors (conditions) of particular concern in exodontia that may cause a difficult extraction procedure, may be categorized as follows:

1. Systemic factors are related to
   a. Psychology of the patient
   b. Systemic condition of the patient
2. Local factors are related to the operative field

Systemic Factors

A. **Psychology of the Patient**

Dental phobia is the most important psychological disorder that may be involved in dental extraction and may create challenges intra-operatively.

• Adverse patient reaction to an unknown procedure is referred to as dental anxiety. It is common and very natural to have anxiety, in particular when they are going to have a treatment, which is a new experience for them. In short, fear of the unknown is known as *anxiety* (Card **5.1**).

Card 5.1. Dental phobia.

Dental phobia

Precautions: Stress reduction protocol

1. Early morning appointment
2. Short appointment
3. Short waiting time
4. Create a good relationship with the patient
5. Provide a good explanation of the procedure
6. Reassure the patient
7. Apply profound local anaesthesia within the recommended dose

Monitor:
BP
O_2 by using pulse oximeter
Heart rate

Management:
If stress reduction protocol is unlikely to manage stress and phobia:

1. A hypnotic agent may be administered to help relax a patient prior to surgery. (Ambien 10 mg)
2. A sedative agent may be administered to control anxiety two hours before surgery is due.
3. Try to have an appointment in the morning with very less or almost no waiting.
4. Regular verbal reassurances should be given and involve in conversations unrelated to the surgery to distract the patient.
5. The patient should be cautioned against discomforting activities.
6. Keep needles and surgical instruments out of sight of the patient.
7. Nitrous oxide-oxygen should be administered.
8. Local anaesthesia should be administered with care and usage should be according to intensity and duration required.
9. Using Epinephrine 1:100,000. However, it should not be greater than 4 ml, dose for an adult is a total of 0.04 mg in any period of 30-minute.
10. Give intravenous sedation if possible and accessible, this should be carefully monitored and administered by a licensed personnel.
11. Postoperative care instructions should be provided verbally and in written form, as well after the surgery.
12. Prescribe effective analgesics.
13. Reassurance should be provided and give information about whom to contact in case of a problem.
14. In the evening after the surgery calls the patient at home to check his/her progress and to see if he/she has any problems or queries.

Conscious sedation may require a consult who is specialized in dental sedation

- ***Dental fear:*** Reaction to anxiety involving a fight-or-flight response when aggressive stimulus is faced.
- Reaction similar to fear, but only more intense is known as ***dental phobia***. In this case, if 1) a dangerous situation is just reminded or even 2) thought of, the fight-or-flight response occurs. A person experiencing ***dental phobia*** would try at all costs to keep away from dental treatment unless either the physical problem becomes unbearable or the ***phobia's*** psychological burden becomes overpowering.

Dental Phobia's Predisposing Factors:

1. **Bad experiences:** Around 80% to 85% of dental phobias cases are due to a bad experience and in worst cases, horrific dental experiences.
2. **Abuse history:** People, who have the unfortunate experience of sexual assault, especially in their childhood, commonly show dental phobia. The experience of being tormented (built in) previously or abused physically or emotionally by a person who has been in charge may lead to the development of dental phobia, and this is worsened if one has bad dental experiences as well.
3. **Uncaring dentist:** The main reason for this is fear of pain. Pain that a dentist inflicts is thought as authoritative and cold which has an immense psychological impact.
4. **Humiliation:** Insensitive remarks and intense feelings of humiliation may be a reason for dental phobia as well. Negative social evaluation will upset most people. For sensitive people, negative evaluation may be overwhelming.
5. **Vicarious learning:** Observational learning can also be a reason for dental phobia. At times when parents are scared of dentists, their offspring may observe this attitude and develop a fear of dentists even though they themselves have not experienced a bad dental situation. Moreover, when children hear bad dental experiences of other people, they may themselves get frightened.
6. **Preparedness:** In a traditional sense a few of the dental phobia subtypes can be regarded as "irrational." Some phobias are inherently present in a person, or they are more "prepared" to learn them, for example, the needle phobia.

Precautions

Stress reduction protocol:

1. Early morning appointment
2. Short appointment
3. Short waiting time
4. Create a good relationship with the patient
5. Provide a good explanation of the procedure
6. Reassure the patient

7. Apply profound local anesthesia within the recommended dose

Management

If the stress reduction protocol is unlikely to manage the stress and phobia:

- A hypnotic agent can be taken to help relax the night prior to surgery (Ambien 10 mg).
- A sedative agent can be taken to control for anxiety two hours earlier to the time surgery.
- Try to have an appointment in the morning with very less or almost no waiting.
- Regular verbal reassurances should be given and involve in conversations unrelated to the surgery to distract the patient.
- The patient should be cautioned before doing any uncomfortable thing.
- Keep needles and surgical instruments out of sight of the patient.
- Nitrous oxide-oxygen can be administered.
- Local anesthetics should be administered with care and usage should be according to intensity and duration required.
- Epinephrine 1:100,000: However, it should not be greater than 4 ml, the dose for an adult is a total of 0.04 mg in any period of 30-minutes.
- Give intravenous sedation if possible and accessible, this should be carefully monitored and administered by licensed personnel.
- Postoperative care instructions should be given verbally and written as well after the surgery.
- Prescribe effective analgesics.
- Reassurance should be provided and give information about whom to contact in case of a problem.
- In the evening after surgery calls the patient at home to check his/her progress and to see if he/she has any problems or queries.

Syncope: A momentary, self-limited unconsciousness in which the person is unable to maintain postural tone, and spontaneous recovery follows it (as well, is called as faint) (Card **5.2**).

The kind of syncope that occurs in dental chairs is considered a physiological response to fear and pain associated with over-activity of the vagus nerve. Pathological syncope is not common in the dental chair, and causes of pathological syncope may be summarized as follows:

1. Pumping of the blood stops for a moment or so;
2. Tone required to maintain blood pressure by the blood vessels is not sufficient to supply blood to the brain;
3. There is not sufficient fluid or blood in the blood vessels (hypovolemia due to

insensible water loss as in sweating); or

4. A combination of one, two, or three reasons mentioned above.

Card 5.2. Syncope.

Syncope

Clinical Features
- dizziness
- nausea
- pallor
- cold, moist skin (clammy)
- pulse initially slow and weak

Precipitating factors
- Anxiety
- Pain
- Fatigue
- Fasting
- High temperature

Monitor:
BP
O$_2$ by using pulse oximeter
Heart rate

Tim
Management
- Lower patient's head (supine position)
- +/- smelling salts
- Rapid recovery (within seconds) usually not lasting more than 2 minutes.

Causes of Pathological syncope:
Cardiac:
- Coronary Artery Diseases

- Hypertension
- Infective endocarditis
- Heart failure
- Artificial valves/transplants

Endocrine:
- Diabetes
- Thyroid dysfunction:
- Hyperthyroidism
- Hypothyroidism
- Patients on long-term steroids
- Pregnancy

Blood disorders:
- Disorders of hemostasis:
- Hemophilia
- Patients on anticoagulants, antiplatelet drugs

Allergy:
- Asthma

Neurological:
- Epilepsy

Systemic conditions that may cause syncope (Pathological Syncope):

A. **Cardiac:**
   - Coronary Artery Diseases
   - Hypertension
   - Infective endocarditis
   - Heart failure
   - Artificial valves/transplants

B. **Endocrine:**
   - Diabetes
   - Thyroid dysfunction:
   - Hyperthyroidism
   - Hypothyroidism
   - Patients on long-term steroids
   - Pregnancy

C. **Blood disorders:**
   - Disorders of hemostasis:
   - Hemophilia
   - Patients on anticoagulants, antiplatelet drugs

D. **Allergy:**
   - Asthma

E. **Neurological:**
   - Epilepsy

F. **Others:**
   - Patients undergoing radiotherapy
   - Others

Physiological syncope (Vasovagal syncope, faint) that happens in during dental procedures is one of the most common causes of loss of consciousness. In this condition, the balance of activity between the chemicals, adrenaline and acetylcholine, are disturbed. Adrenaline activates the body, making the heart pump quicker and veins smaller thereby, increasing pulse rate.

Acetylcholine has an inverse reaction. Over-activation of vagus nerve results in over discharge of acetylcholine, slows the heart rate, and the veins widen, these result in polling of the blood in venous compartment which making the venous blood return to the heart less. This means that the amount of blood ejected by the heart will be lower than normal (low stroke volume). The results are a temporary decrease in the blood supply to the brain causing transient cerebral ischemia and temporary loss of consciousness. This is called syncope.

Clinical Features

- Dizziness
- Nausea
- Pallor
- Cold, moist skin (clammy)
- Pulse initially slow and weak

Precipitating Factors

- Anxiety
- Pain
- Fatigue
- Fasting
- High temperature

Management

- Lower patient's head (supine position)
- +/- Smelling salts
- Rapid recovery (within seconds) usually not lasting more than 2 minutes.

Diabetes

Diabetes mellitus is a syndrome, which features the changes in the metabolism of carbohydrates mainly associated with metabolic changes in protein and lipid. The reason for this is abnormalities in insulin secretion, mechanism and functions.

In a normal individual:

1. Immediately or some while after the meal: insulin secretions are increased, leading to fatty acids being synthesized/stored, causing glycogen storage and synthesis of protein.
2. After an overnight fast: insulin level is low, and glucagon level is high, which leads to the breakdown of glycogen, lipolysis, and hepatic gluconeogenesis.
3. After a prolonged fast: insulin levels are extremely low, and also glucagon is also low; this leads to lipolysis to take over. Main fuel source is the lipids. Minimization of gluconeogenesis since it leads to wastage of nitrogen, building-up of ammonia, and muscle mass loss.

Pathophysiology

The main function of insulin:

- It increase glucose uptake by the cell by the opening of the glucose gates.

- It stimulates the food energy to be stored as glycogen in skeletal muscle and hepatocytes.
- Furthermore, hepatocytes are stimulated through insulin to produce triglycerides and store them in adipose tissue.

	Liver	Adipose or Fat Tissue	Muscle
High insulin	Glycolysis Glycogenesis	Triglyceride synthesis	Amino acid uptake
Low insulin	Gluconeogenesis Glycogenolysis	Lipolysis	Protein synthesis

Effect lipid metabolism: In uncontrolled insulin-dependent diabetes Mellitus (IDDM), the triglycerides rapidly move leading to plasma free fatty acids level to rise. These free fatty acids are metabolized done in order to provide energy. When insulin is not present, there is a drop in malonyl-CoA levels (Malonyl-CoA is a coenzyme, a derivative of malonic acid. Malonyl-CoA is co-enzyme, formed by carboxylation of acetyl-CoA by using enzyme called acetyl-CoA carboxylase. Each molecule of acetyl-CoA uses energy from ATP to join with a molecule of bicarbonate). This has a major function in fatty acid biosynthesis and transport of fat into the mitochondria. When fatty acids are oxidized inside mitochondria, it generates acetyl-COA whose further oxidization can be done in the citric acid cycle – which is also called as Krebs cycle or tricarboxylic acid (TCA) cycle. Nevertheless, a major part of acetyl-CoA inside hepatocytes is metabolized into the ketone bodies (b-hydroxybutyrate and acetoacetate) instead of being oxidized by the TCA cycle. These ketone bodies are employed by the skeletal, heart and brain muscle to produce energy. In IDDM, since ketone bodies and free fatty acids are readily available in high amounts this intensifies the reduced glucose utilization, which enhances the resulting hyperglycemia. Excess ketone bodies production, as compared to the ability of the body, to utilize those results in ketoacidosis. Acetone is produced because of the spontaneous breakdown of acetoacetate, and when it is exhaled by the lungs, it gives breath a distinctive odor.

Effects on protein: Protein metabolism is also affected by the insulin, protein degradation rate is reduced, and synthesis rate is raised. Hence, deficiency of insulin would result in increased protein catabolism. The high proteolysis rate also results in high level of amino acids concentration in plasma. Glucogenic amino acids act as precursors for renal and hepatic gluconeogenesis, enhancing the hyperglycemia observed in IDDM.

Hormones

Blood sugar level is raised by the following hormones:

- Cortisol
- Glucagon
- Growth hormones *etc.*
- Epinephrine and norepinephrine

Causes of Diabetes

Non-insulin dependence diabetes (type 2 diabetes):

The causes of this condition are:

1. **A Relative Deficiency:** The body fails to produce the required amount of insulin to fulfil its need.
2. **Decrease in the Affinity of the Tissue's Insulin Receptors**: is one of the most commonly seen reasons of diabetes type 2. Yalow and Berson (1960) prismatic [27] demonstration notes that, the presence of insulin resistance factors can be considered as the most likely cause of type 2 diabetes, the decrease in receptors sensitivity result in hyperinsulinism in response to increased glucose level. This may explain the development of weight in the pre-diabetic phase. However, recent research questions the primacy, specificity, and insulin resistance contribution to the disease state.
Insulin secretion and actions are inhibited in chronic hyperinsulinemia (feedback action), result in impairment the insulin secretion in response to glucose (hyperglycemia) along with deceased cellular insulin sensitivity is hyperglycemia at the receptors level. Pancreatic atrophy has been approved by Philippe *et al.* through CT-Scans in diabetic patients with a history of 15-years [28].
3. **Destruction of B-cell:** Ferrannini E. (2010) and Talchai C. *et al.* (2012) confirmed that the B-cell destruction occurs in the early phase of the disease and not necessarily follow a period of insulin resistance [29, 30].
4. **Insulin Resistance:** The following are considered as causes for the resistance of the body to insulin:
   - Obesity/overweight (especially excess visceral adiposity)
   - Polycystic ovary disease
   - Excess glucocorticoids (Cushing's syndrome or steroid therapy)
   - Lipodystrophy (acquired or genetic, linked to liver lipid accumulation)
   - Excess growth hormone (acromegaly)
   - Pregnancy and gestational diabetes

5. **Autoantibodies to the Insulin Receptor**
6. Peroxisome proliferators' activator receptor γ (PPAR γ) *mutation*
7. Insulin receptor *mutation*
8. *Mutations* leading to genetic obesity (*e.g.*, melanocortin receptor mutations)
9. *Hemochromatosis* (a hereditary disease that results in iron accumulation in tissues)
10. Pancreatic βcells' *autoimmune destruction* is perhaps a factor in a minute subset of type 2 diabetic patients, and it is also defined as the symptom of latent autoimmune diabetes in adults. In 10% of Scandinavian type 2 diabetes patients, this has been reported and also the latest United Kingdom study identified this as well.
11. There could be *changes in the configuration* of the chemical structure of the insulin.
12. **Genomic Factors**:
    Changes in different single-nucleotide polymorphisms (SNPs), after the age of 40, are a causative factor in certain diabetic patients. Several subsides of single-nucleotide polymorphisms (SNPs) may undergo such changes.

Insulin dependence diabetes (type 1 diabetes)

- Autoimmune: In this disease, the beta cells found in of the pancreas that produces insulin are damaged by the body's own immune system. Consequently, there is a beta cell deficiency, which leads to complete insulin deficiency. Hence, when anti-islet-cell or anti-insulin antibodies are present in the blood, it is called as an autoimmune disease. This results in pancreas islets destruction and lymphocytic infiltration.

Symptoms and Signs

- Increased thirst or *Polydipsia* is a result of the high blood glucose level, raising the blood osmolality and making it more concentrated.
- Increased frequency of urination or *Polyuria* is a result of the extra amount of fluid intake and glucose-induced urination.
- Due to the calories lost in urine, weight loss occurs.
- Increased hunger or *Polyphagia* is a result of the excess or loss of glucose in urine, leading to a higher craving of glucose by the body.

Type 1 and Type 2 diabetes mellitus (Clinical characteristics):

Features	Type 1	Type 2
Age of onset	Usually less than 20 years	Usually greater than 30 years
Body mass	Low (wasted) to normal	Obese

Contd.....

Features	Type 1	Type 2
Plasma insulin	Low or absent	Normal to high initially
Plasma glucagon	High, can be suppressed	High, resistant to suppression
Plasma glucose	Increased	Increased
Insulin sensitivity	Normal	Reduced
Therapy	Insulin	Weight loss, thiazolidinedione, metformin, sulfonylureas, insulin

Guyton and Hall (2006).

Blood sugar levels Table 5.:

Plasma glucose test	Normal	Prediabetes	Diabetes
Random	Below 11.1 mmol/l Below 200 mg/dl	N/A	11.1 mmol/l or more 200 mg/dl or more
Fasting	Below 6.1 mmol/l Below 108 mg/dl	6.1 to 6.9 mmol/l 108 to 125 mg/dl	7.0 mmol/l or more 126 mg/dl or more
2 hour post-prandial	Below 7.8 mmol/l Below 140 mg/dl	7.8 to 11.0 mmol/l 140 to 199 mg/dl	11.1 mmol/l or more 200 mg/dl or more

Random Plasma Glucose Test

A random plasma glucose test is the blood glucose test that can be taken at any time without much planning and is therefore used in the diagnosis of type 1 diabetes when time is of the essence.

Fasting Plasma Glucose Test

A fasting plasma glucose test is taken after at least eight hours of fasting and is usually taken in the morning. It may be affected seriously by pattern of sleeping.

Oral Glucose Tolerance Test (OGTT)

An oral glucose tolerance test involves taking a first taking a fasting sample of blood and then taking a very sweet drink containing 75g of glucose. The amount of glucose taken prior to test may significantly affect the result. The medications have significant input in the result in particular the medication and herbs that accelerate or inhibit the metabolic process.

After having this drink you need to stay at rest until a further blood sample is taken after 2 hours.

HbA1c Test for Diabetes Diagnosis

The term *HbA1c* refers to glycated haemoglobin. It develops when haemoglobin, a protein within red blood cells that carries oxygen throughout the body with glucose in the blood, becoming 'glycated' by measuring glycated haemoglobin (HbA1c), it become possible to get an overall picture of what our average blood sugar levels have been over a period of weeks/months (usually 3 months). This is mean that the HbA1c test does not directly measure the level of blood glucose, however, the result of the test is influenced by how high or low your blood glucose levels have tended to be over a period of 2 to 3 months. This test is unreliable in patients who are with abnormal haemoglobin (haemoglobinopathies – like sickle cell anemia or thalassemia)

Indications of diabetes or prediabetes are given under the following conditions:

- **Normal:** Below 42 mmol/mol (6.0%)
- **Prediabetes:** 42 to 47 mmol/mol (6.0 to 6.4%)
- **Diabetes:** 48 mmol/mol (6.5% or over)

Dental Approach for Diabetic Patients

- It is important to have a latest blood glucose test. This test is easy to perform using a glucometer (an electrical, portable device) before the surgery or any other the dental treatment.
- A history of previous blood glucose tests for the previous 10 days is more important than a recent test, as complications of diabetes (impairs the healing process and increases other relevant cardiovascular diseases – ischemic heart diseases) result from long-standing high glucose levels.

Special Precautions

1. The appointment should be in the morning.
2. Breakfast should be taken, and the usual daily insulin dose must be taken.
3. The patient should not wait for a long time in the waiting area

Diabetic patients that lost consciousness in the dental chair should be immediately treated as hypoglycemic. A ketotic coma (hyperglycemia) is unlikely to develop in a dental chair because it is an accumulative, long-standing disease in which patients become critically ill and dehydrated.

Hypoglycemia is a common emergency condition that may develop in diabetic patients. It requires immediate management (Card **5.3**).

Card 5.3. Hypoglycemia.

Hypoglycemia

Clinical features:
- Rapid onset
- Drowsiness
- Disorientation
- Irritability or aggression
- Warm, moist skin
- Pulse full and rapid
- The patient rarely loses consciousness

Precipitating factors:
- Lack of food
- Too much insulin
- Excessive exercise
- Stress and related factors such as insomnia the night before dental treatment, a late appointment, or a long wait time before the appointment

Monitor:
BP
O$_2$ by using pulse oximeter
Heart rate

Management
- Lie the patient flat
- If possible, give glucose orally (glucose drink/juices) or through IV
- 50ml 50% glucose, especially if the patient loses consciousness

Diabetic patients that loss consciousness in the dental chair should be immediately treated as hypoglycemic. A ketotic coma (hyperglycemia) is unlikely to develop in a dental chair because it is an accumulative, long-standing disease in which patients become critically ill and dehydrated.

Clinical Features

- Rapid onset
- Drowsiness
- Disorientation

- Irritability or aggression
- Warm, moist skin
- Pulse full and rapid
- The patient rarely loses consciousness

Precipitating Factors

- Lack of food
- Too much insulin
- Excessive exercise
- Stress and related factors such as insomnia the night before dental treatment, a late appointment, or a long wait time before the appointment

Management

- Lie the patient flat
- If possible, give glucose orally (glucose drink/juices) or through IV
- 50ml 50% glucose, if the patient loses consciousness

Most common medication for treatment of diabetes (categories and trade name):

- Metformin (Glucophage, Glumetza, and others): Usually, the first medicine prescribed in type 2 diabetes is the metformin. The function of this is to improve the body tissues sensitivity to insulin in order to make the body use insulin in an effective manner. Liver glucose production is adversely affected by this. On its own, metformin may not be able to lower blood sugar as required. The patient's lifestyle should change, for example by increasing the exercise level and losing weight.
- Sulfonylureas: This type of medicines aids in more insulin secretion by the body. Medications examples belonging to this class are glipizide (Glucotrol), glimepiride (Amaryl) and glyburide (DiaBeta, Glynase). Possible side effects could be reduced blood sugar level and excess weight gain.
- Meglitinides: Similar to function in sulfonylureas, these medications also stimulate the pancreas to increase insulin secretion but act more quickly, and their effect in the body remains for a shorter duration. They might also result in low blood sugar, but lower risk as compared to sulfonylureas. It is possible to gain weight by using this class of medications too (*e.g.* nateglinide (Starlix) and repaglinide (Prandin)).
- Thiazolidinediones: These medications also make the tissues of the body more sensitive to insulin, as the metformin do. However, side effects of this class of medications are more diverse for example, gaining weight, and ones that are more serious include a higher risk of heart failure and bone fractures. Due to the serious nature of the side effects, doctors do not prefer these medications as a

first-choice treatment. A few example of thiazolidinedione is pioglitazone (Actos) and rosiglitazone (Avandia).

- Inhibitors of dipeptidyl peptidase 4 (DPP-4 inhibitors): These medications have a modest effect in reducing the blood sugar levels. These do not cause weight gain. A few examples are linagliptin (Tradjenta), sitagliptin (Januvia) and saxagliptin (Onglyza). Blood glucose levels increase by glucagon; the functioning of DPP-4 inhibitors is to reduce the glucagon and hence to decrease the glucose levels in the blood. The DPP-4 inhibitors function is to cause a rise in incretin (GLP-1 and GIP), and inhibiting the release of glucagon, leading to rising in levels of insulin secretion and decreased gastric emptying and hence causes a drop in the blood glucose levels.
- Glucagon-like peptide-1 receptor agonists (GLP-1 receptor agonists): GLP-1 receptor agonists: The use of this class of medications slows down the process of digestion and aids in lowering blood sugar levels however, it is not as effective as sulfonylureas. The use of this medicine results in weight loss. An example of GLP-1 receptor agonists is liraglutide (Victoza) and exenatide (Byetta). Side effects include a higher risk of pancreatitis and nausea.
- Sodium-glucose transport protein 2 (SGLT2 inhibitors) SGLT2 inhibitors: The most recent class of diabetes drugs on the market are this one. Their function is to stop the re-absorption of sugar into the bloodstream by the kidneys. As an alternative, sugar excretes in the urine. Examples of SGLT2 inhibitors are dapagliflozin (Farxiga) and canagliflozin (Invokana). Associated side effects could be urinary tract infections, yeast infections, hypotension and increased urination.
- Any individual suffering from Type-II diabetes must undergo insulin therapy. Previously, insulin therapy was not very much preferred and employed as a last option, but presently, it's often advised at early stages since it has proven beneficial.

Insulin has several types each having a distinct specialized function. Some of the examples are:

Insulin glulisine (Apidra), isophane (Humulin N, Novolin N), Insulin detemir (Levemir), Insulin glargine (Lantus), Insulin Aspart (Novolog), Insulin and Insulin lispro (Humalog).

Hyperglycemia: patients with hyperglycemia should not be operated, and it is advisable to control the blood glucose level a physician is referred; avoidance of the development of ketotic coma is more important than dental treatment for saving a patient's life. Dental treatment should be restricted to the relief of pain (***emergency dental treatment only***).

Card 5.4. Angina.

Coronary Artery Diseases
Angina

Signs and symptoms of unstable angina:
- Occurs mostly while the patient may be sleeping, resting, or doing light physical activity
- It is almost always sudden
- The duration maybe longer as compared to stable angina
- It is not relieved by resting or taking medicine
- It can possibly get bad over time
- May result in a heart attack

Causes of angina:
- Atherosclerosis
- Stenosis of the coronary artery
- Significant increase in cardiac afterload (systemic blood pressure)

Predisposing factors:
- exercise, anxiety, cold.

Precautions:
1. Treatment should be oriented towards prevention of an angina attack.
2. Prophylactic nitroglycerin may be given sublingually prior to any injection or stressful procedure.
3. Administer oxygen by nasal cannula during the procedure.
4. Consider use of oral or IV sedation to reduce anxiety.

Monitor:
BP
O_2 by using pulse oximeter
Heart rate

Management of angina in the dental chair:
1. All stimulation and treatment of the patient should be stopped immediately.
2. Make the patient's position comfortable; it is preferred to sit upright.
3. Call the ambulance
4. Oxygen should be administered *via* mask at 10-15l/min.
5. Vital signs should be monitored and recorded; monitors should be used if available.
6. Take a tablet of nitroglycerin 0.4 mg sublingual or one metered dose spray. While administrating the tablets, use gloves, do not touch them with hands. Nitroglycerin is easily absorbed through the skin.
7. Nitroglycerin should be repeated if after two minutes there is still no relief. The nitroglycerin administration can be repeated for a third time as well incase patients feels no relief.
8. Blood pressure should be monitored after every dose; and the dose should not be repeated if systolic BP drops below 100.
9. Call for medical assistant.

- Patients with unstable angina,
- Patients with coronary artery bypass graft surgery (less than three months),
- Patients with Recent myocardial infarction (less than six months)

Coronary Artery Diseases

Angina (Card **5.4**): Angina is the pain in the chest (substernal pain) or the feeling of discomfort arising when the heart is deprived of oxygen because of coronary arteries being narrowed due to atherosclerosis which may or may not results in a higher heart rate. Typically, it is expressed as a squeezing or crushing feeling in the chest that may go up to shoulders, jaw, back or arm. Commonly it is a signal for heart disease.

Causes of Angina

- Atherosclerosis
- Stenosis of the coronary artery
- Significant increase in cardiac afterload (systemic blood pressure)

Unstable angina, which is also called as acute coronary syndrome, causes unexpected pain in the chest, and this usually happens while the person is at *rest*. A major reason for this is a flow of blood to the cardiac muscle is decreased because of coronary arteries narrowing, due to:

- Stenosis of the coronary artery,
- Atherosclerosis,
- or A significant increase in cardiac afterload (systemic blood pressure).

Physiology

The most important variable for the coronary blood flow regulation and control is:

- Dilatation or constriction degree of coronary arteriolar vascular smooth muscle
- Cardiac wall's extravascular pressure is a consequence of cardiac contraction and relaxation. Around eighty percent of the flow of blood into the heart takes place in the diastolic phase when there is decreased pressure over the cardiac wall. This means that
  - Increasing the heart rate,
  - or Increasing in the pressure over the cardiac wall significantly decreases cardiac blood flow.

Similar to systemic vascular beds, the coronary arteriolar smooth muscle tone extent is controlled by multiple independent negative feedback loops, under normal circumstances. The following are included in these mechanisms:

- Hormonal
- Various neural,
- Local metabolic and non-metabolic regulators.

For coronary flow regulation, the local metabolic regulators of arteriolar tone play a very important role; these feedback systems are dependent on the demand of oxygen by the local cardiac myocytes (myocardial muscle cells). At any single point in time, generally, the coronary blood flow is made up of integrating the various controlling feedback loops into one response (which induces either arteriolar smooth muscle dilation or constriction). A common observation is that a few of these feedback loops work antagonistically to one another. It is interesting to note that coronary arteriolar vasodilation from the state of rest to intense exercise may lead to raising the mean coronary blood flow from around 0.5 to 4.0 ml/min/gram.

Signs and Symptoms of Unstable Angina

- Occurs mostly while the patient may be sleeping, resting, or doing light physical activity
- It is almost always sudden
- The duration may be longer as compared to stable angina
- It is not relieved by resting or taking medicine
- It can possibly get bad over time
- May result in a heart attack

In the following patients:

- *Patients with unstable angina,*
- *Patients with coronary artery bypass graft surgery (less than three months),*
- *Patients with Recent myocardial infarction (less than six months)*

If dental treatment optional and not urgent, it should be delayed. In case it is necessary to treat, the appropriate way should be implemented, including the following:

- Stress-reduction protocols along with sedative agents,
- And use of vasoconstrictor-containing anesthesia should be strictly limited to one to two cartridges,
- After consulting the physician properly (follow the general precaution for angina patients and the recommendation of the patient's physician and be ready for emergency management.

Clinical Features of Angina

- Chest pain (substernal pain) - tightness, heaviness, crushing.
- Radiation - left and right arms, lower jaw.

Predisposing Factors

- Exercise, anxiety, cold.

Precautions

1. Treatment should be oriented towards prevention of an angina attack.
2. Prophylactic nitroglycerin may be given sublingually prior to any injection or stressful procedure.
3. Administer oxygen by nasal cannula during the procedure.
4. Consider use of oral or IV sedation to reduce anxiety.
5. Conscious sedation need trained dental practitioner in these special procedure.

Emergency Management of Angina in the Dental Chair

1. All stimulation and treatment of the patient should be stopped immediately.
2. Make the patient's position comfortable; it is preferred to sit upright.
3. Call the ambulance.
4. Oxygen should be administered *via* mask at 10-15l/min.
5. Vital signs should be monitored and recorded; monitors should be used if available.
6. Take a tablet of nitroglycerin 0.4 mg sublingual or one metered dose spray. While administrating the tablets, use gloves, do not touch them with bare hands. Nitroglycerin is easily absorbed through the skin.
7. Nitroglycerin should be repeated after two minutes if there is still no relief. The nitroglycerin administration can be repeated for the third time as well in case patient feels no relief.
8. Blood pressure should be monitored after every dose, and the dose should not be repeated if systolic BP drops below 100.
9. Call for medical assistant.

Myocardial Infarction (MI)

Myocardial infarction (Card **5.5**) is the heart muscle's necrosis (death) due to sudden coronary artery blockage by a blood clot. Contemporary studies indicate that most myocardial infarctions occur due to significant increases in afterload (systemic pressure); leading to a build-up of pressure in the cardiac muscle wall and diminished coronary artery blood flow.

Pathophysiology

Myocardial infarction (heart attack) is the heart muscle's necrosis, irreversible in nature, second to prolonged ischemia. This usually occurs due to oxygen demand and supply imbalance, the common reason for which is thrombus formation in a coronary vessel following plaque rupture, resulting in blood supply being critically reduced to some of the parts of the myocardium.

Card 5.5. Myocardial Infarction (MI).

Coronary Artery Diseases
Myocardial Infarction (MI)

Clinical features:
- Malaise
- Chest discomfort
- Fatigue

It has been reported that over 70% of all recurrences take place in the first month after the initial vascular event

In acute myocardial infarction, the typical chest pain is observed to have following features:
- It is *very severe*, furthermore for 30-60 minutes it is constantly unrelenting
- Expressed commonly as a *substernal pressure feeling* that can be explained as a aching, squeezing, burning or an even sharp sensation
- *Retrosternal and frequently radiates up to the jaw, neck and shoulder*, and goes down to the ulnar aspect of the left arm
- Symptoms may be described as *epigastric* by some patients with an indigestion feeling or sensation of fullness and gas

Precautions:
1. Treatment should be oriented towards prevention of an angina attack.
2. Prophylactic nitroglycerin may be given sublingually prior to any injection or stressful procedure.
3. Administer oxygen by nasal cannula during the procedure.
4. Consider use of oral or IV sedation to reduce anxiety.

Monitor:
BP
O$_2$ by using pulse oximeter
Heart rate

Management of myocardial infarction in the dental chair:
1) Comfortable position for the patient
2) Oxygen (4 to 6 liters/minute flow rate)
3) Vital signs (BP, pulse)
4) Nitroglycerin 0.2 to 0.6 mg sublingually, every five minutes, up to three times
5) Aspiring 160 to 325 mg if the patient is not allergic.
6) Activate EMS.
7) Summon medical assistant.

During a myocardial infarction the key signals the patient might show are the following:
- Irregular pulse may be observed because of atrial fibrillation or flutter, an accelerated idioventricular rhythm, ventricular tachycardia, ventricular ectopy, or other supraventricular arrhythmias. Bradyarrhythmias may be present.
- The heart rate of patient is usually raised secondary to sympathoadrenal discharge.
- Usually, the blood pressure of patient is initially increased due to the vasoconstriction of peripheral arterial because of the ventricular dysfunction and adrenergic response to pain.
- Nevertheless, hypotension is observed with severe left ventricular dysfunction or right ventricular myocardial infarction.
- There is an increase in the respiratory rate due to anxiety or pulmonary congestion.
- Wheezing, coughing and the frothy sputum production may occur.

Within 24 to 48 hours fever is commonly experienced, with the temperature curve typically parallel to the time course of elevations of blood creatine kinase (CK) levels. The temperature of the body may exceed 102°F at times.

The myocardial injury range is not just dependent on the impaired myocardial perfusion intensity but it also upon the metabolic demand level and duration, at in time event occurs. The myocardium injury is effectively due to the response of tissue including inflammatory changes and apoptosis (cell death). Hence, the patients who have sudden death from acute coronary events, their hearts, at autopsy, may not demonstrate many indications of myocardium injury.

Initially, coagulation necrosis is evidenced by a common myocardial infarction that is eventually led by myocardial fibrosis. In several patients with ischemia, contraction band necrosis is also observed. The result of this is reperfusion, or it shows massive adrenergic stimulation, usually with concomitant myocytolysis.

Currently, for cardiac biomarkers, there exists a point-of-care testing (POCT) for measurement of cardiac biomarkers at saliva, and would hopefully enhance early diagnosis and the dentist will be assisted by having a definitive diagnosis of MI in the dental chair. Salivary markers are more significant than ECG in early stage of myocardial infarction.

Biomarkers

- Myoglobin
- Creatine phosphokinase–myocardial band (CPK-MB)
- Troponins

Challenges

It is highly likely that the markers are not being identified instantly and at an early stage of MI.

- From the starting of chest pain, there is a rise in serum levels within 3-12 hours, which attains a maximum at 24-48 hours, and the baseline is restored over 5-14 days.
- Formerly, regular measurements of CK-MB isoenzyme levels were the standard criteria for myocardial infarction diagnosis. From starting of chest pain CK-MB levels raises within 3-12 hours, attains a maximum at 24 hours, and the baseline is restored 48-72 hours later.
- Myoglobin, which is a low-molecular-weight heme protein found in skeletal and cardiac muscle, is quickly released from infarcted myocardium as compared to troponin. Myoglobin levels in urine are rising within 1-4 hours from the chest pain onset. Myoglobin levels are not specific but highly sensitive; they can prove beneficial within other studies context and in the myocardial infarction early detection in the emergency department (ED). It is not necessary that myocardial infarction show change on the surface ECG, including T-wave

changes or ST-segment depression/elevation. The emergence of cardiac markers in the circulation typically is indicative of myocardial necrosis, and it is a beneficial add-on to the diagnosis. This means that the history of the patient and the signs and symptoms that may develop in the dental chair are the most helpful keys for the diagnosing of MI.

Clinical Features

- Malaise
- Chest discomfort
- Fatigue

In acute myocardial infarction, the typical chest pain is observed to have following features:

- It is *very severe*, furthermore, for 30-60 minutes it is constantly unrelenting
- Expressed commonly as a *substernal pressure feeling* that can be explained as an aching, squeezing, burning or an even sharp sensation
- *Retrosternal and frequently radiates up to the jaw, neck, and shoulder*, and goes down to the ulnar aspect of the left arm
- Symptoms may be described as *epigastric* by some patients with an indigestion feeling or sensation of fullness and gas

During a myocardial infarction the key signals, the patient might show the following:

- The irregular pulse may be observed because of atrial fibrillation or flutter, an accelerated ventricular rhythm, ventricular tachycardia, ventricular ectopy, or other supraventricular arrhythmias. Bradyarrhythmias may be present.
- The heart rate of the patient is usually raised secondary to sympathoadrenal discharge.
- Usually, the blood pressure of the patient is initially increased due to the vasoconstriction of peripheral arterial because of the ventricular dysfunction and adrenergic response to pain.
- Nevertheless, hypotension is observed with severe left ventricular dysfunction or right ventricular myocardial infarction.
- There is an increase in the respiratory rate due to anxiety or pulmonary congestion.
- Wheezing, coughing and the frothy sputum production may occur.
- Within 24 to 48 hours fever is commonly experienced, with the temperature curve typically parallel to the time course of elevations of blood creatine kinase (CK) levels. The temperature of the body may exceed 102°F at times.

Management of Myocardial Infarction in the Dental Chair

- Comfortable position for the patient
- Oxygen (4 to 6 liters/minute flow rate)
- Vital signs (BP, pulse)
- Nitroglycerin 0.2 to 0.6 mg sublingually, every five minutes, up to three times
- Aspiring 160 to 325 mg if the patient is not allergic.
- Activate EMS.
- Summon medical assistant.

Hypertension

Hypertension or High blood pressure (HBP) signifies high pressure (tension) in the arteries.

Definition and Physiology

Systolic pressure (P. systolic): When blood is pumped by the left ventricle into the aorta, the aortic pressure increases. Systolic pressure is the maximal aortic pressure followed by this pumping of blood and contraction of left ventricle.

The diastolic pressure (P. diastolic): As the left ventricle relaxes and refills, the pressure drops in the aorta. The diastolic pressure is the minimal pressure in the aorta, occurring right before the ventricle ejects blood into the aorta.

The sphygmomanometer is the device used for measurement the blood pressure; the lower value is the *diastolic pressure,* and the upper value is the *systolic pressure*. The standard range of systolic pressure is <120 mmHg, and normal range of diastolic pressure is <80 mmHg. The *aortic pulse pressure* is the difference between the systolic and diastolic pressures, the normal range for which is between 40 and 50 mmHg.

$$\text{Pulse Pressure} = \text{Systolic Pressure} - \text{Diastolic Pressure}$$

The Mean Arterial Pressure (MAP) is determined by:

- Systemic Vascular Resistance (SVR),
- Cardiac Output (CO), and
- Central Venous Pressure (CVP)

$$\text{MAP} = (\text{CO} \times \text{SVR}) + \text{CVP}$$

Since the value of CVP is usually equal to 0 mmHg, the above equation can be written as:

$$MAP \text{ approx.} = CO \times SVR$$

Determinants of Cardiac Output (CO) are:

1. Stroke volume
2. Heart rate

$$\text{Stroke volume (SV): } SV = EDV - ESV$$

The End-Diastolic Volume (EDV): After atrial contraction is over, there is a fall in atrial pressure, causing the pressure gradient to reverse across the AV valves. Due to this, the valve floats upward (pre-position) prior to closure. The ventricular volumes are at their highest level at this point, which is called as the end-diastolic volume (EDV). The normal value is 120 ml for the left ventricular EDV (LVEDV), which represents the ventricular preload, and is linked to the end-diastolic pressures of 3 to 6 mmHg and 8 to 12 mmHg in the right and left ventricles, respectively.

End-Systolic Volume (ESV): Even though the ventricular pressures reduce in this phase since all valves are closed. Hence, the ventricles' volumes remain same. The blood volume that is there in the ventricle is called the end-systolic volume, and in the left ventricle, it is ~50 ml. The difference in the end-diastolic volume and the end-systolic volume, signifying the stroke volume, is ~70 ml.

Vascular Resistance (tone): Controlling factors of vascular tone are:

Intrinsic Factors

- Myogenic functions are naturally built-in to the smooth muscle blood vessels, especially in arterioles and small arteries. When the blood flow increases within a vessel suddenly, the vessel would constrict in response. The reducing blood flow inside the vessel causes it to relax and vasodilation to occur.
- Endothelial factors, such as endothelin and nitric oxide (NO), can either increase or decrease tone, respectively.
- The amino acid L-arginine, synthesize NO by the enzymatic action of nitric oxide synthase (NOS). Endothelial has two forms of NOS: inducible NOS (iNOS; type II) and constitutive NOS (cNOS; type III). Co-factors for NOS include NADPH, oxygen, flavin adenine nucleotides, and tetrahydrobiopterin. There is a neural NOS (nNOS; type I) besides endothelial NOS, the function of

which is acting as a transmitter in various nerves of the peripheral nervous system and in the brain.

A vascular action of NOS has the following:

- *Direct vasodilation (receptor-mediated and flow dependent)*
- *Indirect vasodilation (by inhibiting vasoconstrictor influences - that inhibits angiotensin II and sympathetic vasoconstriction*
- *The anti-proliferative effect, which slows down smooth muscle hyperplasia*
- *The anti-thrombotic effect, which slows down platelet adhesion to the vascular endothelium*
- *The anti-inflammatory effect, which slows down leukocyte adhesion to vascular endothelium and scavenges superoxide anion*
- The ET (Endothelin also known as preproendothelin) showed a significant vasoconstriction in vascular beds *in vitro* and caused sustained elevated blood pressure *in vivo* (when animals was injected intravenously with ET), ET-1 was thought as an important contributor in the maintenance of BP (blood pressure). Therefore, the pharmaceutical industries became interested in ET inhibitors as modality for treatment of hypertension. The vascular endothelium synthesizes endothelin (ET-1) which is a 21-amino acid peptide, by acting upon an endothelin converting enzyme (ECE) that is present on the endothelial cell membrane. The angiotensin II (AII), antidiuretic hormone (ADH), and other intrinsic factors stimulate the development and release of ET-1.

The ET-1 is not a circulating hormone; it is rather a local releasing hormone. There are two mediators (receptors) mediate the local action of ET-1. The ET_A, in the underlying vascular smooth muscles inducing vasoconstriction and the ET_B, in endothelial cells stimulate releasing of relaxing factors, such as prostacycline and nitric oxide. This is meaning that the ET-1 is non-specific local hormone. It may induce both constriction and relaxation depending on the mediators ET_A or ET_B. The current researches have demonstrated that endogenous ET-1 is involved in the peripheral blood flow regulation via ET_A on the vascular smooth muscle causing vasocontriction and on the ET_B in endothelial cells stimulate releasing of prostacyclin and nitrous oxide (causing relaxation) Fig. (**5.0**).

Metabolic products: metabolic by-products or hypoxia causes Vasodilation and decreased vascular tone.

Extrinsic Factors

1. **Neuro-Humoral such as a Sympathetic Nerve**
   Neural mechanisms mainly involve parasympathetic cholinergic and sympathetic adrenergic branches of the autonomic nervous system. Generally,

the function of the sympathetic system is to constrict the blood vessels and stimulate the heart, leading to an increase in arterial pressure. The function of the parasympathetic system is to dilate selected vascular beds and slow down cardiac functions.

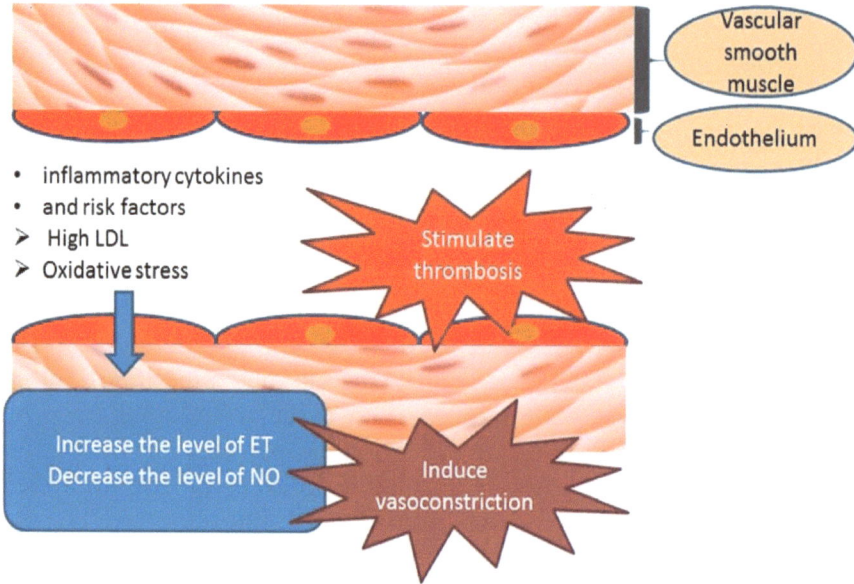

Fig. (5.0). Endothelin also known as preproendothelin.

2. Circulating Catecholamines

Circulating catecholamines, norepinephrine, and epinephrine originate from two sources. The adrenal medulla releases the epinephrine when the preganglionic sympathetic nerves innervating this tissue are activated. Usually, during stress times, this activation occurs (*e.g.*, hemorrhage, heart failure, exercise, pain, excitement or emotional stress). The adrenal medulla also releases norepinephrine (norepinephrine comprises about 20% of its total catecholamine release). The basic source of circulating norepinephrine is overrun from sympathetic nerves innervating blood vessels.

3. The Renin-Angiotensin System

The juxtaglomerular (JG) cells secrete renin in response to low blood pressure (local hypoxia and decrease in renal blood flow). The renin acts upon a circulating substrate, called angiotensinogen, and cause proteolytic cleavage to form the angiotensin I. The enzyme, angiotensin converting enzyme (ACE), which is released mainly by the vascular endothelium of the lung, cause cleavages off two amino acids of the angiotensin I to form the octapeptide, angiotensin II (the active form).

Functions of angiotensin II

- Constricts resistance vessels thus this increases the arterial pressure and systemic vascular resistance.
- The adrenal cortex is stimulated by this to secrete aldosterone, a hormone which activates the kidneys to raise the fluid and sodium retention levels.
- Accelerates sodium transport (reabsorption) at various renal tubular locations hence it raises the level of sodium and water retention by the body.
- Activates vasopressin release (antidiuretic hormone, ADH) from the posterior pituitary, which also acts on kidneys to raise fluid retention.
- Thirst centers are stimulated inside the brain.
- Assisting in release of norepinephrine from sympathetic nerve endings and reuptake of norepinephrine by nerve endings hence, improving the function of sympathetic adrenergic.
- Stimulates cardiac hypertrophy and vascular hypertrophy.

4. **A Few of the Circulating Factors (*e.g.*, Atrial Natriuretic Peptide-NPs)**
   Atrial natriuretic peptide-NPs cause a drop in the vascular tone that is a 28-amino acid peptide, which is produced, released and stored by atrial myocytes because of atrial distension. The NPs function by directly dilating the veins (raise venous compliance) and hence they reduce central venous pressure, which in turn decreases cardiac output by decreasing ventricular preload. Another function of NPs is to cause the arteries to dilate; that results in a reduction in vascular resistance and systemic arterial pressure. Unremitting elevations of NPs apparently cause a decline in the arterial blood pressure mainly by reducing systemic vascular resistance.

Hypertension

Hypertension can be mainly categorized into two types:

- Primary
- Secondary

Most of the patient around 90% to 95%, diagnosed with hypertension suffer from primary hypertension. In contrasting to secondary hypertension, the cause of primary hypertension is not known. Hence, the primary hypertension diagnosis is made after ruling out known causes that make up secondary hypertension.

The frequent and major reasons for secondary hypertension are listed below:

• Chronic renal disease
• Sleep apnea
• Pheochromocytoma
• Hyper- or hypothyroidism
• Preeclampsia
• Stress
• Primary hyperaldosteronism
• Renal artery stenosis
• Aortic coarctation

Chronic Renal Disease: Pathologic processes (*e.g.*, glomerulonephritis or diabetic nephropathy) in various amounts may cause harm to the nephrons in the kidney. If this happens, the kidney may not be able to excrete typical sodium quantity, resulting in water and sodium retention, higher cardiac output and increased volume of blood.

Sleep Apnea: In this disorder, people frequently stop breathing for a short time duration (like 10-30 seconds) while they are asleep, hypertension is more common in these persons. The hypertension mechanism may be associated with hormonal changes and sympathetic activation that are linked with frequent periods of apnea-induced hypercapnia and hypoxia and stress resulting from loss of sleep.

Pheochromocytoma: Catecholamine-secreting tumors present in the adrenal medulla (hyperplasia of Adrenal Modella) may result in circulating catecholamines (both norepinephrine and epinephrine) elevated levels. Resulting in beta-adrenoceptor mediated cardiac stimulation and alpha-adrenoceptor mediated systemic vasoconstriction, the effect of both of which is very high arterial pressure. The catecholamines increase the heart rate (causing tachycardia) which is due to the direct effects of the catecholamines on the vasculature and heart. Extreme beta-adrenoceptor stimulation in the heart usually leads to arrhythmias. Urine or plasma catecholamine levels and their metabolites should be measured (vanillylmandelic acid and metanephrine) to diagnose pheochromocytoma.

Hyper- or hypothyroidism: Both hypothyroidism and hyperthyroidism may result in hypertension, although this functionality is not well understood. High levels of thyroxine result in higher blood volume by activating the renin-angiotensin-aldosterone system, increasing the ventricular contractility and increasing the heart rate. Latest research shows that the cardiac changes are not dependent on sympathetic adrenergic activity. Subnormal levels of thyroxine may decrease the tissue metabolism, which in turn may reduce the endothelial synthesis of nitric oxide and tissue vasodilator metabolites production and hence causing arterial pressure to rise and vasoconstriction. The arterial stiffness also increases (reduced arterial compliance).

Preeclampsia: This condition develops at times in the third trimester of pregnancy and results in hypertension because of the tachycardia and increased blood volume. The former raises cardiac output *via* the Frank-Starling mechanism.

Stress: the sympathetic nervous system is activated by emotional stress, leading to norepinephrine-increased release from sympathetic nerves present in the blood vessels and heart, resulting in higher cardiac output and systemic vascular resistance. In addition to this, more catecholamines (norepinephrine and epinephrine) are secreted by the adrenal medulla. Activation of sympathetic nervous system elevates circulating aldosterone, vasopressin and angiotensin II that may, in turn, elevated systemic vascular resistance. Elevated levels of angiotensin II and catecholamines for a longer duration of time can lead to vascular and cardiac hypertrophy; both are possible factors for sustained blood pressure rise.

Primary Hyperaldosteronism: High levels of aldosterone secretion generally are due to adrenal hyperplasia or adrenal adenoma. Elevated levels of circulating aldosterone may result in renal retention of water and sodium and increase the arterial pressure and blood volume. Usually, there is a reduction in plasma renin levels when the effort is exerted by the body to suppress the renin-angiotensin system; hypokalemia is also linked with elevated aldosterone levels.

Renal Artery Stenosis (Renovascular Disease): Narrowing of the vessel lumen (stenosis) can be caused by renal artery disease. The pressure at the afferent arteriole and renal perfusion are lowered within the kidney by reducing the lumen diameter. Renin release, because of this, is stimulated by the kidney, causing a rise in circulating aldosterone and angiotensin II (AII). The function of these hormones is to raise the blood volume by improving renal reabsorption of water and sodium.

Aortic Coarctation: Aorta coarctation (or narrowing) is a defect by birth that is most commonly found just distal to the left subclavian artery in the arch of the aorta. The distal arterial pressure is lowered, and arterial pressures in the arms and the head region are increased when the aorta is blocked at this point. The systemic arterial pressure when reduced stimulates the renin-angiotensin-aldosterone system, causing a rise in blood volume. Hence, arterial pressures in the upper body are further elevated, and a decrease in lower body arterial pressures is largely offset by this. To identify this condition (arterial pressures measurements) of the arms and legs can be easily compared. Normally, the pressures in arms and legs are almost same, but with contractions, there can be a big difference in arterial pressures in the arms and legs, with pressure in the arm being much higher. The baroreceptors are desensitized as a result of the chronic nature of this condition, and arterial pressures in the upper body remain high since the cardiac output to these body parts is increased.

Treatment of Hypertension: Drugs Used.

Below is a classification of drugs that is used to treat hypertension:

- Vasodilators
  - Renin inhibitors
  - Angiotensin receptor blockers (ARBs)
  - Direct acting arterial dilators
  - Nitrodilators
  - Alpha-adrenoceptor antagonists (alpha-blockers)
  - Angiotensin-converting enzyme inhibitors (ACE inhibitors)
  - Potassium channel openers
  - Calcium channel blockers
  - Ganglionic blockers
- Diuretics
  - Potassium-sparing diuretics
  - Thiazide diuretics
  - Loop diuretics
- Cardioinhibitory drugs
  - Calcium channel blockers
  - Beta blockers
- Centrally acting sympatholytics

Diuretics

The urine output is increased by the kidney by this class of drug (*i.e.* promoting diuresis), to bring about this, the way kidney handles sodium is altered. If more sodium is excreted by the kidney, then more water will be excreted as well. The majority of diuretics synthesize diuresis by slowing down the sodium reabsorption at various segments of the renal tubular system.

Generic name	Common brand names
Chlorthalidone	Hygroton*
Chlorothiazide	Diuril*

Generic name	Common brand names
Furosemide	Lasix*
Hydrochlorothiazide	Esidrix*, Hydrodiuril*, Microzide*
Indapamide	Lozol*
Metolazone	Mykrox*, Zaroxolyn*

Potassium-sparing Diuretics

- Aldosterone actions (acting as aldosterone receptor antagonists) are hindered, by few of the drugs belonging to this class, at the distal tubule's distal segment. This results in greater amount of sodium (and water) to go into the collecting duct, and then in urine, they are excreted. Since unlike loop and thiazide diuretics, they do not produce hypokalemia, they are called as K+ sparing diuretics. This happens because when aldosterone-sensitive sodium reabsorption is inhibited, this transporter exchanges a few hydrogen and potassium ions in place of sodium. Hence urine has a lesser amount of hydrogen and potassium being excreted.
- Other potassium-sparing diuretics act by inhibiting the sodium channels directly which are linked with the aldosterone-sensitive sodium pump, and so they produce effects similar to the aldosterone antagonists on hydrogen and potassium ions. Their functioning is dependent upon renal prostaglandin production. Since the effects on overall sodium balance by this diuretics class are comparatively weak, they are mostly used in combination with loop diuretics or thiazide in order to avoid hypokalemia.

Generic name	Common brand names
Amiloride hydrochloride	Midamar*
Spironolactone	Aldactone*
Triamterene	Dyrenium*

Loop Diuretic

Sodium-potassium-chloride cotransporter in the thick ascending limb is inhibited by loop diuretic (see above figure). Under normal circumstances, 25% of the sodium load is reabsorbed by this transporter hence; if this pump is slowed down, it may result in a significant rise in the distal tubular concentration of sodium, less water reabsorption in the collecting duct and decreased hypertonicity of the neighboring interstitium. The changes in managing of water and sodium results in both natriuresis (increased sodium loss) and diuresis (increased water loss). Loop diuretics are very powerful diuretics since they act upon the thick ascending limb that is managing sodium reabsorption in a larger amount. This class of medication also induces renal production of prostaglandins, contributing to their renal action, which includes the redistribution of renal cortical blood flow and rise in renal blood flow.

Generic name	Common brand names
Bumetanide	Bumex*

Thiazide Diuretics

The most frequently used diuretic are the Thiazide diuretics, which inhibit the sodium-chloride transporter found in the distal tubule. Since only about 5% of filtered sodium is reabsorbed by these transporters, these diuretics are not much effective as compared to loop diuretics in producing natriuresis and diuresis.

Generic name	Common brand names
Amiloride Hydrochloride + Hydrochlorothiazide	Moduretic*
Spironolactone + Hydrochlorothiazide	Aldactazide*
Triamterene + Hydrochlorothiazide	Dyazide*, Maxzide*

Beta-Blockers

Beta-blockers are medications that attach to beta-adrenoceptors and hence the binding of epinephrine and norepinephrine to these receptors is blocked. This results in slowing down of normal sympathetic effects that take place through these receptors. Therefore, beta-blockers are sympatholytic drugs.

Generic name	Common brand names
Acebutolol	Sectral*
Atenolol	Tenormin*
Betaxolol	Kerlone*
Bisoprolol Fumarate	Zebeta*
Carteolol Hydrochloride	Cartrol*
Metoprolol Tartrate	Lopressor*
Metoprolol Succinate	Toprol-XL*
Nadolol	Corgard*
Penbutolol Sulfate	Levatol*
Pindolol*	Visken*

Contd.....

Generic name	Common brand names
Propranolol Hydrochloride*	Inderal*
Solo to the Hydrochloride	Betapace*
Timolol Maleate*	Blocadren*

Alpha-Blockers

Alpha-Blockers acts by blocking the sympathetic nerves effect on blood vessels by attaching to alpha-adrenoceptors found in the vascular smooth muscle. A majority of these drugs function as competitive antagonists to the attaching of norepinephrine, which the sympathetic nerves are synapsing on smooth muscle release. Hence, we call these drugs as sympatholytics at times, because they upset the sympathetic activity.

Generic name	Common brand names
Doxazosin	Cardura
Prazosin	Minipress
Alfuzosin	Uroxatral
Terazosin	Hytrin
Tamsulosin	Flomax
Silodosin	Rapaflo

Angiotensin-Converting Enzyme Inhibitors (ACE)

The ACE inhibitors create vasodilation by slowing down the angiotensin II formation. This vasoconstrictor is produced by the proteolytic action of renin (released by the kidneys) whose function is to circulate angiotensinogen to form angiotensin I. Angiotensin I is then changed by the angiotensin converting enzyme to angiotensin II.

Generic name	Common brand names
Captopril	Capoten
Zofenopril	Zofenopril
Enalapril	Vasotec/Renitec
Ramipril	Altace/Prilace/Ramace/Ramiwin/Triatec/Tritace
Quinapril	Accupril
Perindopril	Coversyl/Aceon/Perindo
Lisinopril	Listril/Lopril/Novatec/Prinivil/Zestril

Contd.....

Generic name	Common brand names
Benazepril	Lotensin
Imidapril	Tanatril
Cilazapril	Mavik/Odrik/Gopten
Fosinopril	Trandolapril
Captopril	Inhibace

Angiotensin II Receptor Blockers (ARBs)

This class of medication works in a similar way to angiotensin-converting enzyme (ACE) inhibitors, and we employ them for the same symptoms (heart failure, hypertension, post-myocardial infarction). The way they act is, however, very distinct from ACE inhibitors, which function by inhibiting the angiotensin II formation. ARBs are receptor antagonists that function by blocking type 1 angiotensin II (AT1) receptors located on blood vessels and other tissues and organs, for example, the heart.

Generic name	Common brand names
Candesartan	Atacand*
Eprosartan Mesylate	Teveten*
Irbesarten	Avapro*
losartan Potassium	Cozaar*
Telmisartan	Micardis*
Valsartan	Diovan*

Calcium Channel Blockers

Presently the CCBs that are approved attach to L-type calcium channels found in the cardiac myocytes, cardiac nodal tissue (atrioventricular and sinoatrial nodes) and vascular smooth muscle. Regulation of the calcium influx into muscle cells is the function of these channels, resulting in stimulation of cardiac myocyte contraction and smooth muscle contraction. CCBs decrease systemic vascular resistance, lowering the arterial blood pressure by producing vascular smooth muscle relaxation. The main effect of these drugs on arterial resistance vessels, with very little effects on venous capacitance vessels.

Generic name	Common brand names
Amlodipine Besylate	Norvasc*, Lotrel*

Contd.....

Generic name	Common brand names
Bepridil	Vasocor*
Diltiazem Hydrochloride	Cardizem CD*, Cardizem SR*, Dilacor XR*, Tiazac*
Felodipine	Plendil*
Isradipine	DynaCirc*, DynaCirc CR*
Nicardipine	Cardene SR*
Nifedipine	Adalat CC*, Procardia XL*
Nisoldipine	Sular*
Verapamil Hydrochloride	Calan SR*, Covera HS*, Isoptin SR*, Verelan*

Hypertensive emergency is rare (Card **5.6**). It mostly occurs:

- When an individual does not treat hypertension,
- When a patient skips his/her medication for blood pressure,
- The patient takes in over-the-counter medication that aggravates high blood pressure.

Complications that may occur because of hypertensive crisis:

- Bleeding into the brain (cerebral stroke)
- Mental status altered, such as confusion
- Chest pain (unstable angina)
- Heart attack
- Pulmonary edema
- Heart failure
- Rupture of the body's main artery (aorta)
- Kidney failure

Predisposing factors for a sudden increase in BP:

- Pain or stress
- Light or improper anesthesia
- Hypercarbia
- Hypoxia
- Myocardial infarction (MI)

Signs and Symptoms

- Nausea and vomiting
- Severe anxiety
- Seizure
- Increasing chest pain

- A headache or blurred vision
- Edema (Swelling - fluid buildup in the tissues)
- Increasing shortness of breath
- Increasing confusion or level of consciousness

Card 5.6. Hypertension.

Hypertension

Signs and symptoms:
- Nausea and vomiting
- Severe anxiety
- Seizure
- Increasing chest pain
- A headache or blurred vision
- Edema (Swelling or edema - fluid buildup in the tissues)
- Increasing shortness of breath
- Increasing confusion or level of consciousness

Predisposing factors for a sudden increase in BP
- Pain or stress
- Light or improper anesthesia
- Hypercarbia
- Hypoxia
Myocardial infarction (MI)

Hypertensive emergency is rare. It mostly occurs:
- When an individual does not treat hypertension,
- When a patient skips his/her medication for blood pressure,
- The patient takes in over-the-counter medication that aggravates high blood pressure.

Monitor:
BP
O_2 by using pulse oximeter, Heart rate

Hypertensive Crisis Management:

1) Terminate treatment
2) Terminate (D/C) N_2O if in use and administer O_2
3) If BP is not back to normal in a few minutes, summon medical assistant
4) Furosemide (Lasix) should be administered (40 mg, *via* the oral route).
5) If this proves insufficient to control pressure, captopril should be administered (25 mg *via* the oral or sublingual route).

The following medications can be used for lowering high blood pressure (BP) but are not advisable for use in dental clinics, as they may cause uncontrolled lowering of BP and cerebral ischemia:

- Nitroglycerin (NTG),
- Nifedipine,
- Labetalol,
- Sodium nitroprusside and hydralazine

Complications that may occur because of hypertensive crisis:
- Bleeding into the brain (cerebral stroke), Mental status altered, such as confusion, Chest pain (unstable angina), Heart attack, Pulmonary edema, Heart failure, Rupture of the body's main artery (aorta), Kidney failure

Hypertensive Crisis Management

- Terminate treatment
- Terminate (D/C) N_2O if in use and administer O_2
- If BP is not back to normal in a few minutes, summon medical assistant
- Furosemide (Lasix) should be administered (40 mg, *via* the oral route).
- If this proves insufficient to control pressure, captopril should be administered (25 mg *via* the oral or sublingual route).

The following medications can be used for lowering high blood pressure (BP) but are not advisable for use in dental clinics, as they may cause uncontrolled lowering of BP and cerebral ischemia:

- Nitroglycerin (NTG),
- Nifedipine,
- Labetalol,
- Sodium nitroprusside and hydralazine

Hypotension (Card 5.7)

Predisposing Factors

- Excessive medications
- Overdose of sedatives
- Vascular absorption of local anesthetics
- Positional changes of the patient
- Hypoxia and hypercarbia
- Adrenocortical deficiency
- Myocardial infarction
- Cardiac arrest
- Anaphylaxis
- Infections

Signs and Symptoms

- Fainting (syncope)
- Confusion
- Nausea or vomiting
- Blurry vision
- Sleepiness
- Dizziness
- Lightheadedness
- Weakness

Card 5.7. Hypotension.

Hypotension

Signs and symptoms:
- Fainting (syncope)
- Confusion
- Nausea or vomiting
- Blurry vision
- Sleepiness
- Dizziness
- Lightheadedness
- Weakness

predisposing factors:
- Excessive medications
- Overdose of sedatives
- Vascular absorption of local anesthetics
- Positional changes of the patient
- Hypoxia and hypercarbia
- Adrenocortical deficiency
- Myocardial infarction
- Cardiac arrest
- Anaphylaxis
- Infections

Monitor:
BP
O_2 by using pulse oximeter
Heart rate

Management of hypotension:
1) Discontinue N_2O/O_2 if it is being used
2) Terminate dental treatment
3) Lay the patient flat, elevating the legs if possible
4) Establish IV line
5) Summon medical assistant. If possible, give crystalloid bolus, 10 ml/kg, and continue as necessary.
6) In the hospital, the patient may be given a vasopressor, metaraminol bolus 0.005-0.01 mg/kg. If severe, give adrenaline; for a child, 0.001 mg/kg IV very slowly and for an adult, 0.1 mg IV bolus very slowly. Titrate to clinical response followed, if necessary, by an infusion of adrenaline. For children, 1 mg in 1000 ml (1 mcg/ml), starting at 0.1 mcg/kg/minute and for adults, 1 mg in 100 ml burette starting at 60ml/hr.

Management of Hypotension

- Discontinue N_2O/O_2 if it is being used
- Terminate dental treatment
- Lay the patient flat, elevating the legs if possible

- Establish IV line
- Summon medical assistant.
- If possible, give a crystalloid bolus, 10 ml/kg, and continue as necessary.
- At the hospital, patients are given a vasopressor, metaraminol bolus 0.005-0.01 mg/kg.
- If severe, give adrenaline; for a child, 0.001 mg/kg IV very slowly and for an adult, 0.1 mg IV bolus very slowly. Titrate to clinical response followed, if necessary, by an infusion of adrenaline. For children, 1 mg in 1000 ml (1 mic.g/ml), starting at 0.1 mcg/kg/minute and for adults, 1 mg in 100 ml burette starting at 60ml/hr.

Hypertension and Local Anesthesia

In the United States, approximately more than 50 million people are suffering from high blood pressure or taking antihypertensive drugs, and dental anesthesia is received by about 70% of these patients as a minimum one time in their life.

- A usual worry that the dental practitioners face is to decide whether a vasoconstrictor-containing local anesthetic agent should be given to a patient with a cardiovascular disorder such as hypertension or not.
- A logical answer to the above query is to bear in mind the functioning and effects of vasoconstrictors.
- One benefit and an important effect of adrenal vasoconstrictors in dental local anesthetics are:
  - *Slow down the anesthetic absorption into the systemic circulation.*
  - *Increase the anesthesia duration*
  - *And increase the anesthesia depth*
  - *The risk of toxic reaction is decreased: by implying that the safety of the local anesthesia is raised by the use of the adrenal vasoconstrictor.*
- Vasoconstrictor present in a local anesthesia generally raises the efficacy of the anesthesia and reduces the chances of a large rise in blood pressure due to anxiety with experiencing the pain.
- Can we conclude by the above arguments that giving a patient suffering from hypertension an epinephrine-containing L.A. is fine?
  The answer is: yes, we may conclude this, because of the afore-mentioned reasoning. Since in L.A. the epinephrine quantity is very low, normally 1:200000 or 1:100000. A few research studies suggest that a local anesthesia with epinephrine in high intensity should not be given to patients suffering from hypertension, such as1:50000 or 1:20000.
- The American Dental Association along with the American Heart Association, in 1964, accomplished in a joint conference that, the normal vasoconstrictors concentrations in local anesthetics are not contraindicated with cardiovascular

disease if aspiration is practiced at the beginning, the slow injection of agent is done, and the minimum dose to produce the required effect is given. The above suggestions play an important role in handling the hypertensive patients since then.

- It is recommended that the total epinephrine dosage in patients with cardiac risk should be limited to 0.04 mg. This is around equal to two cartridges of 1:100,000 epinephrine contained in a local anesthetic.

- Efficacy of felypressin as a vasoconstrictor is approximated as one-fifth when compared to epinephrine. Hence, it is used in a 1:20,000 concentration. In the given concentration, risk associated with levonordefrin is same as 1:100,000 epinephrine.

- Many of the studies conclude that using one to two 1.8 ml cartridges of vasoconstrictor-containing local anesthetic is not risky for the majority of hypertensive patients or other cardiovascular patients.

- Nonetheless, using greater than two cartridges of vasoconstrictor-containing local anesthetic is relatively risky rather than contraindicated.

- When the first dose of one to two cartridges of local anesthetic having vasoconstrictor is administered using slow injection and careful preliminary aspiration, and the patient does not show any signs or symptoms of changes in cardiac output, if required additional local anesthetic is not containing epinephrine or vasoconstrictor-containing local anesthetic may be administered.

- Initial anesthesia by some physicians is opted using an anesthetic agent not containing vasoconstrictor, for example, 4% prilocaine plain or 3% mepivacaine, and later use local anesthetic containing a vasoconstrictor in a little amount to supplement for the inadequacy of anesthesia.

- In the case of serious uncontrolled hypertension, if the dental treatment is not urgent it should be postponed until the patient's physician is able to control his/her blood pressure.

- Nevertheless, in the case of dental treatment being urgently required, the dentist may use Valium to sedate the patient and to complement it one to two cartridges of local anesthetic having vasoconstrictor can be used.

- The dental practitioner may face another concern, which is the chance that an undesirable interaction may occur between antihypertensive drug of the patient and the local anesthetic agent; this is more probable in the case of nonselective beta-adrenergic and the adrenergic-blocking agent's medications, for example, propranolol (Inderal). There is lesser risk of reaction involved in cardioselective beta-blockers (*e.g.* Lopressor, Tenormin). Due to the competitive reduction of hepatic clearance, serum levels of anesthetic solutions may be increased by both classes of beta-blockers. These considerations are though confined to theory, but the small risk exists of a reaction if the total dose of anesthetic, containing 1:100,000 epinephrine or equal to that, is limited to two cartridges of 1.8 ml.

- The central sympatholytic drugs, such as methyldopa (Aldomet) and clonidine, and peripheral adrenergic antagonists for example reserpine used with direct vasodilators, may increase the sensitivity of the adrenergic receptor to sympathomimetics, leading to an elevated systemic response to vasoconstrictor-containing anesthetics.
- Still, we repeat, that these drugs have no major risk given that the anesthetic containing a vasoconstrictor is confined to one to two 1.8 ml cartridges.

While using the local anesthetic containing a vasoconstrictor, a further reminder is to inject it slowly so to avoid the hazard of having injection site ischemia that results from the potentiated localized vasoconstrictor effect.

Cardiac Arrhythmias

Any abnormal heart rate or rhythm is termed as cardiac arrhythmia. The classification of cardiac arrhythmias according to their origin is:

- The supraventricular arrhythmias;
- The ventricular arrhythmias (originating in the ventricles);

It can be classified according to how they affect the heart rate as well:

- Tachycardia, indicating a heart rate of more than 100 beats per minute
- Bradycardia, indicating a heart rate of fewer than 60 beats per minute

Causes

1. Sinus node dysfunction: Heart rate is reduced (bradycardia), resulting in a heart rate of 50 beats per minute or less. Sinus node dysfunction may result from:
   ○ Hypothyroidism
   ○ Severe liver disease,
   ○ Coronary artery disease
   ○ Hypothermia,
   ○ Scare replace sinus node
   ○ Typhoid fever or other conditions. Vasovagal hypertonia may also cause this, which is an active vagus nerve.
2. Supraventricular tachyarrhythmias: This is a diversified collection of cardiac arrhythmias resulting in rapid heartbeat (tachycardias) occurring in parts above heart ventricles. The problem in majority of the cases is either
   ○ A pathway that is abnormal and is bypassing the normal heartbeat signals route; or
   ○ An abnormality in the A-V node
3. Atrial fibrillation – a kind of supraventricular arrhythmia is resulting in heartbeats that are irregular and rapid, during which the atria quiver or

"fibrillate" instead of beating normally. During atrial fibrillation, heartbeat signals begin in many different locations in the atria rather than in the sinus node. In the atrial fibrillation, the heart becomes unable to eject blood out of the heart effectively. The result of this is that blood begins to pool inside the chambers of the heart, hence, increasing the risk of formation of a blood clot inside the heart. The atrial fibrillation main risk factors are:

- ○ Thyrotoxicosis.
- ○ hypertension,
- ○ coronary artery disease,
- ○ diabetes,
- ○ rheumatic heart disease (caused by rheumatic fever),
- ○ and age

4. A-V block or heart block – This class of arrhythmias, deals with the heartbeat transmission problems, from the sinus node to the ventricles. A-V block can be categorized into three degrees:

    a. First-degree A-V block, in this type signal transmission, takes place but time taken is usually longer to transmits signals from the sinus node to the ventricles

    b. Second-degree A-V block, in this type few of the heartbeat signals, are lost between the atria and ventricles

    c. Third-degree A-V block, in this type signals, is not transmitted at all to the ventricles, hence beating of ventricles on their own with no control from above and it is slow too. For A-V block a few common reasons are:

       ▪ An overdose of the heart medication Digitalis,

       ▪ Heart attack,

       ▪ Coronary artery disease.

5. Ventricular tachycardia (VT) is an irregular heart rhythm starting in either the left or the right ventricle. It may

    ○ for several minutes or even hours (sustained VT) or

    ○ last for just some seconds (non-sustained VT),

6. Ventricular fibrillation - In this type of arrhythmia, there is ineffective trembling of the ventricles, which produces no real heartbeat. Consequently, the person becomes unconscious and commonly leads to brain damage and death within minutes. Ventricular fibrillation is regarded as a cardiac emergency.

7. The causes of ventricular fibrillation can be:

    ○ A lightning strike, or drowning.

    ○ An electrical accident,

    ○ A heart attack,

Predisposing Factors in Dental Clinic

- Local anesthesia toxicity
- Stressful events in dental clinic

Signs and Symptoms

- Weakness
- Fainting
- Shortness of breath
- Dizziness
- Angina
- Palpitations (awareness of rapid heartbeat)

Dental Management

1. Summon medical help
2. Record and monitor the vital signs
3. Sublingual nitrates administered to manage chest pains.
4. The patient should be placed in the Trendelenburg position
5. Massage in the carotid pulse region (vagal maneuvering where necessary - Valsalva maneuver).
6. The dental team should be prepared for basic cardiopulmonary resuscitation.

Infective Endocarditis

An infective illness that involves a few parts of the endocardium is termed as infective endocarditis (The endocardium is the tissue lining the inner side of the chambers of the heart). More than one heart valves are generally engrossed by this infection that is endocardium component. It is a severe illness, which can lead to death even.

Antibiotic prophylaxis guidelines (published in April 2007 in the Journal of the ADA) clearly state that if a person has regularly taken prophylactic antibiotics previously but now does not require it includes patient with the following diseases:

- Calcified aortic stenosis
- Rheumatic heart disease
- Mitral valve prolapsed
- Bicuspid valve disease
- Congenital heart conditions, for example, atrial septal defect, hypertrophic cardiomyopathy, and ventricular septal defect. The recent guiding principles are in particular, designed for highest risk patient of a terrible outcome in the case of

heart infection development. It is suggested that in the case of any of the following conditions it is better that the concerned person takes preventive antibiotics before a dental procedure:

- Infective endocarditis in the past
- Artificial heart valves
- A problem in a heart valve for a cardiac transplant patient.
- Some definite, severe innate heart conditions, which include:
  - ○ Untreated or partially treated cyanotic congenital heart disease, which includes those with palliative conduits and shunts.
  - ○ The first six months after the surgery for an innate heart defect that is fully treated using a prosthetic material or device, placed either by catheter intervention or by surgery
  - ○ A treated heart defect by birth which has some defect left near the prosthetic device or a prosthetic patch site *(for further details about prophylactic antibiotic read page: 251 – complication of exodontia).*

Hemophilia

This is an X-linked congenital (present at birth) bleeding disorder which occurs in about one of 10,000 births. Deficiency of coagulation factor IX (FIX) is the cause of (hemophilia B) and factor VIII (FVIII) (hemophilia A) which links to clotting factor gene mutations.

Clotting Mechanism

• The Platelets Function:

The contribution of platelets to the hemostatic process is made in two ways:

1. Firstly, by their cohesive and adhesive nature leading to a hemostatic plug formation.
2. Second, coagulation mechanisms can be stimulated by them through:
   - ○ performing the role of a catalytic site for the coagulation development
   - ○ coming into contact with an adequate phospholipidic surface,
   - ○ the consolidating the hemostatic plug is an important step for hemostasis is the attachment of platelets in the beginning onto vascular subendothelium. Many factors affect the platelet-subendothelium interactions: plasma subendothelial adhesive proteins, their receptors on platelet membrane, and rheological factors. Changes in any coagulation factors may result in physiologic hemostasis disorders, which may lead to bleeding episodes or thrombosis.

The main components of subendothelial structures:

- Von Willebrand factor,
- Fibronectin,
- Laminin,
- And collagen of various kinds. Studies have established that for platelet attachment to subendothelial parts, it is vital that the attachment of Von Willebrand factor to platelet glycoprotein and subendothelium Ib takes place. The platelet glycoprotein IIb-IIIa mediates the aggregate formation and successive platelet spreading.

The activation of platelet happens after the events of adhesion and attachment take place or after other stimuli that prompt activation mechanisms, platelet activating factor:

- Thrombin
- ADP,
- Thromboxane A2,
- Endothelial cells, PMN (polymorphonuclear leukocytes) or monocytes secreting PAF (platelet activating factor).

1. During the initial step of activation, platelets undergo:
    - Organelle centralization,
    - Cytoskeleton rearrangement,
    - Shape change.
    - The release of serotonin and dense granule contents (ADP and ATP).
2. There is an alpha granule release of the following during the second step:
    - Fibronectin;
    - vWF;
    - Fibrinogen; Fibronectin and fibrinogen receptors come in contact on the platelet surface.
    - Arachidonic acid releases, and changes to thromboxane A2, which plays a strong mediating role in platelet aggregating response. Cyclooxygenase is a vital enzyme accountable for the thromboxane A2 production in platelets. Aspirin and other anti-inflammatory drugs obstruct prostaglandin pathways in its initial stages, and formation of pro-aggregatory cyclic endoperoxides , which are precursors of thromboxane A2. The platelets contribution to hemostasis is not solely dependent upon cohesive and adhesive functions mediated by membrane receptors. A catalytic phospholipid surface is provided by the activated human blood platelets plasma membranes on which the gathering of the "prothrombinase" complex (factor Xa-factor Va) and c complex (factor IXa-factor VIIIa) can activate the Coagulation process.

Coagulation Factors

Fibrinogen (factor I) have three polypeptide chains: alpha, beta, and gamma. Thrombin (factor IIa) converts it to fibrin (factor Ia). A mesh is formed surrounding the wound by fibrin ultimately leading to the formation of a blood clot. The hereditary disorders because of mutations in fibrinogen are hyperfibrinogenemia (dysfunctional fibrinogen), afibrinogenemia (complete lack of fibrinogen) and hypofibrinogenemia (reduced levels of fibrinogen).

Prothrombin (factor II) can be classified as a vitamin K-dependent serine protease. Its cleavage to thrombin is done by the enzymatic action of activated factor X (FXa). The thrombin converts fibrinogen from soluble to insoluble fibrin, and the thrombin stimulation of factors V, VIII, XI, and XIII as well. Thrombin, in combination with the thrombomodulin, found on surfaces of endothelial cell, by making a complex that changes protein C to activated protein C (APC). Prothrombin deficiency individuals have hemorrhagic diathesis, and in the case of female patients, they may suffer from menorrhagia. Individual may also have hypoprothrombinemia (dysfunction of prothrombin) or hypoprothrombinemia (reduced levels of prothrombin).

The tissue factor (factor III) termed as a platelet tissue factor as well, is present on the side blood vessels outer wall, remaining unexposed to the bloodstream. An extrinsic pathway at the injury location is started by it. It plays the role of a high-affinity receptor for factor VII. It functions as a cofactor in the factor VIIa-catalyzed activation of factor X to FXa.

Factor V termed as the labile factor, or proaccelerin is not active enzymatically and plays the role of a cofactor to the serine protease FXa, which, in the occurrence of calcium ions and a suitable phospholipid (PL) membrane surface, improves prothrombin to activated thrombin. Parahemophilia or factor V deficiency is resulted by a mutation in factor V Leiden, which is an uncommon bleeding disorder. It may also result in myocardial infarction and deep vein thrombosis.

Factor VII is a vitamin K-dependent serine protease. By activating tissue factor along with factors IX and X in the extrinsic pathway, it starts the process of coagulation. The deficiency of this may result in menorrhagia, epistaxis, hemarthrosis, hematomas, and cerebral or digestive tract hemorrhages.

Factor VIII which is also called as an anti-hemophilic factor (AHF) acts as a cofactor in factor X activation to FXa, and factor IXa acts as a catalyst in the existence of phospholipids and calcium. Factor VIII gene mutations lead to the disorder of hemophilia A. Another name for this is classical hemophilia, an X-linked recessive coagulation disorder. This type of hemophilia is the most commonly occurring. Individuals that suffer may show clinical symptoms in their early childhood; traumatic and spontaneous bleeds may be present throughout the life of the patient.

Factor IX called as Christmas factor is a proenzyme serine protease that in occurrence calcium triggers factor X. The deficiency of this results in Christmas disease or hemophilia B. For hemophilia A, and B, clinical symptoms might be similar, but the severity of hemophilia A is more as compared to hemophilia B. There is a higher risk of thromboembolism when factor IX has a high activity or antigen levels.

Factor X, which is also termed as Stuart-Prower factor, functions in both extrinsic and intrinsic blood coagulation pathways when calcium and phospholipids are present. Factors IX and VII stimulate Factor X to FXa. For the common pathway of blood coagulation, it is the first member. Thrombin is cleaved to prothrombin by FXa. The deficiency of this results in hemorrhages and bleeding diathesis. Gastrointestinal bleeds, epistaxis, and hemarthrosis are commonly seen in patients. Women suffering from a deficiency of Factor X are more likely to have miscarriages.

Factor XI termed as plasma thromboplastin antecedent is activated by factor XIIa to factor Xia, and it can be classified as serine protease zymogen. Injury-related bleeding is a consequence of deficiency of this factor. Hemophilia C is another name for this disorder. People are having severe deficiency suffer from hemorrhage after trauma or surgery and generally, do not show excessive bleeding conditions. Menorrhagia and prolonged bleeding after childbirth are experienced by female patients.

Factor XII, termed as Hageman factor, is a plasma protein. It is factor XIIa, zymogen form, which stimulates prekallikrein and factor XI. Because of the factor XIIa lack of involvement in thrombin formation, excessive hemorrhage is not caused by its deficiency. However, the risk of thrombosis may rise due to fibrinolytic pathway inadequate activation.

Factor XIII, -Fibrin stabilizing is a plasma transglutaminase proenzyme form made up of two subunits: alpha (α) and beta (β). In the presence of calcium, it is stimulated by thrombin to convert into factor XIIIa. The ε-(γ-glutamyl)-lysyl bonds are formed by it between the fibrin chains and the blood clot is stabilized by this. Hence, the clot's sensitivity to degradation by proteases is decreased. Factor XIII gene's genetic defects can lead to permanent bleeding diathesis. Intracranial bleeding and even death are common among patients.

Antithrombin that is also known as antithrombin III plays a vital role in acting as a natural inhibitor of the coagulation system has activated serine proteases. It's significant function is inhibiting thrombin, factors IXa and Xa. It also acts as an inhibitor for factors XIa, XIIa, tissue factor and the complex of factor VIIa. The presence of heparin enhances its activity. Based on the immunological and functional assays, antithrombin deficiency can be categorized into two types: type I and type II. In the type I deficiency the antithrombin level present to inactivate the coagulation factors are decreased. Antithrombin quantity is normal in the type II deficiency, but it is not performing its function effectively. Pulmonary embolism and recurrent venous thrombosis are seen in patients.

Protein C is a serine protease enzyme. The role played by this is inactivating factors VIIIa and Va. Thrombin activates it into activated protein C (APC). APC in combination with protein S degrades factors VIIIa and VA The deficiency of protein C is an uncommon genetic disorder resulting in venous thrombosis. There is two types of Protein C deficiency: type I and type II. The consequence of too little amount of protein C is the type I deficiency and defective protein C molecules is seen in type II deficiency. Patients may have venous and arterial thrombosis.

Protein S is classified as vitamin K-dependent plasma glycoprotein. It plays the role of a cofactor to protein C. Hence it enhances factors VIIIa and Va inactivation. Protein S deficiency may result from PROS1 gene mutations, raising thrombosis risk. Protein S deficiency can be classified into three types: type I, type II and type III. Insufficient quantity of both total and free protein S levels are typical features of type I deficiency. The level of protein is normal in type II deficiency, but the functional activity of protein S reduces. A small amount of free protein S is a typical feature of type III deficiency.

Protein Z has a function in factor Xa degradation.

Engaged in hemostasis, the **vonWillebrand factor (vWF)** is a multimeric glycoprotein. Platelets' binding is assisted to the injury site by a bridge formation between the platelet surface receptor complex and collagen matrix. The von Willebrand disease is a result of genetic or acquired defects in vWF. Gastrointestinal bleeding, menorrhagia, and bleeding diathesis may be experienced by the patients.

Plasminogen can be classified as a glycoprotein that flows as a proenzyme. The tissue plasminogen activator (tPA or PLAT) converts it in into plasmin in the occurrence of a fibrin clot. The dissolving of the blood clots' fibrin is the key function of plasmin. Significant functions of plasminogen are the maintenance of liver homeostasis and healing of the wound. The plasmin deficiency may result in thrombosis because the clots are not degraded sufficiently.

Heparin cofactor II can be classified as a serine protease inhibitor. It acts as an inhibitor of factor X and thrombin and as a cofactor for dermatan sulfate and heparin. Gene mutations, in this case, are related to heparin cofactor II deficiency, which may result in a hypercoagulable state and increased thrombin generation.

Kallikrein found in an inactive form known as prekallikrein is a serine protease. It is transformed by factor XIIa to its active form. Kallikrein cleaves kininogen-releasing bradykinin.

High-molecular-weight kininogen (HMWK) is also classified as the Williams-Fitzgerald-Flaujeac factor. Enzymatically it is inactive and plays the role of factor XII activation and as a cofactor for the kallikrein. Kinins, for example, the bradykinin are secreted by kininogen upon plasma kallikrein activation.

Clinical features: Serious
   ○ Muscle/soft tissue
   ○ Joints (hemarthrosis)
   ○ Hematuria
   ○ Mouth/gums/nose
Life threatening
   ○ Gastrointestinal (GI)
   ○ Severe trauma
   ○ Neck/throat
   ○ Central nervous system (CNS)
The incidence of different sites of bleeding:
   ○ Hemarthrosis: 70% to 80%
   ○ Muscle/soft tissue: 10% to 20%
   ○ Other major bleeds: 5% to 10%
   ○ Central nervous system (CNS) bleeds: < 5%
Guiding principle for regular dental treatment of individuals suffering from bleeding disorders is as follows:
   ○ Prior to going for any surgical procedure, it is important to consult with a physician.
   ○ Children suffering from bleeding disorders should be given dental appointments, along with providing education in preventive dentistry for children and caregivers, as soon as the baby teeth start erupting.
   ○ Surgical procedures and deep injections – especially one which regional, local anesthetic blocks or involve bone (extractions and dental implants) should be administered after the raising suitably the level of clotting factors.
   ○ Treatment of oral infections should be done using antibiotics prior to

performing the surgical procedure.

○ A detailed dental assessment should be done around age 12 or 13 for future planning and find the most suitable way to overcome difficulties from misplaced third molars or other teeth or overcrowding.

○ For mild or moderate hemophilia patients, non-surgical dental treatment can be performed under cover of antifibrinolytic (epsilon-aminocaproic acid or tranexamic acid), but it is important to consult hematologist prior to other procedures.

○ For individuals suffering from severe hemophilia, it is vital to have factor replacement prior to surgery, scaling or regional block injections (It is suggested to consult Patient's physician in those cases).

○ For individuals suffering from mild hemophilia A (FVIII > 5%), some minor surgery and scaling is achievable under desmopressin (DDAVP desmopressin acetate tablets), a synthesized product similar in function to the natural pituitary hormone 8-arginine vasopressin (ADH), that belongs to antidiuretic hormone class that affects the renal water conservation. Intranasal or Intravenous desmopressin administration to healthy individuals results in an increase in levels of both VWF and its precious cargo, FVIII. As expected, a person with a deficiency of V2 receptors—*i.e.*, nephrogenic diabetes insipidus patients—do not illustrate this rise in FVIII and VWF levels.

○ Local applications of swish-and-swallow rinses of tranexamic acid and fibrin glue once prior to and later following dental extractions are shown as secure and productive methods to overcome bleeding.

○ Use of tranexamic acid topically reduces bleeding significantly; 10 ml of a 5% solution used for rinsing mouth for two minutes, four times in a day, and for a complete week is recommended. Individuals may use it in combination with oral tranexamic acid tablets for up to five days.

○ Painkillers (analgesics) like NSAIDs may worsen the bleeding. Paracetamol/acetaminophen and codeine can be used safely as alternative analgesics.

Oral Anticoagulants

Appropriate laboratory tests should be in knowledge of dentists when minor oral surgery is recommended for anticoagulated patients, so they may order and interpret it. The most regularly used tests are the international normalized ratio (INR) and prothrombin time (PT).

The efficacy of the extrinsic and common pathways is determined by PT test. The range for the normal value is 10 to 15 seconds as estimated. Since there is a lot of inconsistency in PT values that various laboratories report, this test is not considered sufficient to monitor the anticoagulation level, the INR test was introduced which is a reliable test for assessing anticoagulation status. INR has less variability and is a more dependable measure. The normal value of INR is 1.0.

INR

Prothrombin time result (in seconds), when applied to any normal individual, varies according to the analytical system type being used. The reason for these variations is the difference among various batches of tissue factor that the company manufactures use as a reagent for performing the test. The purpose of finding INR test is so that the results can be standardized. Every manufacturer assigns a particular ISI value (international sensitivity index) for the manufacturers' tissue factor. A tissue factor from a particular batch can be compared to an international reference tissue factor. The value for ISI lies between 1.0 and 2.0 normally. The INR value is the prothrombin time for a patient ratio the normal (control) sample, raised to the power, which is the ISI value for the employed analytical system.

$$INR = \left(\frac{PT_{test}}{PT_{normal}} \right)^{ISI}$$

Interpretation of PT and PTT

Result of pt	Result of ppt	Conditions
Prolonged	Not affected (Normal)	Decreased vitamin K, Prolonged Normal Liver disease chronic low-grade disseminated intravascular coagulation (DIC), Decreased or defective factor VII, anticoagulation therapy (warfarin)
Not affected (Normal)	Prolonged	Deficiency or defective in factor VIII, IX, XI, or XII, von Willebrand disease, autoantibody against a specific factor such as factor number VIII
Prolonged	Prolonged	Deficiency or defective factor number I, II, V or X, presence of autoimmune disease (the most important of them is lupus anticoagulant), liver disease (severe state), DIC (acute), anticoagulant (overdose)
Normal	Normal (or slightly prolonged)	Possibly indicative of normal hemostasis; nevertheless, PTT and PT may show normal value in the case such as mild forms of von Willebrand disease and mild deficiencies in coagulation factor(s), to diagnose these conditions, a further test may be needed.

The most commonly used oral anticoagulants:

- Warfarin
- Acenocoumarol
- Phenindione
- Dabigatran
- Etexilate
- Rivaroxaban

Target dose and Indications of warfarin:

High dose (high Intensity) of Warfarin Therapy (INR of 2.5 to 3.5, with a target of 3.0 - 7-10mg/day, long term)	Low dose (low Intensity) of Warfarin Therapy (INR of 2.0 to 3.0, with a target of 2.5 - 5-7mg/day for 3-6 months)
• Prevention of systemic embolism • Tissue heart valves in mitral or aortic position for a trimester • Atrial fibrillation • Tissue valves with a history of pulmonary embolism • Treatment of pulmonary embolism • Valvular heart disease • Tissue's heart valves with atrial fibrillation • Prophylaxis of venous thrombosis (high-risk surgery) • Mitral valve prolapse with an embolism or atrial fibrillation in past • Acute MI	• Prevention of recurrent MI • Mechanical prosthetic heart values • Thrombosis treatment that is linked to antiphospholipid antibodies

Dental Management

The patient should be referred to a hematologist to adjust the INR to a level that allows for a safe extraction procedure. Medical care:

1. **Withdrawal of anti-coagulant:** The dental practitioners are advised by the present literature not to stop the warfarin therapy because there are chances that a thromboembolic event might occur, which may increase the patient's mortality risks and morbidity.
2. **Modification of Oral-anticoagulant**

Low-intensity INR 2.0-3.04:

- Recent INR laboratory results should be acquired before initiating the invasive dental procedure and physician of the patient should be consulted.
- If the range of INR is 2.0-3.0: while simple surgical procedures or most invasive

non-surgical is performed, the procedure can be carried out given that INR is within the therapeutic range of 2.0 to 3.0. (Non-surgical invasive procedures may comprise of subgingival debridement with slight to moderate inflammation.) Standard local hemostatic measures should be carefully adopted in order to control the bleeding.

- If the INR value is above 2.5: When the subgingival debridement with severe inflammation or complex surgical procedures is to be performed, the physician of the patient should be consulted so that the INR drifts down to a safe INR range, between 2 to 2.5. Standard local hemostatic measures should be carefully adopted in order to control the bleeding. Physician of the patient should be consulted regarding any concerns that are transiently interrupting the anticoagulation therapy.

High-intensity INR 2.5 to 3.5:

- Physician of the patient should be consulted, and latest INR laboratory results should be obtained before the invasive dental procedure is commenced.
- While simple surgical and non-surgical (subgingival debridement with slight to moderate inflammation) procedures are performed, INR should be maintained in the 2.5 to 3.5 range; standard local hemostatic measures should be approached carefully to limit and control bleeding.
- It is better that physician of the patient is consulted when subgingival debridement with severe inflammation and complex surgical procedures are to be carried out; keeping in mind the local hemostatic measures, one can safely continue in the lower ranges of INR 2.5 to 3.0. It is better to discuss with patient's physician if there are concerns for briefly interrupting the anticoagulation therapy. Generally interrupting the anticoagulation therapy is not advisable as this may result in thromboembolic phenomena.
- Low molecular weight heparin preparations should be considered in order to bridge the patient by using the invasive procedure, as an alternative anticoagulant.
- Substitute with standard and high molecular weight heparin (LMWHs): Standard heparin functions as the catalyst inhibiting plasma thrombin along with plasmin and coagulation factors IX, X, XI, and XII, hence stopping the conversion of fibrinogen to fibrin, though itself standard heparin is not considered an anticoagulant. The potentiating anticoagulant effects of LMWHs are exerted more over the factor Xa.2. The use of these drugs is done for treating thromboembolic disorders functioning as prophylaxis anti-thrombotic agent. Treatment using standard heparin generally contains IV infusions in a hospital environment; an aPTT laboratory test is essential to monitor it. Preparations for LMWH are administered on an outpatient basis and subcutaneously. Based on the body weight of the patient their dosage is computed and is administered

every 12-hour. Usually, the physician suggests his/her patient to be admitted to the hospital for this procedure.

Dental Care

- The patient should be referred to haematologist to adjust the INR to a level that allows the surgical procedure.
- It is better that a surgical procedure that seems potentially problematic are performed in the morning time, hence time for hemostasis is sufficient before nightfall, and preferably at the beginning of the week, so there are no problems over the weekend, as at that time staff is less.
- Surgery should be carried out with 2% lidocaine (lignocaine) with 1:80,000 or 1:100,000 epinephrine (adrenaline).
- The performance of surgery should be done with such as care that strain to soft tissues and bones is minimized. It is essential to take local measures for protecting the soft tissues and area operated furthermore the risk of postoperative bleeding should be minimized as well.
- In difficult extractions scenario, when raising mucoperiosteal flaps is important, the lingual tissues in the lower molar regions not disturbed if possible, since planes may be opened up by trauma into which hemorrhage may track and endanger the airway.
- Hence, to lower third molar removal, it is safer to use the buccal approach.
- Bones removal should be as less as possible, and sectioning of teeth should be done if possible, for removal. Thoroughly done curettage of the site of extraction is important in order to prevent excessive bleeding (in case the postoperative bleeding takes place, the reason may be a local infection and not be the prolonged INR).
- Usually, the postoperative bleeding is not occurring in all sites of extraction, in the multiple extractions scenario, instead, it mostly occurs at a single site, and generally, is a location that is linked with severe periodontitis.
- Bleeding assessment should be done intraoperatively, and an absorbable hemostatic agents such as, collagen (synthetic or microcrystalline or porcine), oxidized regenerated cellulose, cyanoacrylate; re-absorbable gelatin sponge, or fibrin glues should be placed in the extraction site in case of concern. Which is primarily composed of thrombin and fibrinogen, presenting tissue sealing, adhesion, and quick hemostasis (the recombinant fibrin products are more favorable). The advantage of suturing is that it aids in stabilizing gum flaps and preventing postoperative trouble in wounds by eating. It is preferred to use the resorbable suture since it retains less plaque. Removal of non-resorbable sutures should be done at four to seven days.
- Applying gauze pressure (a tranexamic acid-soaked gauze aids) is advised and, after biting on gauze for10 minutes, assessment of hemostasis should be done.

The patient may be discharged if bleeding is controlled, and a seven-day follow-up appointment should be given, along with the contact of the office, which can provide guidelines in case of bleeding. The treating clinician should be careful in case of incidence of bleeding and take preventive measures (*i.e.*, placing sutures and prescribing medication in advance), using an antifibrinolytic agent. For example, topical 4.8% tranexamic acid, for a week.

Patients on Long-Term Steroids

Two hormones are produced by the cortex of the adrenal gland: sex hormone (androgens) and corticoid hormone, the later one is divided into glucocorticoid (cortisol) and mineralocorticoid (aldosterone) steroids. The primary function of glucocorticoids is related to metabolism of glucose, and they have a "permissive role" in affecting many physiological processes. This class of hormones has limited mineralocorticoid effect that changes the fluid and electrolyte balance by raising water and sodium retention. A significant role is played by glucocorticoids in the response of the body to stress. Cytokines are released due to stress, especially the cytokine interleukin-1 that results in a rise in cortisol levels hence causing mobilization in glycogen and fat stores of the body. The hypothalamic-pituitary-adrenal (HPA) axis controls the release of cortisol, whereby corticotrophin-releasing hormone (CRH) being secreted from the hypothalamus modulates the anterior pituitary gland to release adrenocorticotropic hormone (ACTH). The release of cortisol is directly a response to the action of ACTH. The function of cortisol, along with exogenous glucocorticoids is to provide a negative feedback on CRH release from the hypothalamus and, hence, ACTH. This negative feedback results in atrophy of the adrenal gland and a significant reduction in the adrenal gland hormone required during stress processes that may develop during tooth extractions. A life-threatening condition acute adrenal crisis occurs when the cortisol quantity is not sufficient, a hormone that adrenal glands produce.

Adrenal crisis risk factors are:

- Stopping the corticosteroid treatment too early
- Injury to the adrenal or pituitary gland
- Dehydration
- Surgery
- Trauma
- Infection and other physical stress
- Stressful events Precaution: If the patient is currently taking steroid therapy or if the steroid has been given during last three months in a dose of 10mg or more, supplementation should be given as a 25mg IV. There is no need for a high dose

(200mg. IV).

Indication for supplementary dose in dental practice:

Time since the last course	Dose of prednisolone	Type of Surgery	Cover Needed
> 3 months	Not needed	N/A	N/A
< 3 months	<10 mg/day	Not needed	Not needed
< 3 months	>10 mg/day	Restorative or single extraction	The daily dose or 25mg HCSS
		Multiple extraction	25mg HCSS IV +Daily Dose
		Moderate Surgery under GA	100mg/day for 24 h. and for 72 h. for major Max. Fax. *e.g.* Oncology

Symptoms of Adrenal Crisis

- Dizziness or light-headedness
- Shaking chills
- Confusion or coma
- Headache
- Abdominal pain
- Dehydration
- Loss of consciousness
- Skin rash or lesions
- Nausea
- Unusual face or palms excessive sweating
- Profound weakness
- Slow, sluggish movement
- Fatigue
- Rapid heart rate
- Darkening of the skin
- Rapid respiratory rate
- Low blood pressure
- Vomiting

Management of Adrenal Crisis

- Lay patient flat, with legs raised
- Give methylprednisolone 500mg/hydrocortisone 500mg IV
- Give oxygen
- Summon medical assistance

Asthma

- Atopy
  - IgE against common antigens
  - *e.g.* grass pollen, house dust mites
- Increased responsiveness of the airways
  - Fall in FEV1 in bronchial provocation tests

Dental products and materials that may worsen asthma should be in knowledge of the dentist. These items include:

- Dentifrices
- Methyl methacrylate
- Tooth enamel dust
- Fissure sealants
- Cotton rolls and fluoride trays are also likely to promote asthmatic events.
- People suffering from corticosteroid-dependent asthma may have a greater likeliness of having an adverse reaction to sulfites.

Precautions

1. Make sure that patient has taken the most recent scheduled medication dose. The purpose of inhaled corticosteroids is maintenance therapy, and they do not help in avoidance of an acute attack.
2. At every visit patient's metered-dose inhaler, bronchodilator should be readily available as to lower the attack risk.
3. The appointment time should be preferably in the late afternoon or late morning.
4. If a bronchodilator is not used by an asthmatic patient, it is necessary that the emergency kit has included a bronchodilator as well as oxygen.
5. Prevention of diminished lung function during dental treatment could be done by a prophylactic dose of an agonist bronchodilator. It is shown that the H1-blocking antihistamines also play a good role in blunting the bronchoconstrictor response with a pretreatment dose. Diphenhydramine and promethazine are advantageous as antiemetic and sedative in addition to being antihistaminic.
6. Anxiety triggers asthma very usual in the dental environment; an acute asthmatic attack might occur. So it is necessary that the latest anti-asthma medication according to schedule is taken by the patient before coming for the treatment.
7. Furthermore, substantive stress-management techniques are to be employed.
8. Using N_2O for the mild-to-moderate asthmatic patient may help to avoid acute stress-related symptoms. Due to the chances that N_2O might cause airway irritation, its use is contraindicated in severe asthma patients. Medical advice is

recommended prior to administering N_2O to these particular patients.

9. Patient with severe persistent asthma should be treated in the hospital-based dental clinic because the risk of severe acute episodes is high.

Management of an Acute Asthmatic Attack

- Dental procedure should discontinue immediately, and the patient should take a relaxing position.
- Start and maintain an unobstructed airway and give b2 agonists *via* nebulizer or inhaler.
- Provide oxygen at 6 to 10 liters *via* nasal hood, cannula or face mask. In case it does not get better and symptoms seem to get worse, administer epinephrine subcutaneously (0.01 mg per kg, to a maximum dose of 0.3 mg).
- Register the event initiation in the time from call for medical help.
- A good oxygen level should be maintained till the wheezing is finished by the patient and/or medical help arrives.
- Start the basic life support activity as required.
- In case, it seems necessary to transfer the patient to the hospital.

Local Anesthesia and Asthmatic Patient

- Preventing an acute asthma attack is the primary focus of dental management of asthmatic patients, keeping in mind that stress acts as a precipitating factor for asthma attacks.
- Based on the Food and Drug Administration's warnings, it is advised that sulfites contained drugs may result in allergic reactions by the susceptible individuals. It is suggested by 23 Studies that an antioxidant agent, sodium metabisulfite, used in dental vasoconstrictors-containing local anesthetic solutions inhibits the vasoconstrictor breakdown and may provoke extrinsic, asthma attacks or cause allergy. However, the data on this problem's frequency is inadequate, and might be an uncommon reaction, even in patients that are sulfite-sensitive, as only a small amount of metabisulfite is used during dental anesthetics.
- It is estimated that around 96% of asthma, patients are not sensitive to sulfites, and patients who susceptible are mostly severe, steroid-dependent.
- It is believed by Awe. *et al.* that a vasoconstrictor-containing local anesthetic may be safe to be employed in non-steroid-dependent asthmatics. Nonetheless, until clear knowledge regarding sulfite sensitivity threshold is attained, it is suggested that vasoconstrictors-containing local anesthetic should not be preferably given to corticosteroid-dependent asthma patients, as they are more prone to sulfite allergy, and there is a risk that a severe and abrupt asthmatic reaction might result from accidental intravascular injection in a sensitive patient.

Epilepsy

The majority of the reader are aware that epilepsy, which is a neurological condition, occasionally causes small disturbances in the brain's normal electrical activity. A person suffering from epilepsy has the normal pattern interrupted by irregular bursts of electrical energy that are stronger than standard.

Predisposing factors include:

- Epileptogenic drugs: tricyclic, phenothiazines, alcohol, enflurane, methohexitone
- Fatigue
- Starvation/hypoglycaemia
- Stress
- Infection
- Flickering lights
- Menstruation

Management

- Maintain airway and oxygenation and protect the patient from injuring himself or herself.
- If the patient has not recovered within five minutes, give diazepam 0.1mg/kg IV or midazolam 2mg IV every minute.
- If status is epileptics, give up to 800mg chlormethiazole IV (60 to 150 drops per minute)

Anaphylaxis (Card 5.8)

Instant hypersensitivity is a rapid IgE- and mast cell-mediated vascular and smooth muscle response happening in genetically susceptible persons when exposed to certain environmental antigens to which they have been recently exposed. We also term these reactions as allergies, and the antigens are prompting these reactions are usually known as allergens. These reactions symptom may range in severity from mild hay fever or allergies to pet dander to severe anaphylaxis triggered by drugs ingestion, such as penicillin or injection with insect venoms. One of the most common disorders of the immune system are allergies and may around 20% of the population is affected by them. Normally they result in a few of the following: throat or tongue swelling, low blood pressure, vomiting, an itchy rash, lightheadedness, and shortness of breath. These manifestations are apparent over minutes to hours normally.

Card 5.8. Anaphylaxis.

Anaphylaxis

Clinical features:
Cold, clammy skin
Pulse weak and rapid
Oedema / urticaria / wheeze
Acutely falling blood pressure

Monitor:
BP
O_2 by using pulse oximeter
Heart rate

Management
1. Lay patient flat
2. Give oxygen (High O_2 flow)
3. Establish the IV line
4. Give Chlorphenamine
5. Give 1:1000 adrenaline IM
6. Give hydrocortisone sodium succinate 200-500mg IM or methylprednisolone 500mg IV
7. Summon medical assistance

Adrenaline in patients with life-threatening anaphylactic shock is to give intramuscular adrenaline:
In an adult, use 0.5mg or 0.5 mls undiluted adrenaline
For children > than 6 years give 0.3 ml and for those < 6 give 0.15 ml

Chloramphenamin IV:
In an adult, use 10mg
For children > than 6 give 0.5mg and for those < 6 give 2.5mg

IV solution: for the adult give 500 – 1000ml and for children 50ml /Kg until the signs of anaphylaxis start to disapear

Chloramphenamin IV OR IM:
In an adult, use 200mg
For children > than 6 years give 100mg and for those < 6 give 50mg

Pathophysiology

Anaphylaxis which is a term used for severe allergic reaction with a quick onset and many body systems are affected by it. The reason for this at times is the release of cytokines and inflammatory mediators from basophils and mast cells, due to an immunologic reaction mostly however at times it could be due to a non-immunologic response. The division of T-helper cell (Th) can be done into two subsets. Th1 cells, which synthesize tumor necrosis factor (TNF)-beta, interleukin (IL)-2, and interferon (IFN)-gamma, phagocyte-dependent inflammation and evoke cell-mediated immunity. Th2 cells, which synthesize IL-4, IL-5, IL-6, IL-9, IL-10, and IL-13, induce strong responses by eosinophil accumulation and antibody (including those of the IgE class) however, several functions of phagocytic cells (phagocyte-independent inflammation) are inhibited by it. 1-Primary exposure: The allergen stimulates the Th-2 cells, `then secretes IL-4, IL-5, IL-9, and IL-13. The role played by IL-5 is in development, recruitment, and activation of eosinophil, which functioning, as a regulator of the mast cell activation is the IL-9. The role of IL-4 and IL-13 is to act on B cells in order to promote the antigen-specific IgE antibodies production`. Production of antigen-specific IgE antibodies: Binding of B cells to the allergen is necessary to make this happen, *via* allergen-specific receptors.

Formation of the major histocompatibility (MHC) is also called the human leukocyte antigen (HLA).

1- For the antigen to be presented to the B cells, the antigen and its peptides from are internalized by binding to the major histocompatibility Class II molecules that are present on B-cell surfaces and are then presented the antigen receptors on TH2 cells. It is important that B cell also binds to the T-helper 2 (TH2) cell, and this is done by binding the CD40 communicated on its surface to the CD40 ligand on the surface of the TH2 cell. TH2 cells secrete the IL-4 and IL-13 that cause the B cell to promote class switching to antigen-specific IgE production from immunoglobulin M production.

2- Sensitization and re-exposure: Binding of antigen-specific IgE antibodies can be done to high-affinity receptors that are placed on the surfaces of basophils and mast cells. Antigen exposure may cause antigen binding to and cross-link the bound IgE antibodies on the basophils and mast cells. As a result from these cells, secretion and formation of chemical mediators are done. These mediators comprise of cytokines, newly synthesized mediators, and preformed mediators. The chemical mediators can be categorized as preformed mediators and newly formed mediators. These include the following:

Mechanism

1- Trigger Events

The trigger of anaphylaxis are:

a. Immunologically mediated (anaphylactic and lgE):
   Most cases of anaphylaxis are lgE, or rarely lgG4, mediated. Following previous exposure to an antigen, the plasma cells responsible for releasing of lgE reagin antibodies into the circulation by derived from B-lymphocytes, under the influence of helper T-cells. These antibodies bind to glycoprotein receptors on tissue mast cells or blood-borne basophils, thereby sensitizing them. Subsequent re-exposure to the antigen cross-links the Fab portions of two surface-bound lgE molecules, triggering the release of:
   - **Chemical Mediators**: including histamine, Leukotrienes produced *via* the lipoxygenase pathway, Cyclooxygenase products, Cytokines and others
   - and **Activating the Cell**: Specific lymphocyte subtypes (CD4), (T-helper cell 2 -Th2 T-cells) responsible for releasing of Cytokines (interleukins), (B-cell) responsible for the synthesis of lgE and IgG
b. Non-immunoglobulin mediated (anaphylactoid): Anaphylactoid reactions are non-immunoglobulin mediated and caused by mediator release triggered independently of reagin antibodies. These reactions do not require prior exposure, and patients may not react on every occasion. The reactions may be due to complement activation and chemical mediators.

2- Complement Activation

Complement activation *via* the classical pathway or alternate pathway leads to the formation of anaphylatoxins C3a, C4a, and C5a. These anaphylatoxins stimulate mast cells and basophils to degranulate, releasing mediators that cause local and systemic reactions. C3a and C5a also directly induce increased vascular permeability, smooth muscle contraction, and neutrophil chemotaxis.

Chemical Mediators

Preformed Mediators

Histamine is the most important inflammatory chemical mediator in this group. The function of this mediator is to activate histamine 1 (H1) and histamine 2 (H2) receptors which result in the, increased vaso-permeability, vasodilation, contraction of the smooth muscles of the GI tract and airway, cutaneous vasodilation, enhanced mucus production, and gastric acid secretion, pruritus.

Newly Formed Mediators

Arachidonic acid metabolites:

A. Leukotrienes produced *via* the lipoxygenase pathway: Leukotrienes are inflammatory mediators produced in leukocytes other immune cells (including mast cells, eosinophils, neutrophils, monocytes, and basophils). This occurs by the oxidation of arachidonic acid and the essential fatty acid eicosapentaenoic acid (EPA) under the action of an enzyme known as arachidonate 5-lipoxygenase.

1. Leukotrienes C4 and D4 - Cause arteriolar constriction, raise vascular permeability, and potent bronchoconstrictors.
2. Leukotriene B4 - Augmentation of vascular permeability; neutrophil chemotaxis and activation.
3. Leukotrienes C4, D4, and E4 - Contain what was known before as the slow-reacting substance of anaphylaxis.
4. Leukotriene E4 - Raises vascular permeability and improves bronchial responsiveness.

B. Cyclooxygenase products:
1. Prostaglandin F2-alpha - peripheral vasodilator, bronchoconstrictor, platelet aggregation inhibitor and coronary vasoconstrictor.
2. Prostaglandin D2 - Mainly synthesized by mast cells;
   - it is a peripheral vasodilator,
   - coronary and pulmonary artery vasoconstrictor,
   - bronchoconstrictor,
   - enhancer of histamine release from basophils,
   - neutrophil chemoattractant,
   - platelet aggregation inhibitor.
3. Thromboxane A2 - Causes platelet aggregation, bronchoconstriction, and vasoconstriction.
4. Adenosine: This belongs to the class of bronchoconstrictor that also potentiates IgE-induced mast cell mediator release.
5. Platelet-activating factor (PAF): Made from membrane phospholipids through a different pathway from arachidonic acid is the PAF, aggregating the platelets and functions as a powerful mediator in allergic reactions. It raises vascular permeability, bronchoconstriction, chemotaxis, and lastly, degranulation of eosinophils and neutrophils.
6. Bradykinin: Kininogenase secretes through the mast cell and in order to produce bradykinin it acts upon plasma kininogens. An alternative (or additional) route of kinin generation, involving activation of the contact system *via* factor XII by heparin-released mast cell. Bradykinin raises smooth muscle contraction, vaso-permeability, hypotension, vasodilation, pain, and activation of arachidonic acid metabolites. Nevertheless, the role played by IgE-mediated allergic reactions are inadequately illustrated.

C. Cytokines:
1. IL-4: TH2 cell proliferation is stimulated and maintained by IL-4, and B cells are switched to IgE synthesis.

2. IL-5: An important role in the maturation, chemotaxis, activation, and survival of eosinophils is undertaken by IL-5. In addition, IL-5 primes basophils for histamine and leukotriene release.

3. IL-6: Mucus production is promoted by IL-6.

4. IL-13: This has many functions similar to IL-4.

5. Tumor necrosis factor-alpha: This is a pro-inflammatory cytokine which plays a role in activating eosinophils and neutrophils and increasing monocyte chemotaxis. Binding of SummaryImmunoglobulin E (IgE) is done to the antigen (the foreign material that provokes the allergic reaction). Antigen-bound IgE then FcεRI receptors are activated by IgE on leukocyte basophils and mast cells. Causing the inflammatory mediators, for example, histamine, to be released. These mediators subsequently trigger vasodilation, cause heart muscle depression, increase bronchial smooth muscles contractions is amplified and raise the leakage of fluid from blood vessels. An immunologic mechanism exists, not relying on IgE, but whether this occurs in humans is still not known.

Clinical Features

- Cold, clammy skin
- Pulse weak and rapid
- Oedema/urticaria/wheeze
- Acutely falling blood pressure

Management

1. Lay patient flat
2. Give oxygen (High O_2 flow)
3. Establish the IV line
4. Give Chlorphenamine
5. Give 1:1000 adrenaline IM
6. Give hydrocortisone sodium succinate 200-500mg IM or methylprednisolone 500mg IV
7. Summon medical assistance

PART 2: LOCAL FACTORS CONTRIBUTE TO COMPLEXITY OF DENTAL EXTRACTIONS

The Complex extraction technically is the extraction which can't be achieved by using a forceps alone and may need using of elevators or/and roots separation or even surgical intervention.

Limited mouth opening is one of the most important challenges in dental extraction and contributes widely to difficulty because the accessibility is one of an important factor in all types of surgical procedure.

1. Limitation of mouth opening: may relate to:
   ○ Muscular
   ○ Skeletal
   ○ TMJ
2. Limitation in the mouth opening could be due to one of the following:
   1. Trismus
   2. Pseudo ankylosis
   3. True ankylosis

Causes of Trismus

- Odontogenic: Myofascial pain, Malocclusion, tooth eruption
- Infection: pteryogomandibular Space, Lateral pharyngeal Space, Temporal Space or any other masticatory spaces.
- Trauma: mandibular fractures, Muscles contusion
- Tumor: Nasopharyngeal tumor, tumors invading the muscles of mastications
- Psychologic: hysterical trismus
- Pharmacologic: Phenothiazines
- Neurologic: Tetanus

(Extra-Capsular) Causes

- Depressed zygomatic arch fracture
- Fracture dislocation of the condyle
- Adhesion of the coronoid process
- Hypertrophy of the coronoid process
- Fibrosis of temporalis muscle
- Myositis ossifications
- Scare contracture following injuries
- Tumor of condyle or coronoid process

(Intra-Capsular) Causes

- Infection: Otitis Media, Suppurative arthritis
- Inflammation: Rheumatic arthritis, Still disease, ankylosing spondylitis, Marie Strumpell disease,
- Surgical: post – operative complications of orthognathic surgery, TMJ surgery
- trauma: intracapsular condylar fracture, medial displaced condylar fracture, obstetric trauma, intracapsular fibrosis and ankylosis

Clinical evaluation of the tooth to be extracted usually consisted of two parts:

1. Clinical evaluation
2. Radiographic evaluation

Clinical Evaluation

- The site of the tooth
- The size of the tooth
- Remaining of tooth structures:
  1. Full sound crown
  2. Remaining root, if it is a remaining root -is the roots above the alveolar ridge or below the alveolar ridge? If the remaining roots below the alveolar ridge, the closed extraction should not be tried since this tooth should be approached as a surgical extraction.
  3. Is it a badly carious? The badly carious tooth usually lost large amount of tooth structure which makes it easily to crush under the forceps pressure (Fig. **5.1**).
  4. Is there a large filling? Large filling makes the tooth structure less resistant to pressure applied during dental extraction. The breakdown is not uncommon event during extraction (Fig. **5.2**).
  5. Is it endodontic treated tooth? The endodontic treated tooth becomes brittle after root canal treatment. There are two opinions regarding the cause of tooth brittleness. A) Some endodontists believe that removing of the pulp results in loss of the fluid circulation through the dental tubules. The fluid in dental tubules considers as an important deterrent for maintaining of tooth structure resiliency and relative elasticity of this hard tissues. B) Other endodontists believe that the amount of tooth structure that removed during the root canal access cavity is critically enough to cause this brittleness (Fig. **5.3**).
  6. Is there a periodontal problem? The periodontally involved tooth usually become mobile due to loss of the surrounding periodontium (the bone and periodontal attachment) which make the tooth mobile and easily to extract.

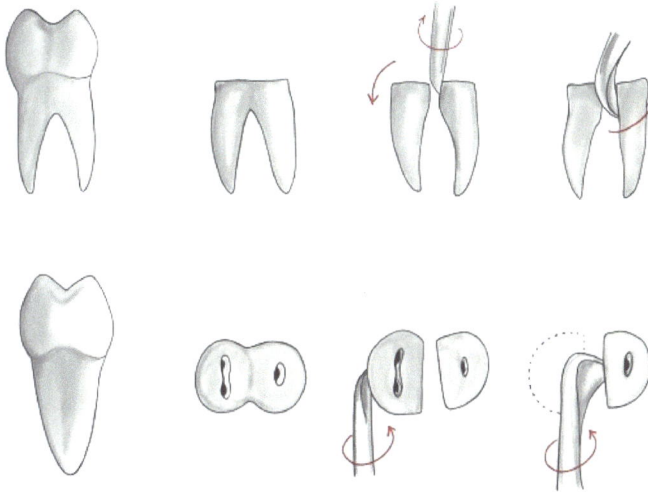

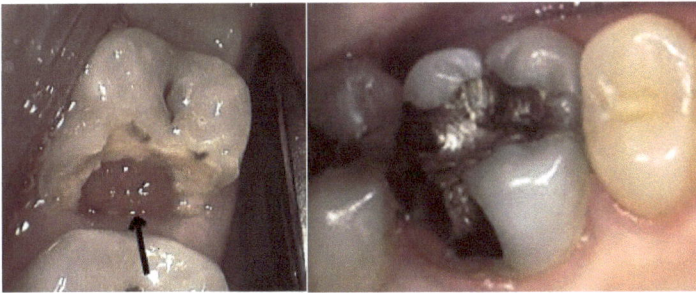

Fig. (5.1 and 5.2). Remaining of tooth structures: extraction of the sound full crown tooth usually easier than the extraction of badly carious tooth or tooth with a large filling.

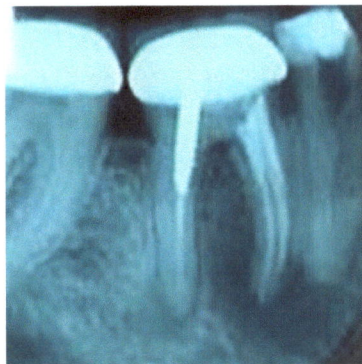

Fig. (5.3). Root canal (endodontic) treated tooth usually brittle in nature and easily fracture during extraction while the weak periodontal tooth is easier in the extraction procedure.

- Is it an isolated tooth (no adjacent teeth)? The interseptal bone is a piece of bone that located between the teeth, during extraction of adjacent teeth, the socket is healed by bone formation. The interseptal bone becomes a part of the healing process. The bone formation at adjacent area results in atrophy of the periodontal ligament (PDL) at the tooth near the healing area. As the periodontal space become narrower as the extraction, become difficult. The complete loss of PDL is called ankyloses (Fig. **5.4**). The ankyloses may result in absolute difficulty in extraction as the tooth structure become part of the bone (this depend on the degree on ankyloses.
- Is it a mal-posed tooth, Is it located in teeth crowding area? Mal-posed tooth or tooth in the crowded area usually carries a risk of A) accidental extraction of the adjacent tooth. B) difficulty in application and adaptation of the extraction's instruments to the tooth structure.
- The site: as the posterior teeth more difficult in extraction than anterior teeth: the surgical accessibility is the most important factor in all surgical procedures. As the tooth need extraction become more posterior, the accessibility significantly decreased, so the extraction becomes relatively difficult.
- The size of the tooth: If the tooth larger in size than normal usually associated with more difficult extraction. Abnormal tooth morphology like dental gemination or dental fusion is considered as local causes for difficulty.

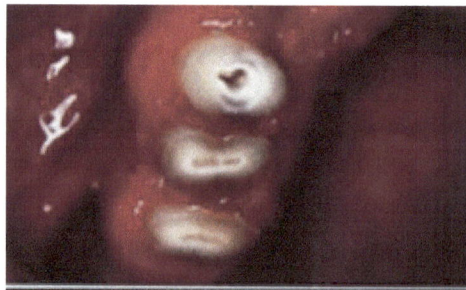

Fig. (5.4). Bony exostosis (the isolated tooth in the alveolar ridge) mean the tooth is surrounded by dense sclerotic bone and narrow periodontal ligament space such as the tooth in area of previous extraction for adjacent teeth.

Radiographic Evaluation

In all cases of extraction it is mandatory to take OPG and Peri-apical radiograph.

- Roots – shape, size, pathology
- Bone
- The periodontal ligament space
- Relation to vital structures

The following may contribute to difficult extraction:

1. Tooth with abnormal number of roots
2. Tooth associate with pathology, *e.g.*, periapical dilacerations (Fig. **5.6**), dental gemination or dental fusion (Fig. **5.7**), hypercementosis (Fig. **5.8a**) and (List 5.1), periapical cementoma (Fig. **5.8b**).
3. Condensing osteitis: occurs, as a result, to low-grade chronic inflammation: The low-grade inflammation (infection) (due to large amalgam restoration adjacent to a pulp or in the case of improper root canal treatment), result in stimulation of osteoblasts and osteocytes, which result in more production of osteoid deposition. The over activity of the osteoblasts and osteocytes is considered as a local defense mechanism to localized the inflammation. When the balance between the defense mechanism (local and systemic) and the inflammatory process is broken down due to lowering of the defense of increasing in inflammation, this will result in abscess formation (Fig. **5.8c**).
4. Narrow periodontal ligament space, absence periodontal space and fusion of the roots to the bone is called ankylosis which are the most important local factor contribute to the difficulty in dental extraction (Fig. **5.9**) and (List: 5.2).
5. Bone sclerosis (age-related or pathological) and bony exostosis (List 5.3)
6. Abnormal position of vital structures *e.g.* maxillary sinus, mandibular canal (Fig. **5.10**)

Endodontic treated tooth with a large filling (Fig. **5.5**), such a tooth become brittle because of:

1. Tooth preparation for endo. Treatment remove large a mount of tooth structure.
2. Dehydration of Dentin because of loss of the blood supply of the pulp result in loss of dentinal fluid circulation.
3. The large filling in endodontic treated tooth makes the situation worst.

The low grade inflammation (infection) (due to large amalgam restoration adjacent to pulp or in case of improper root canal treatment), result in stimulation of osteoblasts and osteocytes, which result in more production of osteoid deposition. The over activity of the osteoblasts and osteocytes is considered as a local defense mechanism to localized the inflammation. when the balance between the defense mechanism (local and systemic) and the inflammatory process is break down due to lowering of the defense of increasing in inflammation, this would result in abscess formation.

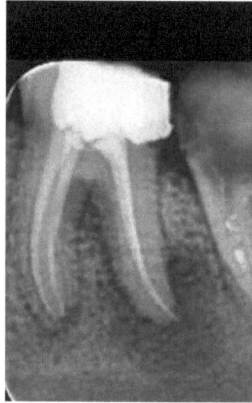

Fig. (5.5). Shows endodontic treated tooth with a large filling, such a tooth become brittle.

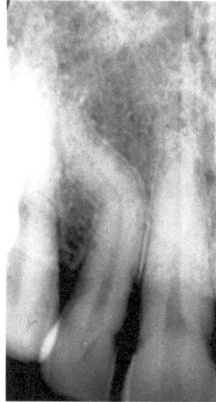

Fig. (5.6). Radiograph: showed dilacerated root: Difficulty and fracture of the apical one third should be suspected during tooth extraction. The proper choice to avoid these highly possible risk is starting the case as surgical extraction since such cases end with surgery.

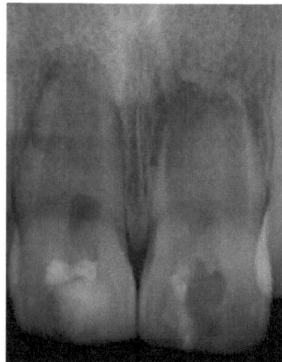

Fig. (5.7). Radiograph: showed gemination which usually associated with difficult extraction.

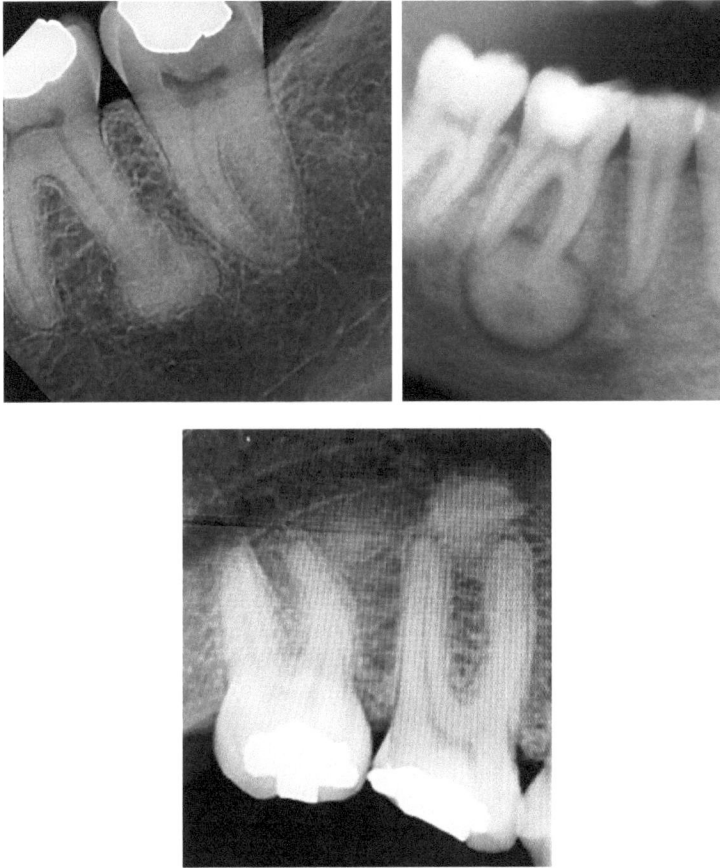

Fig. (5.8). (a) Hypercementosis periapical cementoma, (b) Hypercementosis: is a continuous deposition of the cementum result in large bulbous roots especially at the apical one third. (Paget's disease create unusual resistance during tooth extraction and the apical one third have wider diameter than the cervical third make the root delivery difficult, (c) Condensing osteitis: occurs as a result to low grade chronic inflammation.

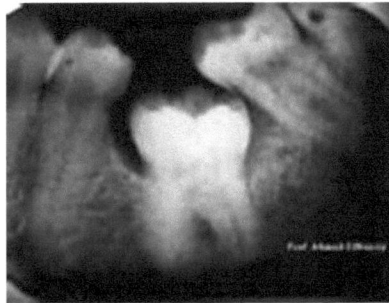

Fig. (5.9). Ankylosis: The tooth is fused to alveolar bone. There are no periodontal ligament space. In ankylosed tooth the extraction without fracture of the tooth or alveolar process is impossible.

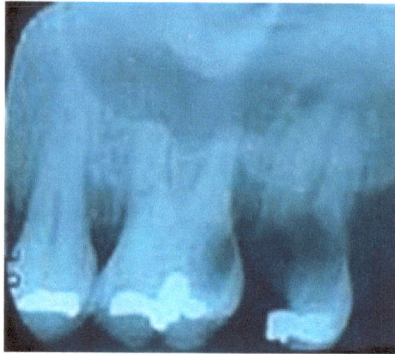

Fig. (5.10). This radiograph shows root which is almost inside the sinus and separated with a thin layer of bone, Oro-antral communication may be developed during extraction. Great care with atraumatic extraction should be used. The elevators are advisable to be avoided. Surgical extraction in some cases may be used to avoid excessive force (traumatic extraction). The surgical extraction also helps greatly in root sectioning and making the extraction easier with less force application and better visualization.

(List: 5.1): Causes of Hypercementosis

Systematic Factors

- Idiopathic
- Bone diseases: Paget's Disease
- Endocrine: Pituitary Gigantism, Calcinosis and Acromegaly
- Auto-immune: Arthritis and Rheumatic fever
- Periapical granuloma

Local Factors

- Chronic long standing Occlusal Trauma
- Unopposed tooth
- Non-functional tooth

(List: 5.2): Causes of Ankylosis

- Genetics
- Abnormal local metabolism of the Periodontal ligaments PDL
- Retained deciduous teeth
- Clinically, the ankylosed tooth can be diagnosed by the level of the occlusal surface which is located below the occlusal plane of other teeth.
- Radiographically, the narrowing of PDL space is a good indictor for diagnosis of ankyloses. In sever case the PDL space becomes absent, and the root becomes fused to surrounding bone.

The Bone Sclerosis

One of a local cause for difficult exodontias is the bone sclerosis. The most common causes for it are the following:

Systemic Causes (List: 5.3)

1. Physiological:
   - ○ It may also be present as a normal finding in old patient
2. Pathological:
   - a. Hormonal:
     - ▪ Hyperparathyroidism
     - ▪ Others
   - b. Autoimmune:
     - ▪ Sclerosis of phalangeal tufts may be noted in systemic lupus erythematosus,
     - ▪ Rheumatoid arthritis
     - ▪ Late stage of Pagets disease
   - c. Inflammatory:
     - ▪ Calcium pyrophosphate dihydrate crystal deposition disease
     - ▪ Sarcoidosis
     - ▪ Tuberculous spondylitis
   - d. Tumor and tumor like lesions:
     - ▪ Local:
       - • Fibrous Dysplasia
       - • Cemento-Osseous Dysplasias: **Includes -** Periapical Cemental Dysplasia (PCD), - Florid cemento-osseous dysplasia , - Focal Cemento-osseous dysplasia
       - • Cemento-ossifying fibroma
       - • Plasmacytoma
     - ▪ Systemic:
       - • Some forms of plasma cell myeloma
       - • Lymphoma
       - • Hodgkins disease
   - e. Others:
     - ▪ Ankylosing spondylitis
     - ▪ Renal osteodystrophy
     - ▪ POEMS syndrome (polyneuropathy, organomegaly, endocrinopathy, monoclonal gammopathy, and skin changes)

PART 3: PRINCIPLES OF ELEVATORS IN DENTAL EXTRACTIONS

Definition

Elevators are one end bladed instruments for extraction of roots mainly and teeth.

Introduction

In the extraction of teeth, there is no dispute that forceps are the the most reliable instruments for extraction. It is therefore absolutely mandatory to become skillful in the use of forceps before any trial to master the use of elevators. The elevators could be very harmful instruments in the inexpert hand. Elevators are primary associate to the forceps.

Design of the Elevators

Basically, there are two essential designs of elevators, the use of which should be skilled by every dental surgeon:

1. Straight
2. Curved (offset)

It is essential to Develop expertness and proficiency in the use of few elevators rather than attempt to use of many of them.

Each manufacture has his particular designs and names, but many of them are of the same kind and work on the same principles which are:

1. Lever fulcrum principle
2. Wedge principles
3. Wheal and axle principle

Indications for Elevators

1. To reflect mucoperiosteal membrane
2. To luxate teeth
3. To remove teeth:
    a. When the use of forceps is impossible due to abnormal position
    b. Crowded & Malposed teeth with lingualy, labially, buccally placed teeth. When it is impossible to apply the forceps without impinging on the adjacent teeth.
    c. Badly carious teeth and extensively damaged: very often there is no crown for holding.
4. To remove a roots

5. To loosen teeth prior to forceps application
6. To split teeth in case of roots sectioning
7. To remove intra-radicular bone or apical fractured root fragments

Dangers in the use of Elevators

1. Damaging or even extracting of the adjacent tooth.
2. Fractures of the bone (maxilla, mandible).
3. Fracture of alveolar process.
4. Slipping and plunging of the instrument into the soft tissue – danger of perforating large blood vessels or nerves.
5. Penetration into the maxillary antrum or forcing the root in the antrum.
6. Forcing the apical third of the root of the lower third molar into the mandibular canal.

Rules in the use of the Elevators

1. Never use adjacent tooth as a fulcrum unless that tooth is to be subsequently extracted.
2. Never use the upper border of the buccal or lingual plate as a fulcrum.
3. Never apply the elevator lingual, it should be always applied Mesiobuccally or Distobuccally.
4. The cutting edge (concave surface) of the blade must be in contact with the mesial or distal surface of the tooth to be extracted, and be seated between the tooth and alveolar bone.
5. Always use finger guards to protect the patients in case of using elevators
6. Be certain that the forces is applied by the elevators under control, and the elevators tip is exerting pressure in the correct direction.
7. When cutting though the inter-septal bone, take care not to engage the roots of the adjacent tooth, thus inadvertently forcing it out of its alveolus.

Parts of the Elevators

All elevators have the following parts:

1. Handle: usually bulky, it may be a continuation of the shank or at right angle to it.
2. Shank: this is analogous to the long arm of the lever.
3. Blade: this is the part that engages the crown or root. It is comparable to the short arm of the lever.

How does the elevators work with lever principles?
Generally, the elevators work like a lever, where solid bone acts as fulcrum (Fig. **5.11**).

If the:

Long arm of the elevator is LA.
The short arm SA.
The effort you put in E and the resistance exerted by the tooth is R:

Formula of the levers is (R x SA = LA)

Resistance × distance from resistance to fulcrum = effort × distance from effort to fulcrum× distance from resistance to fulcrum = effort × distance from effort to fulcrum

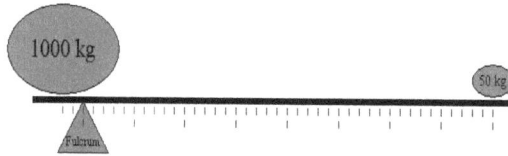

Fig. (5.11). Generally, the elevators work like a lever, where solid bone acts as fulcrum.

In order to gain the mechanical advantage, the effort arm LA must be longer than the resistance arm SA.

If effort E is applied against line of least resistance R, then the tooth will come out. The point at which force must be applied to effect delivery is called point of application of the elevator.

Point of application can be mesial, buccal, or distal. If the tooth moves out of the socket, it must move along a certain path depending on the shape and direction of the root. The path is called the line of withdrawal.

Work principles in the use of Elevators

1. Lever Principle (Fig. **5.11**)
2. Wedge Principle (Fig. **5.12**)
3. Wheel and Axle Principle (Fig. **5.13**)
4. Combination of any of 1, 2, 3

1. **The Elevator as Lever**

Generally, the elevators work like a lever, where solid bone acts as fulcrum.

If the:

Long arm of the elevator is LA.

The short arm SA.
The effort you put in E and the resistance exerted by the tooth is R:

Formula of the levers is (R x SA = LA)

Resistance × distance from resistance to fulcrum = effort × distance from effort to fulcrum× distance from resistance to fulcrum = effort × distance from effort to fulcrum

In order to gain the mechanical advantage, the effort arm LA must be longer than the resistance arm SA.

If effort E is applied against line of least resistance R, then the tooth will come out. The point at which force must be applied to effect delivery is called point of application of the elevator.

Point of application can be mesial, buccal, or distal. If the tooth moves out of the socket, it must move along a certain path depending on the shape and direction of the root. The path is called the line of withdrawal.

2. **The Elevator as Wedge (Fig. 5.12)**

The wedge elevator is forced between the root and the surrounding bone parallel to the long axis of the root.

As the instrument is forced down towards the apex, the root is displaced upwards.

Formula for wedge: R

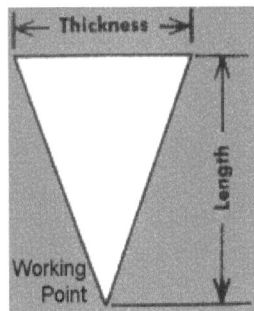
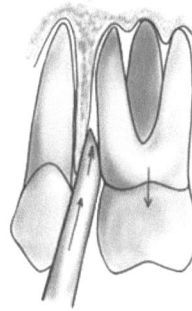

Fig. (5.12). The elevator as wedge.

(E x L x T = R x H)
elevator's thickness x elevator's length = root's length x thickness

OR

$$R/E = L/H$$

R = Resistance
E = Effort
L = Length
H = Height
T = Thickness
Mechanical advantage = L/R

Wedge elevators have mechanical advantage of 2.5. Therefore each pressure applied is multiplied by 2.5

3. Elevators as Wheel and Axle (Fig. 5.13)

Uses in conjunction with a wedge principle and sometimes with lever principle *e.g.* Cryer.

In wheel and axle, the mechanical advantage is obtained through the greater diameter of the handle over the blade.

When inserted horizontally between tooth and the bone the sharp blade engaged the point of application on the cementum with alveolar bone as fulcrum the handle is rotated to left the root out of the socket along it's line of withdrawal.

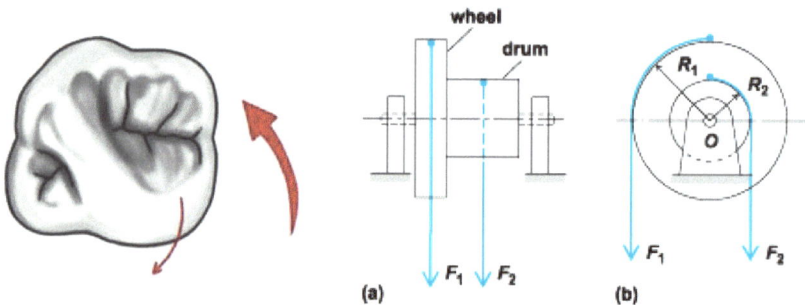

Fig. (5.13). 3 Elevators as wheel and axle.

Formula for wheel and axle:

$$F = E \times D/d$$

E= force applied at the elevator handle
D= Diameter of handle
d= diameter of blade
Mechanical advantage = D/d

The Cryer is constricted in such a way that mechanical advantage is 4.5. Therefore every force applied to the handle is multiplied by 4.5 times.

Classification of the Elevators

1. According to use:
   a. For removal of entire tooth *e.g.* Coupland, Cryer where there is a thick buccal plate to act as a fulcrum.
   b. For removal of roots broken off at gingival margin, *e.g.* Apexo elevator (R., L., Straight).
   c. For removal of root broken halfway to apex *e.g.* hospital pattern.
   d. For removal apical third of the root. *e.g.* apexo, warwich james elevators.
2. According to form:
   a. Straight: the blade, shank, and the handle are in one plane
   b. Angular: right and left
   c. Cross bar: handle at right angle to the shank

Path of removal (Fig. **5.14**):

• Path of removal is a very important determinant in the technique to be used in tooth extraction. The path of removal can be evaluated and determined by using a periapical radiograph, which give a good information about root inclination.

• If the root is inclined distally: this is mean that the force delivered by elevator to the tooth and/or the root should be occlusal and mesial, so the elevator must be applied distobuccally.

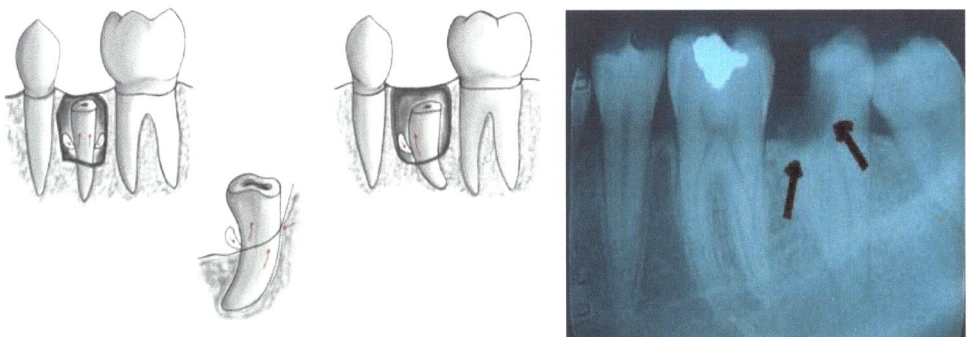

Fig. (5.14). Path of removal.

- If the root is inclined mesially: the force delivered by elevator to the tooth and/or the root should be occlusal and distal, so the elevator must be applied mesiobuccally.

- In multi-rooted teeth such as molars teeth, there are 2 or even 3 paths of removal. In these cases, it becomes recommended to separate the roots (Fig. **5.15**).

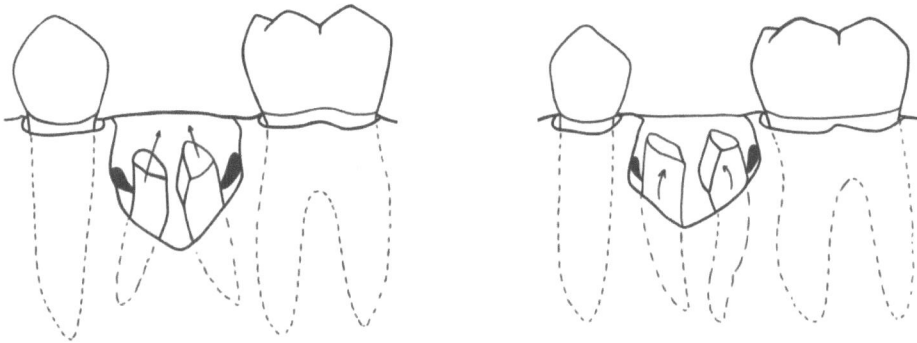

Fig. (5.15). Path of removal.

- The roots of the molar can be separated as following (Fig. **5.16**): The mesial root should be separated from the distal root. Straight fissure bur can be used. The bur should be entered deeply at bifurcation area until the bur drop suddenly due to change in the structures from tooth to bone (the tooth structure is usually harder than the bone surrounding the tooth) and the bleeding from the bifurcation area seen (Fig. **5.17**). The separation can be completed by using an elevator to ensure that the separation achieved. In mandibular molars a great care should be taken to protect the tongue during using of bur in sectioning (Fig. **5.19-5.25**).

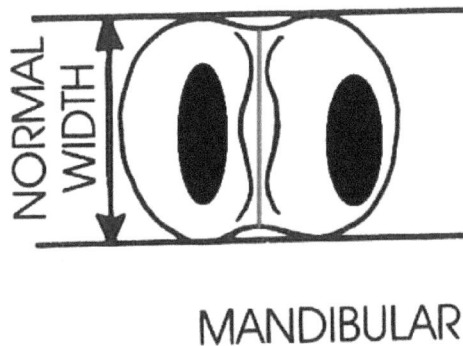

Fig. (5.16). Lower molar sectioning.

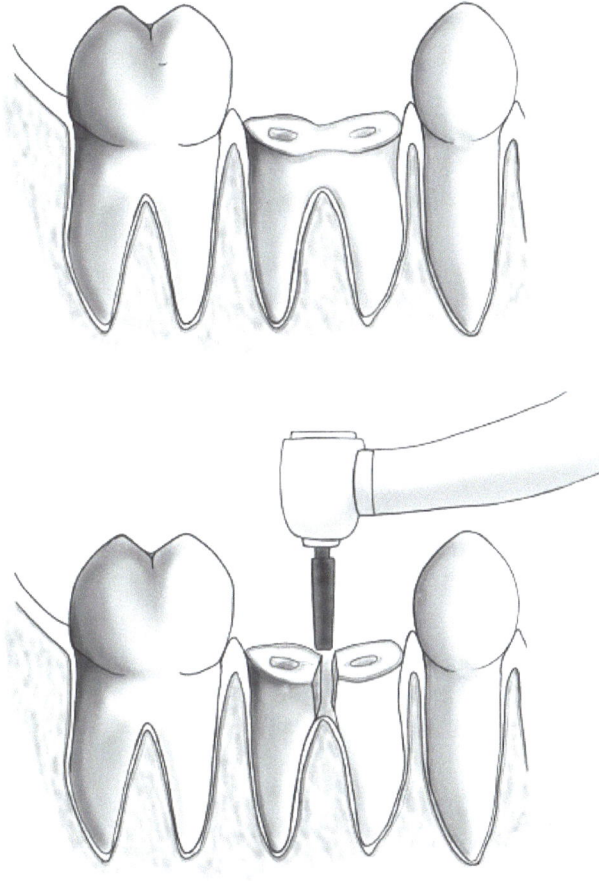

Fig. (5.17). Lower molar sectioning.

MAXILLARY

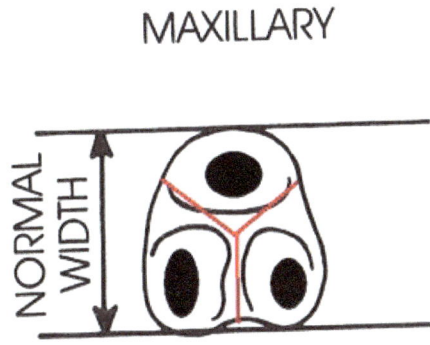

Fig. (5.18). Upper molar sectioning.

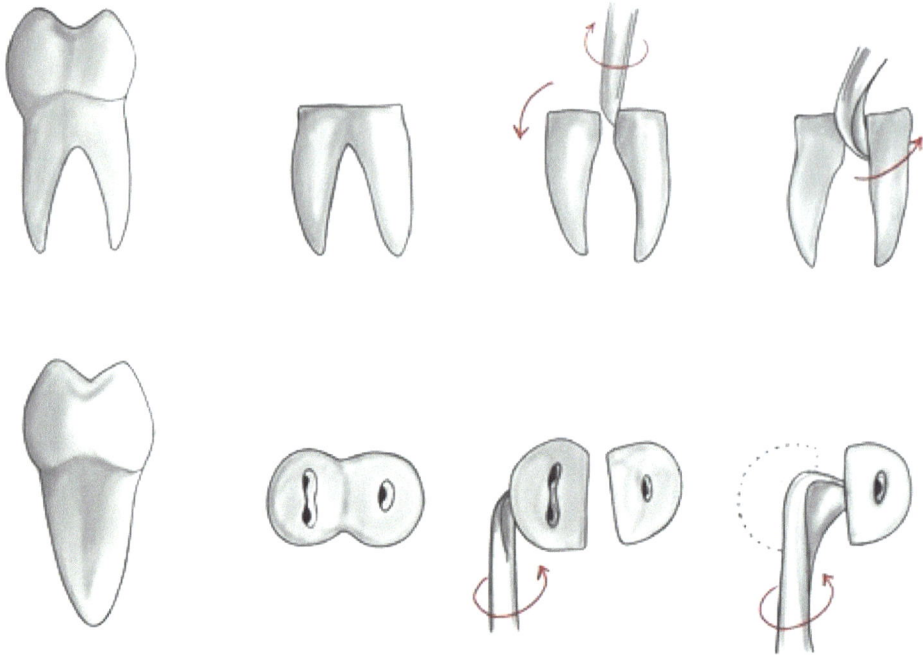

Fig. (5.19). Using of rotation technique in roots removal. Using the elevators usually started by wedging to engage the area below the cement-enamel junction then followed by rotation. The lever principle is rarely used in dental extraction.

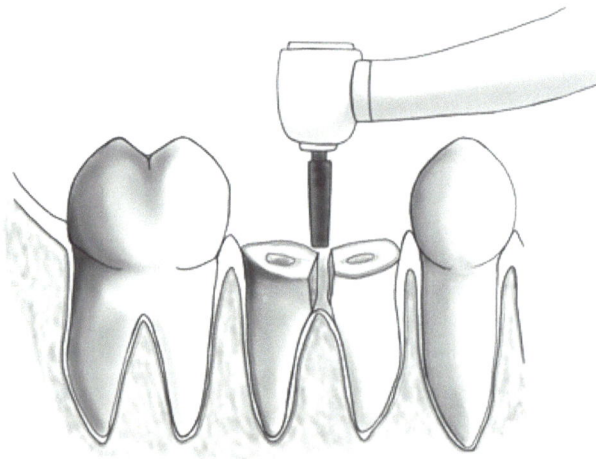

Fig. (5.20). Roots separation, long straight fissure burs should be used. The bur must be placed at bi-furcation area. The sectioning should be from lingual to buccal area and moves down to inter-radicular area where the area start to bleed. Great care and protection for the tongue and cheek should be down during sectioning. The sectioning should separated the roots as in Fig: 5.21.

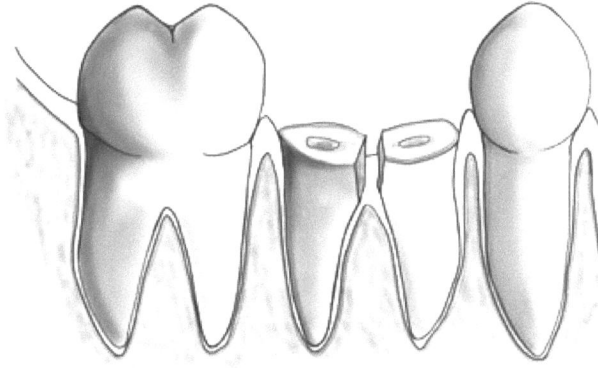

Fig. (5.21). Roots separation.

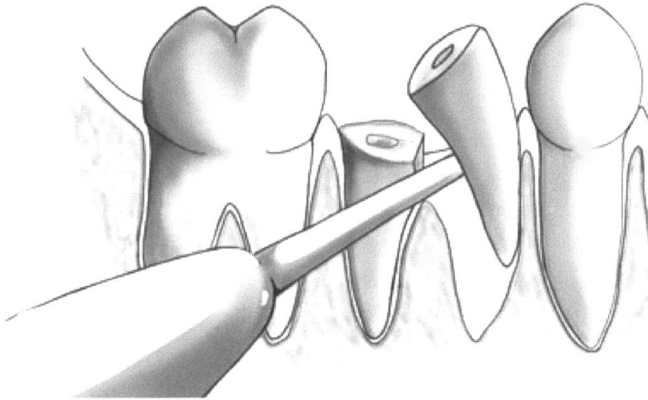

Fig. (5.22). Using of elevator for roots removal.

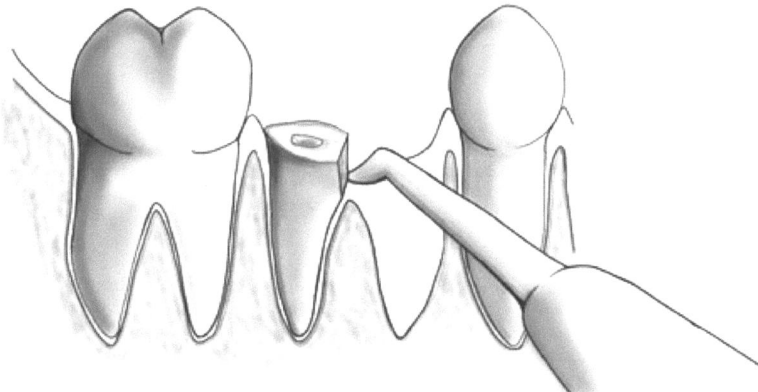

Fig. (5.23). Using of elevator for roots removal.

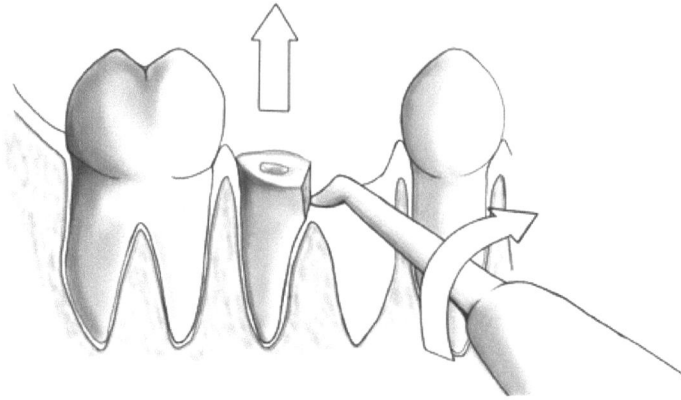

Fig. (5.24). Using of elevator for roots removal.

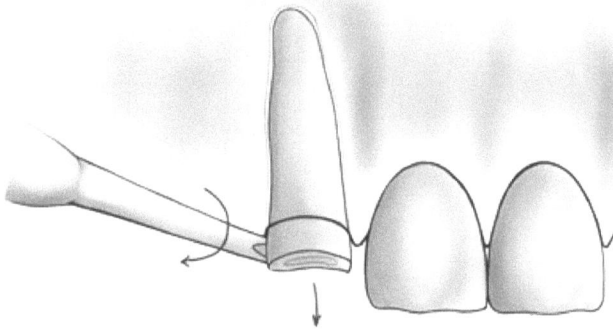

Fig. (5.25). Rotation for removal of Single root tooth, the procedure usually started with wedging.

For roots separation in maxillary molars, the mesial, the distal roots should be separated first by sectioning line extend buccopalataly until the center of tooth,s bifurcation area (area of connection of the three roots at the level of bifurcation). The palatal root is separated by extending of two sectioning line from the bifurcation connection area of the roots to antero-bucco-palatal direction and second to postero-buccao-palatal direction (As seen in the Fig. **5.18**).

BIBLIOGRAPHY

[1]   A Archer WH Oral and maxillofacial surgery. Philadelphia: Saunders 1975.

[2]   Gans BJ. Atlas of oral surgery. Saint Louis: C.V. Mosby Co. 1972.

[3]   Fragiskos FD. Oral surgery. Berlin: Springer 2007.
      [http://dx.doi.org/10.1007/978-3-540-49975-6]

[4]   Hooley JR, Whitacre RJ. A Self-instructional guide to oral surgery in general dentistry. Seattle, Wa.:
      Stoma Press 1979.

[5]   Howe GL. Minor oral surgery. 3rd ed., Oxford: Wright 1997.

[6]   Dimitroulis G. A synopsis of minor oral surgery. Oxford: Wright 1996.

[7]   Kruger GO. Textbook of oral and maxillofacial surgery. St. Louis: Mosby 1984.

[8]   Laskin DM. Oral and maxillofacial surgery. St. Louis: C.V. Mosby 1992.

[9]   Laskin DM, Abubaker AO. Decision making in oral and maxillofacial surgery. Chicago: Quintessence Pub. Co. 2007.

[10]   Kwon PH, Laskin DM. Clinician's manual of oral and maxillofacial surgery. Chicago: Quintessence Pub. Co. 1991.

[11]   Rounds CE, Rounds FW. Principles and technique of exodontia. St. Louis: Mosby 1962.

[12]   Peterson LJ. Contemporary oral and maxillofacial surgery. St. Louis: Mosby 1998.

[13]   Contemporary H. Oral and Maxillofacial Surgery. Elsevier 2014.

[14]   Sailer HF, Pajarola GF. Oral surgery for the general dentist. Stuttgart: Thieme 1998.

[15]   Dym H, Ogle OE. Oral surgery for the general dentist. Philadelphia: Saunders 2012.

[16]   Waite DE. Textbook of practical oral and maxillofacial surgery. 1987.

[17]   Aldrete JA, Johnson DA. Evaluation of Intracutaneous Testing for Investigation of Allergy to Local Anesthetic Agents. Anesth Analg 1970; 49(1.).
       [http://dx.doi.org/10.1213/00000539-197001000-00032]

[18]   Goswami A, Bora A, Kundu G, Ghosh S, Goswami A. Bleeding disorders in dental practice: A diagnostic overview. Journal of the International Clinical Dental Research Organization 2014; 6(2): 143.
       [http://dx.doi.org/10.4103/2231-0754.143529]

[19]   American Dental Association. Patients with pulmonary diseases Oral health care guidelines. Chicago, Ill.: American Dental Association 1982.

[20]   Scully C, Ettinger RL. The Influence of Systemic Diseases on Oral Health Care in Older Adults. J Am Dent Assoc 2007; 138.

[21]   American Dental Association Council on Dental Therapeutics. Accepted dental therapeutics. 40th ed. Chicago: American Dental Association Ill 1984; Vol. 5: pp. 203-9.

[22]   Angelopoulos AP, Spyropoulos ND. Oral diagnostics. 2nd ed., Athens: Litsas 1988.

[23]   Assem ES, Punnia-Moorthy A. Allergy to local anaesthetics: an approach to definitive diagnosis. A review with an illustrative study. Br Dent J 1988; 164(2): 44-7.
       [http://dx.doi.org/10.1038/sj.bdj.4806337]

[24]   Association of Hemophilia Clinic Directors of Canada. Hemophilia and von Willebrand's disease. 1. Diagnosis, comprehensive care and assessment. Can Med Assoc J 1995; 153: 19-25.

[25]   Bagg J. Tuberculosis, a re-emerging problem for health care workers. Br Dent J 1996; 180(10): 376-81.
       [http://dx.doi.org/10.1038/sj.bdj.4809093]

[26]   Baker PR, Maurer W, Warman J. Perioperative management of diabetes mellitus. Oral Maxillofac Surg Clin North Am 1998; 10(3): 363-71.

[27]   Yalow RS, Berson SA. Immunoassay of endogenous plasma insulin in man. J Clin Invest 1960; 39: 1157-75.
       [http://dx.doi.org/10.1172/JCI104130]

[28]   Philippe MF, Benabadji S, Barbot-Trystram L, Vadrot D, Boitard C, Larger E. Pancreatic volume and endocrine and exocrine functions in patients with diabetes. Pancreas 2011; 40: 359-63.

[http://dx.doi.org/10.1097/MPA.0b013e3182072032]

[29]   Ferrannini E. The stunned beta cell: a brief history. Cell Metab 2010; 11: 349-35210.
[http://dx.doi.org/10.1016/j.cmet.2010.04.009]

[30]   Talchai C, Xuan S, Lin HV, Sussel L, Accili D. Pancreatic beta cell dedifferentiation as a mechanism of diabetic beta cell failure. Cell 2012; 150: 1223-123410.
[http://dx.doi.org/10.1016/j.cell.2012.07.029]

[31]   Bavitz JB. Perioperative hematologic management. Oral Maxillofac Surg Clin North Am 1992; 4(3): 629-37.

[32]   Becker DE. Management of respiratory complications in clinical dental practice. Pathophysiological and technical considerations. Anesth Prog 1990; 37: 169-7.

[33]   Beekmann SE, Henderson DK. Managing Occupational Risks in the Dental Office: HIV and the Dental Professional. J Am Dent Assoc 1994; 125(7): 847-52.
[http://dx.doi.org/10.14219/jada.archive.1994.0210]

[34]   Benoliel LR, Leviner E, Katz J, Tzukert A. Dental treatment for the patient on anticoagulant therapy. Prothrombin time value (what difference does it make?). Oral Surg Oral Med Oral Pathol 1986; 62: 149-51.
[http://dx.doi.org/10.1016/0030-4220(86)90036-8]

[35]   Blair DM. Cardiac emergencies. Dent Clin North Am 1982; 26(1): 49-69.

[36]   Bodnar J. Corticosteroids and oral surgery. Anesth Prog 2001; 48(4): 130-2.

[37]   Borea G, Montebugnoli L, Capuzzi P, Magelli C. Tranexamic acid as a mouthwash in anticoagulant treated patients undergoing oral surgery. An alternative method to discontinuing anticoagulant therapy. Oral Surg Oral Med Oral Pathol 1993; 75: 29-31.
[http://dx.doi.org/10.1016/0030-4220(93)90401-O]

[38]   Boyd DH, Kinirons MJ, Gregg TA. Recent advances in the management of patients with haemophilia and other bleeding disorders. Dent Update 1994; 21: 254-7.

[39]   Braun TW, Demas PN. Perioperative hepatic evaluation. Oral Maxillofac Surg Clin North Am 1992; 4(3): 599-608.

[40]   Brewer AK, Roebuck EM, Donachie M, *et al.* The dental management of adult patients with haemophilia and other congenital bleeding disorders. Haemophilia 2003; 9(6): 673-7.
[http://dx.doi.org/10.1046/j.1351-8216.2003.00825.x]

[41]   Brooks SL. Survey of compliance with American Heart Association guidelines for the prevention of bacterial endocarditis. J Am Dent Assoc 1980; 101: 41-3.
[http://dx.doi.org/10.14219/jada.archive.1980.0361]

[42]   Brownbill JW. Dental extractions and anticoagulants. Aust Dent J 2003; 48(4): 267-8.

[43]   Burke GR, Guyassy PF. Surgery in the patient with renal disease and related electrolyte disorders. Med Clin North Am 1979; 63: 1191-203.
[http://dx.doi.org/10.1016/S0025-7125(16)31635-2]

[44]   Burke JF, Francos GC. Surgery in the patient with acute or chronic renal failure. Med Clin North Am 1987; 71: 489-97.
[http://dx.doi.org/10.1016/S0025-7125(16)30853-7]

[45]   Caldarola F, Tealdi R, Molinatti MP. (INR) in extractive dental surgery in patients treated with oral anticoagulants. Minerva Stomatol 1994; 43: 167-9.

[46]   Campbell JH, Huizinga PJ, Das SK, Rodriguez JP, Gobetti JP. Incidence and significance of cardiac arrhythmia in geriatric oral surgery patients. Oral Surg Oral Med Oral Pathol Oral Radiol Endod 1996; 82(1): 42-6.
[http://dx.doi.org/10.1016/S1079-2104(96)80376-3]

[47]   Campbell RL, Langston WG. A comparison of cardiac rate-pressure product and pressure-rate quotient in healthy and medically compromised patients. Oral Surg Oral Med Oral Pathol Oral Radiol Endod 1995; 80: 145-52.
[http://dx.doi.org/10.1016/S1079-2104(05)80193-3]

[48]   Canfield D, Gage T. Guideline to local anesthetic testing. Anesth Prog 1987; 34: 157-63.

[49]   Caughman WF, McCoy BP, Sisk AL, Lutcher CL. When a patient with a bleeding disorder needs dental work. How you can work with the dentist to prevent a crisis. Postgrad Med 1990; 88: 175-82.
[http://dx.doi.org/10.1080/00325481.1990.11716431]

[50]   Cawson RA. Infective endocarditis as a complication of dental treatment. Br Dent J 1981; 151: 409-14.
[http://dx.doi.org/10.1038/sj.bdj.4804724]

[51]   Cawson RA. The antibiotic prophylaxis of infective endocarditis. Br Dent J 1983; 154: 253-8.
[http://dx.doi.org/10.1038/sj.bdj.4805046]

[52]   Cerrulli M. Management of the patient with liver disease. Oral Maxillofac Surg Clin North Am 1998; 10(3): 465-70.

[53]   Cesareo BV, Pettini M, Soreca G, *et al.* An outpatient regimen for dental improvements in patients with valvular cardiopathies and oral anticoagulant therapy (a preliminary note). Minerva Stomatol 1994; 43: 409-15.

[54]   Council on Dental Therapeutics. Prevention of bacterial endocarditis, a committee report of the American Heart Association. J Am Dent Assoc 1984; 110: 98-100.

[55]   Council on Dental Therapeutics, American Heart Association. Preventing bacterial endocarditis, a statement for the dental professional. J Am Dent Assoc 1991; 122: 87-92.
[http://dx.doi.org/10.14219/jada.archive.1991.0059]

[56]   Cowper TR. Pharmacologic management of the patient with disorders of the cardiovascular system. Infectiveendocarditis. Dent Clin North Am 1996; 40(3): 611-47.

[57]   Cowper TR, Terezhalmy GT. Pharmacotherapy for hypertension. Dent Clin North Am 1996; 40(3): 585-610.

[58]   Crociani P, Bolzan M, Schivazappa L. Sampling study on practitioners' attitude to the prevention of infectious endocarditis. G Ital Cardiol 1994; 24: 853-68.

[59]   Dajani AS. Prevention of bacterial endocarditis. Recommendations by the American Heart Association. JAMA 1997; 277(22): 1794-801.
[http://dx.doi.org/10.1001/jama.1997.03540460058033]

[60]   De Rossi S, Glick M. Dental considerations for the patient with renal disease receiving hemodialysis. J Am Dent Assoc 1996; 127: 211-9.
[http://dx.doi.org/10.14219/jada.archive.1996.0171]

[61]   Dionne R, Phero JC. Management of pain and anxiety in dental practice. New York: Elsevier 1991.

[62]   Doyl KA, Goepferd SJ. An allergy to local anesthetics? The consequences of a misdiagnosis. ASDC J Dent Child 1989; 56: 103-6.

[63]   Dym H. The hypertensive patient. Treatment modalities. Oral Maxillofac Surg Clin North Am 1998; 10(3): 349-62.

[64]   Findler M, Galili D, Meidan Z, Yakirevitch V, Garfunkel AA. Dental treatment in very high risk patients with active ischemic heart disease. Oral Surg Oral Med Oral Pathol 1993; 76: 298-300.
[http://dx.doi.org/10.1016/0030-4220(93)90257-5]

[65]   Findler M, Garfunkel AA, Galili D. Review of very high-risk cardiac patients in the dental setting. Compendium 1994; 15: 58-66.

[66]   Friedman LS, Maddrey WC. Surgery in the patient with liver disease. Med Clin North Am 1987; 71: 453-76.
[http://dx.doi.org/10.1016/S0025-7125(16)30851-3]

[67]   Glick M. Glucocorticoid replacement therapy, A literature review and suggested replacement therapy. Oral Surg Oral Med Oral Pathol 1989; 67: 614-20.
[http://dx.doi.org/10.1016/0030-4220(89)90285-5]

[68]   Goldmann DR, Brown FH, Guarnieri DM. Perioperative medicine: the medical care of the surgical patient. New York: McGraw-Hill, Health Professions Division 1994.

[69]   Gould IM. Current prophylaxis for prevention of infective endocarditis. Br Dent J 1990; 168: 409-10.
[http://dx.doi.org/10.1038/sj.bdj.4807219]

[70]   Goulet JP, Perusse R, Turcotte JY. Contraindications to vasoconstrictors in dentistry. Part III, Pharmacologic considerations. Oral Surg Oral Med Oral Pathol 1992; 74: 692-7.
[http://dx.doi.org/10.1016/0030-4220(92)90367-Y]

[71]   Hall MB. Perioperative cardiovascular evaluation. Oral Maxillofac Surg Clin North Am 1992; 4(3): 577-90.

[72]   Halpern LR, Chase DC. Perioperative management of patients with endocrine dysfunction. Physiology, presurgical, and postsurgical treatment protocols. Oral Maxillofac Surg Clin North Am 1998; 10(3): 491-500.

[73]   Hasse AL, Heng MK, Garrett NR. Blood pressure and electrocardiographic response to dental treatment with use of local anesthesia. J Am Dent Assoc 1986; 113: 639-42.
[http://dx.doi.org/10.14219/jada.archive.1986.0245]

[74]   Hatch CL, Canaan T, Anderson G. Pharmacology of the pulmonary diseases. Dent Clin North Am 1996; 40(3): 521-41.

[75]   Herman WH, Konjelman JL. Angina, an update for dentistry. J Am Dent Assoc 1996; 127: 98-104.
[http://dx.doi.org/10.14219/jada.archive.1996.0037]

[76]   Hirsch IB, McGill JB, Cryer PE, White PF. Perioperative management of surgical patients with diabetes mellitus. Anesthesiology 1991; 74: 346-59.
[http://dx.doi.org/10.1097/00000542-199102000-00023]

[77]   Hirsch J. Oral anticoagulant drugs. N Engl J Med 1991; 324: 1865-75.
[http://dx.doi.org/10.1056/NEJM199106273242606]

[78]   Hodgson TA, Shirlaw PJ, Challacombe SJ. Skin testing after anaphylactoid reactions to dental local anesthetics. A comparison with controls. Oral Surg Oral Med Oral Pathol 1993; 75: 706-11.
[http://dx.doi.org/10.1016/0030-4220(93)90427-6]

[79]   Hollins RR, Lydiatt DD. Evaluation of surgical risk in the oral and maxillofacial surgery patient. Oral Maxillofac Surg Clin North Am 1992; 4: 571-6.

[80]   Huber MA, Drake AJ. Pharmacology of the endocrine pancreas, adrenal cortex, and female reproductive organ. Dent Clin North Am 1996; 40(3): 753-77.

[81]   Hupp JR. Advances in cardiovascular pharmacological therapy. J Oral Maxillofac Surg 1992; 50: 157-62.
[http://dx.doi.org/10.1016/0278-2391(92)90362-4]

[82]   Jackson D, Chen AH, Bennett CR. Identifying true lidocaine allergy. J Am Dent Assoc 1994; 125: 1362-6.
[http://dx.doi.org/10.14219/jada.archive.1994.0180]

[83]   Jastak JT, Yagiela JA. Vasoconstrictors and local anesthesia, a review and rationale for use. J Am Dent Assoc 1983; 107: 623-30.
[http://dx.doi.org/10.14219/jada.archive.1983.0307]

[84] Katz J, Terezhalmy G. Dental management of the patient with hemophilia. Oral Surg Oral Med Oral Pathol 1988; 66: 139-44.
[http://dx.doi.org/10.1016/0030-4220(88)90081-3]

[85] Kelly JP. Perioperative pulmonary evaluation. Oral Maxillofac Surg Clin North Am 1992; 4(3): 591-7.

[86] Kelly MA. Common laboratory tests – their use in the detection and management of patients with bleeding disorders. Gen Dent 1990; 38: 282-5.

[87] Key SJ, Hodder SC, Davies R, Thomas DW, Thompson S. Perioperative corticosteroid supplementation and dento-alveolar surgery. Dent Update 2003; 30(6): 316-20.
[http://dx.doi.org/10.12968/denu.2003.30.6.316]

[88] Knoll-Kohler E, Knoller M, Brandt K, Becker J. Cardiohemodynamic and serum catecholamine response to surgical removal of impacted mandibular third molars under local anesthesia, a randomized double-blind parallel group and crossover study. J Oral Maxillofac Surg 1991; 49: 957-62.
[http://dx.doi.org/10.1016/0278-2391(91)90059-U]

[89] Koerner KR, Taylor SE. Pharmacological considerations in the management of oral surgery patients in general dental practice. Dent Clin North Am 1994; 38: 237-54.

[90] Kouimtzis TA, Oulis CJ. Management of child with bleeding disorder at the dental office. Pedodontia 1995; 9: 134-42.

[91] Kouvelas N, Vierrou AM. Hemophilic patients. Treatment protocol in the dental office. Hell Stomatol Chron 1988; 32(3): 221-7.

[92] Lamster IB, Begg MD, Mitchell-Lewis D, *et al.* Oral manifestations of HIV infection in homosexual men and intravenous drug users. Study design and relationship of epidemiologic, clinical, and immunologic parameters to oral lesions. Oral Surg Oral Med Oral Pathol 1994; 78: 163-74.
[http://dx.doi.org/10.1016/0030-4220(94)90140-6]

[93] Laskaris G, Damoulis D. AIDS and preventive measures for infections at the dental office. Results of points of view, knowledge and behavior of 717 dentists. Hell Stomatol Chron 1993; 37: 88-95.

[94] Little JW, Falace DA. Dental management of the medically compromised patient. 4th ed., St Louis: Mosby 1993.

[95] Little JW, Falace DA, Miller CS, Rhodus NL. Dental management of the medically compromised patient. 5th ed., St Louis: Mosby, St Louis 1997.

[96] Luke KH. Comprehensive care for children with bleeding disorders. A physician's perspective. J Can Dent Assoc 1992; 58: 115-8.

[97] Lyttle JJ. Anesthesia morbidity and mortality in the oral surgery office. Oral Maxillofac Surg Clin North Am 1992; 4: 759-68.

[98] MacKay S, Eisendrath S. Adverse reaction to dental corticosteroids. Gen Dent 1992; 40: 136-8.

[99] Mark AM. Reducing the risk of endocarditis, a review of the AHA guidelines. J Am Dent Assoc 1995; 126: 1148-9.
[http://dx.doi.org/10.14219/jada.archive.1995.0335]

[100] Lipp M. Daubländer Monika, Fuder H Local anesthesia in dentistry. Chicago: Quintessence Pub. Co. 1993.

[101] Martinowitz U, Mazar AL, Taicher S, *et al.* Dental extraction for patients on oral anticoagulant therapy. Oral Surg Oral Med Oral Pathol 1990; 70: 274-7.
[http://dx.doi.org/10.1016/0030-4220(90)90139-J]

[102] McCabe JC, Roser SM. Evaluation and management of the cardiac patient for surgery. Oral Maxillofac Surg Clin North Am 1998; 10(3): 429-43.

[103] McKown CG, Shapiro AD. Oral management of patients with bleeding disorders. Dental

considerations. J Indiana Dent Assoc 1991; 70: 16-21.

[104] Meiller TF, Overholser CD. The dental patient with hypertension. Dent Clin North Am 1983; 27(2): 289-301.

[105] Milam SB, Cooper RL. Extensive bleeding following extractions in a patient undergoing chronic hemodialysis. Oral Surg 1983; 55: 14-6.
[http://dx.doi.org/10.1016/0030-4220(83)90298-0]

[106] Moore PA. Preventing local anesthesia toxicity. J Am Dent Assoc 1992; 123(9): 60-4.
[http://dx.doi.org/10.14219/jada.archive.1992.0239]

[107] Naylor GD, Fredericks MR. Pharmacologic considerations in the dental management of the patient with disorders of the renal system. Dent Clin North Am 1996; 40(3): 665-83.

[108] Niwa H, Sato Y, Matsuura H. Safety of dental treatment in patients with previously diagnosed acute myocardial infarction or unstable angina pectoris. Oral Surg Oral Med Oral Pathol Oral Radiol Endod 2000; 89(1): 35-41.
[http://dx.doi.org/10.1016/S1079-2104(00)80011-6]

[109] Ogle O, Hernandez AR. Management of patients with hemophilia, anticoagulation, and sickle cell disease. Oral Maxillofac Surg Clin North Am 1998; 10(3): 401-16.

[110] Ostuni E. Stroke and the dental patient. J Am Dent Assoc 1994; 125: 721-7.
[http://dx.doi.org/10.14219/jada.archive.1994.0119]

[111] Pallasch TJ. A critical appraisal of antibiotic prophylaxis. Int Dent J 1989; 39: 183-96.

[112] Parkin JD, Smith IL, O'Neill AI, Ibrahim KM, Butcher LA. Mild bleeding disorders. A clinical and laboratory study. Med J Aust 1992; 156: 614-7.

[113] Patton LL, Ship JA. Treatment of patients with bleeding disorders. Dent Clin North Am 1994; 38: 465-82.

[114] Pavek V, Bigl P. Stomatological treatment of patients with artificial heart valves, coagulation control and antibiotic cover. Int Dent J 1993; 43: 59-61.

[115] Phelan JA, Jimenez V, Tompkins DC. Tuberculosis. Dent Clin North Am 1996; 40(2): 327-41.

[116] Pirrot S. Asthmatic crisis. Rev Odontostomatol (Paris) 1991; 20: 381-3.

[117] Prusinski L, Eisold JF. Hyperlipoproteinemic states and ischemic heart disease. Dent Clin North Am 1996; 40(3): 563-84.

[118] Pyle MA, Faddoul FF, Terezhalmy GT. Clinical implications of drugs taken by our patients. Dent Clin North Am 1993; 37(1): 73-90.

[119] Rahn R, Schneider S, Diehl O, Schafer V, Shah PM. Preventing post-treatment bacteremia. J Am Dent Assoc 1995; 126(8): 1145-9.
[http://dx.doi.org/10.14219/jada.archive.1995.0334]

[120] Rakocz M, Mazar A, Varon D, Spierer S, Blinder D, Martinowitz U. Dental extractions in patients with bleeding disorders. The use of fibrin glue. Oral Surg Oral Med Oral Pathol 1993; 75: 280-2.
[http://dx.doi.org/10.1016/0030-4220(93)90135-Q]

[121] Ramstrom G, Sindet-Pedersen S, Hall G, Blomback M, Alander U. Prevention of postsurgical bleeding in oral surgery using tranexamic acid without dose modification of oral anticoagulants. J Oral Maxillofac Surg 1993; 51: 1211-6.
[http://dx.doi.org/10.1016/S0278-2391(10)80291-5]

[122] Recommendations of the American Heart Association. Prevention of bacterial endocarditis. JAMA 1990; 264: 2919-22.
[http://dx.doi.org/10.1001/jama.1990.03450220085028]

[123] Recommendations from the Endocarditis Working Party of the British Society for Antimicrobial

Chemotherapy. Antibiotic prophylaxis of infective endocarditis. Br Dent J 1990; 169: 70-1.

[124] Recommendations from the Endocarditis Working Party of the British Society for Antimicrobial Chemotherapy. Antibiotic prophylaxis of infective endocarditis. Lancet 1990; 335: 88-9.
[http://dx.doi.org/10.1016/0140-6736(90)90549-K]

[125] Report of a Working Conference Jointly Sponsored by the American Dental Association and American Heart Association. Management of dental problems in patients with cardiovascular disease. J Am Dent Assoc 1964; 68: 333-42.
[http://dx.doi.org/10.14219/jada.archive.1964.0104]

[126] Riben PD, Epstein JB, Mathias RG. Dentistry and tuberculosis in the 1900 s. J Can Dent Assoc 1995; 61(6): 492-, 495-498.

[127] Rogerson KC. Hemostasis for dental surgery. Dent Clin North Am 1995; 39: 649-62.

[128] Romriell GE, Streeper SN. The medical history. Dent Clin North Am 1982; 26(1): 3-11.

[129] Rosenberg MB. Risk to the surgeon anesthetist. Oral Maxillofac Surg Clin North Am 1992; 4: 809-13.

[130] Royer JE, Bates WS. Management of von Willebrand's disease with desmopressin. J Oral Maxillofac Surg 1988; 46: 313-4.
[http://dx.doi.org/10.1016/0278-2391(88)90016-X]

[131] Ruggiero SL. Evaluation, treatment, and management of the asthmatic patient. Oral Maxillofac Surg Clin North Am 1998; 10(3): 337-48.

[132] Ruskin JD, Green JG. Perioperative considerations in the immunocompromised patient. Oral Maxillofac Surg Clin North Am 1992; 4(3): 639-49.

[133] Ryan DE, Bronstein SL. Dentistry and the diabetic patient. Dent Clin North Am 1982; 26(1): 105-18.

[134] Sanders BJ, Weddell JA, Dodge NN. Managing patients who have seizure disorders, dental and medical issues. J Am Dent Assoc 1995; 126: 1641-7.
[http://dx.doi.org/10.14219/jada.archive.1995.0112]

[135] Sansevere JJ, Milles M. Management of the oral and maxillofacial surgery patient with sickle cell disease and related hemoglobinopathies. J Oral Maxillofac Surg 1993; 51(8): 912-6.
[http://dx.doi.org/10.1016/S0278-2391(10)80114-4]

[136] Saour JN, Ali HA, Mammo LA, Sieck JO. Dental procedures in patients receiving oral anticoagulation therapy. J Heart Valve Dis 1994; 3: 315-7.

[137] Scully C, McCarthy G. Management of oral health in persons with HIV infection. Oral Surg Oral Med Oral Pathol 1992; 73(2): 215-25.
[http://dx.doi.org/10.1016/0030-4220(92)90197-X]

[138] Shannon ME. Strokes. Dent Clin North Am 1982; 26(1): 99-104.

[139] Shapiro AD, McKown CG. Oral management of patients with bleeding disorders. Part 1: Medical considerations. J Indiana Dent Assoc 1991; 70: 28-31.

[140] Shapiro N. When the bleeding won't stop. A case report on a patient with hemophilia. J Am Dent Assoc 1993; 124: 64-7.
[http://dx.doi.org/10.14219/jada.archive.1993.0238]

[141] Scheitler LE. Unusual allergic reaction follows allergy testing. J Am Dent Assoc 1991; 122: 88-90.

[142] Sheller B, Tong D. Dental management of a child on anticoagulant therapy and the International Normalized Ratio. Case report. Pediatr Dent 1994; 16(1): 56-8.

[143] Sherman RG, Lasseter DH. Pharmacologic management of patients with diseases of the endocrine system. Dent Clin North Am 1996; 40(3): 727-52.

[144] Siefkin AD, Bolt RJ. Preoperative evaluation of the patient with gastrointestinal or liver disease. Med Clin North Am 1979; 63: 1309-20.

[http://dx.doi.org/10.1016/S0025-7125(16)31643-1]

[145] Silverstein KE, Adams MC, Fonseca RJ. Evaluation and management of the renal failure and dialysis patient. Oral Maxillofac Surg Clin North Am 1998; 10(3): 417-27.

[146] Simard-Savoie S. Mechanisms of drug interactions of interest to dentists. Can Dent Assoc J 1987; 53: 43-56.

[147] Sonis ST, Fazio RC, Fang L. Principles and practice of oral medicine. 2nd ed., Philadelphia, Pa: Saunders 1995.

[148] Sowell SB. Dental care for patients with renal failure and renal transplants. J Am Dent Assoc 1982; 104: 171-7.
[http://dx.doi.org/10.14219/jada.archive.1982.0030]

[149] Speirs RL. Haemostasis. Dent Update 1991; 18: 166-71.

[150] Stamler J, Stamler R, Neate J. Blood pressures systolic and diastolic, and cardiovascular risks, US population data. Arch Intern Med 1993; 153: 598-615.
[http://dx.doi.org/10.1001/archinte.1993.00410050036006]

[151] Steinberg MJ, Moores JF. Use of INR to assess degree of anticoagulation in patients who have dental procedures. Oral Surg Oral Med Oral Pathol Oral Radiol Endod 1995; 80: 175-7.
[http://dx.doi.org/10.1016/S1079-2104(05)80198-2]

[152] Stone JD. Perioperative renal evaluation. Oral Maxillofac Surg Clin North Am 1992; 4(3): 609-20.

[153] Stout F, Doering P. The problematic drug history. Dent Clin North Am 1983; 27(2): 387-402.

[154] Svirsky JA, Saravia ME. Dental management of patients after liver transplantation. Oral Surg Oral Med Oral Pathol 1989; 67: 541-6.
[http://dx.doi.org/10.1016/0030-4220(89)90270-3]

[155] Tan SY, Gill G. Selection of dental procedures for antibiotic prophylaxis against infective endocarditis. J Dent 1992; 20: 375-6.
[http://dx.doi.org/10.1016/0300-5712(92)90032-8]

[156] Tealdi R, Caldarola F. Our protocol in outpatient oral surgery interventions on patients in treatment with oral anticoagulants. Minerva Stomatol 1993; 42: 541-6.

[157] Terezhalmy GT, Lichtin AE. Antithrombotic, anticoagulant, and thrombolytic agents. Dent Clin North Am 1996; 40(3): 649-64.

[158] Thoma KH. Oral surgery. 5th ed. St Louis, Mo.: Mosby 1969; Vol. 1.

[159] Tierney LM Jr, McPhee SJ, Papadakis MA. Current medical diagnosis and treatment. 36th ed., London: Prentice- Hall 1997.

[160] Tupputi M, di Martino MR, Mostarda A, Piras V. Anesthesia and pregnancy in oral medicine. Minerva Anestesiol 1992; 58: 1051-6.

[161] Ublansky JH. Comprehensive dental care for children with bleeding disorders – a dentist's perspective. J Can Dent Assoc 1992; 58: 111-4.

[162] Umino M, Nagao M. Systemic diseases in elderly dental patients. Int Dent J 1993; 43: 213-8.

[163] Vicente Barrero M, Knezevic M, Tapia Martin M, *et al.* Oral surgery in patients undergoing oral anticoagulant therapy. Med Oral 2002; 7(1): 63-66, 67-70.

[164] Vlahou A, Kokali A, Oulis C. Dental problems and management of children with chronic renal insufficiency. Pedodontia 1992; 6: 61-7.

[165] Wahl MJ, Howell J. Altering anticoagulation therapy, a survey of physicians. J Am Dent Assoc 1996; 127: 625-38.
[http://dx.doi.org/10.14219/jada.archive.1996.0275]

[166] Weaver T, Eisold JF. Congestive heart failure and disorders of the heart beat. Dent Clin North Am 1996; 40(3): 543-61.

[167] Weibert RT. Oral anticoagulant therapy in patients undergoing dental surgery. Clin Pharm 1992; 11: 857-64.

[168] Weitekamp MR, Caputo GM. Antibiotic prophylaxis, update on common clinical uses. Am Fam Physician 1993; 48: 597-604.

[169] Younai FS, Murphy DC. TB and dentistry. N Y State Dent J 1997; 63(1): 49-53.

[170] Zeitler DL. Perioperative evaluation of the endocrine patient. Oral Maxillofac Surg Clin North Am 1992; 4(3): 621-7.

[171] Zusman SP, Lustig JP, Baston I. Postextraction hemostat in patients on anticoagulant therapy, the use of a fibrin sealant. Quintessence Int 1992; 23: 713-7.

PART 4: THE OUTLINE OF COMPLICATIONS OF EXODONTIAS

Complications of dental extractions can be classified into:

1. Pre-Operative causes of Complications
2. Intra-Operative Complications & Challenges (read chapter 5)
3. Post-Operative Complications

1. **Pre-Operative Causes of Complications**
   a. Systemic Factors
   b. Local Factors
   c. Radiographic Factors
   a. **Systemic Factors**
   - Improper or non-accurate medical history taking (the systemic condition of the patient and psychology). It can be due to lack of the training and/or lack of skill in history taking.
   - Improper assessment of the difficulties: psychology of the patient, attitude, behavior, build, age and gender, systemic condition, past medical and past dental history
   - Lack of training and/or skills in management of critically ill patient and emergencies in dental chair (read the complex extraction page: 131).
   a. **Local Factors**
   - Examination of a wrong patient and/or wrong file (it is uncommon occasion may occur in busy clinic with negligent and loss of regulation/policy and procure).
   - Improper diagnosis and wrong decisions
   - Improper assessment of the local difficulties which including: Size, site, shape and situations of the tooth, relation to surrounding vital structures, bone to tooth relationship (PDL space)
   - Unavailability of proper/sutaible instruments or availability of corroded sets
   a. **Radiographic Factors**
   - No radiograph
   - Improper radiograph
   - Incorrect radiograph
   - Improper interpretation of the radiographic information

2. **Intra-Operative Complications & Challenges (read page 123)** Can be related to one of the following:
   a. Patient's factors (Systemic & Local)
   b. Surgeon's factors (the dentist)
   c. Surgical team factors (surgical nurse or dental assistant)
   d. Equipment's factors (the Dental clinic, Chair, Facilities)

a. **Patient's Factors**
  ▪ Systemic Intra-operative Complications & Challenges have been discussed in details in complex Extractions (page: 130), (both the psychology and Systemic conditions)
  Difficulty in Surgical procedures as have been mentioned chapter (7) is the presence of factor that may create possible Challenges intra-Operatively, and/or may result in development of possible complications post-Operatively which include:
  • Build, age and gender,
  • Psychology, attitude and behavior
  • Systemic condition of the patients
  • Past & Current medications
  ▪ **Local Patient's Factors**
  • Difficulty of accessibility
  • Abnormal resistance
  • Fracture of the tooth where normal and ideal extraction method are used: the tooth may be fracture owning to –advanced caries, -large restoration, -devitalized tooth, periodontal disease, dilaceration, age or when it is associated with certain pathology such as hypercementosis.
  • Fracture of the alveolar process or Fracture of the mandible where normal and ideal extraction method are used: this is most likely to occur in old patients whom the bone loss it's resiliency and become sclerotic. In young patient this may occur with certain pathological lesion which weaken the mandible such as a cysts or tumors.
  • Dislocation of the TMJ: seen in those patients with TMJ hypermobility disorders
  • Oro-antral fistula: most likely seen when the floor of the antrum abnormally low and the roots of the tooth located inside the sinus (normal anatomical variation).
  • Haemorrhage: causes of bleeding (read the post-operative Complications)
a. **Dentist's and Technique Factors** It is a dentist's responsibility to determent and to perform a proper evaluation of each condition.
  Complications related to dentist and technique: mainly occur due to traumatic extraction (excessive force and/or using of short jerky movement, and/or using of wrong instruments).
  The possible complications include the following:
  1. Damaging of the tooth: Damaging of adjacent tooth, extraction of the adjacent tooth, extraction of a wrong tooth, dislocation of the adjacent tooth or adjacent filling.
  2. Fracture of the alveolar process,

3. Fracture of the mandible,
4. Dislocation of the TMJ.
5. Damaging of the inferior alveolar vasa-nervorum,
6. Injuries of the soft tissues,
7. Hemorrhage,
8. Surgical emphysema,
9. Broken instruments,
10. Long surgical procedure,
11. Oro-antral fistula,
12. Root in the antrum
13. Inability to extract
14. Traumatic extraction increase the risks of post-operative complications

b. In cases of Loss of tooth or roots after dental extraction, the following should be examined:
   - The mouth including under the muco-periostium,
   - Suction apparatus,
   - Alimentary tract
   - and Lung by using X-ray,
   - Tissues spaces,
   - Bone cavities.

3. Post-Operative Complications

a. **Post-Operative Systemic Complications** Most of the post-operative systemic complications are related to the patient's factors, but sometimes it may relate to dentist (Iatrogenic) causes, this is true in case of traumatic extraction or because of:
   1. Improper evaluation of the case
   2. Inability to Follow the right technical procedure or/and
   3. Lack of the basic skills or/and
   4. Using of wrong instruments
   5. Inability to follow the aseptic technique

b. Otherwise it is a normal body response to surgical procedure unless there was an underlying local or systemic Condition.
   - Difficulty in Surgical procedures mean factors that may create possible Challenges intra-Operatively, or/and may result in development of possible complications post-Operatively
   - Psychology, attitude, behavior
   - Systemic condition of the patients … cardiac problems
   - Build, age, gender,
   - Medications

c. **Post-Operative Local Complications**
  ◦ Pain
  ◦ Swelling
  ◦ Trismus
  ◦ Infection
  ◦ Dry sockets
  ◦ Antral perforation or root's tip in the antrum
  ◦ Hemorrhage

Infection and Dry Socket

Factors Responsible for developing of infections:

1. Virulence of Micro-organism
2. Integrity of host Defense
3. Anatomical Factor
4. Others local factors:
  ◦ Long surgical procedure,
  ◦ Traumatic extraction,
  ◦ Lost of aseptic technique.

Dry socket, is not potentially life threatening like bleeding or infections, is one of the most painful, common, debilitating and dreaded post extraction problems encountered in dentistry.

Patients often state that they felt fine for a day or two after the extraction, but then the extraction site began to become painful. They may also say they have a bad taste in their mouth and a bad smell.

Dry sockets are more common after the extraction of lower teeth than they are after extraction of upper teeth, this could be due to low blood supply for the mandible in comparing with maxilla. They can happen after even the simplest of extractions.

Factors which increase the risk of dry socket:

• Smoke during the first 48 hours after the extraction
• Contraceptive pills,
• Grind and clench their teeth
• Mouth wash during the first 48 hours after the extraction
• Poor oral hygiene
• Previously infected tooth
• Age it is more common in old patient

- Traumatic extraction is the most common cause for dry socket
- Long surgical procedure and loss of aseptic technique
- A dry socket (**Fig: 5.26**) is a condition in which the blood clot becomes detached from the walls of the extraction site, or dissolves away by the action of hemolytic micro-organism leaving the bare bone exposed to saliva and the foods.
- The bone becomes contaminated with the saliva and inflamed by bacteria. This inflammation is persistent and painful. The dry socket emanate a bad odor.

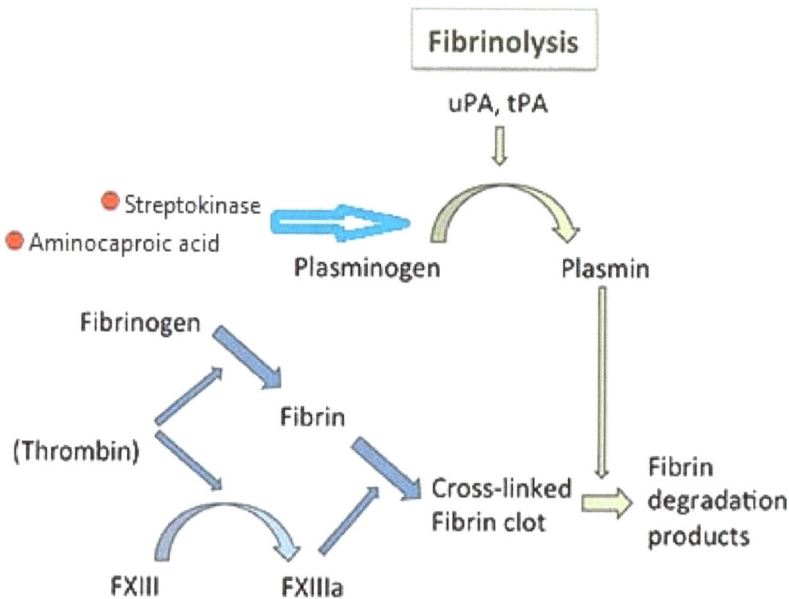

Fig. (5.26). Dry Sockets (Role of Micro-organism).

Some micro-organism release Streptokinase such as Streptococcus pyogenes. This exotoxin stimulates the conversion of plasminogen to plasmin. The plasmin causes a lysis of blood clot and makes the socket empty from it which may result in a dry socket.

Dry sockets would always heal if left alone. It may take a month or more, and the pain is always persistent for the period of curing and healing.

- Medications like:
  - The analgesic (pain killer) are not effective
  - The antibiotics are not recommended and are not useful in healing and curing of dry socket, and the usual

Preventive Measures:
Studies have shown that in office pre-operative and post-operative rinsing with 0.12% chlorhexidine after 24 hours of extraction for 5 days reduces the incidence of dry sockets.

Treating the socket immediately post-operatively with a small amount of tetracycline on a piece of Gelfoam has been shown to reduce the likelihood of dry socket.

In Another clinical trial a metronidazole powder on a piece of Gelfoam has been added with great success.

Management of Dry Socket:
Packing the socket:
This procedure done (usually) without anesthesia even though it can be painful. It does not take too long, and the pain relief is almost complete, beginning a few minutes after the socket is packed. The first packing will provide relief for 12 to 24 hours. At second subsequent visit: old packing is removed, the socket is washed out and a new packing is placed. Each succeeding packing debrides (clean) the socket and renews the pain. A second pack can last for 24 to 48 hours, and good packing may last longer. Within three packing, or sometimes more depending on the severity of the dry socket, the wound starts to heal from the apical to the coronal part.

Retained roots (Pieces of tooth fractured in the socket):

The root tip can be left if:

1. Less than one third of the root
2. and the tooth is not infected
3. And if the tip near a vital structure

Delay in healing process of the socket:

1. **Systemic Factors**
   1. Nutrition: vitamin deficiency and/or Poor nutrition adversely affects healing.
   2. Age: adults usually take longer time for healing of dry socket than children; healing process is decreased with age.
   3. Health: Chronic diseases depresses the healing process (anemia, diabetes, oxidative stress, systemic infection).
   4. Hormonal factors: There are some hormone may enhance healing process and other may depress the process of healing (corticosteroids depress

healing, growth hormone enhances healing).
5. Atherosclerosis: associated with age (as a result of hyperlipidemias and oxidative stress) decreases healing process.
6. Smoking: significantly may decreases healing process.
7. Drugs: Steroidal and Non-steroidal anti-inflammatory medication (*e.g.* ibuprofen) depress healing process.

2. **Local Factors**
1. Degree of local trauma/bone loss: A comminuted fracture with more soft tissue injury is slower to heal.
2. Area of bone affected and bone quality.
3. Abnormal bone (infection, tumour, irradiated).
4. food impinging at the socket site delays healing.

Hemorrhage (Bleeding)

There are three types of bleeding may associated with Exodontias:

• Primary hemorrhage (Intra-operative Complications)
• Reactionary hemorrhage (Post-operatively within 48 hours)
• Secondary hemorrhage (Post-operatively after 48 hours)

Causes of Hemorrhage

1. **Primary Hemorrhage**

a. Systemic Causes:
　1. Pathological (bleeding disorders)
　2. Medication (oral anti-coagulants)
b. Local Causes: The local causes can be
　1. Pathological Causes
　2. Technical Causes

a. The Systemic Causes of primary hemorrhage:
　1. Pathological Causes: Including all bleeding disorders. The most common among them are:
　　▪ Haemophilia A
　　▪ Haemophilia B
　　▪ Von Willebrand's disease
　2. **Medications**: Including all those patients taking Oral Anti-coagulants
b. Local Causes of primary haemorrhage:
　1. Pathological: The most common cause is the hemangiomas, and early stage of fibro-osseous lesions and with some systemic bone lesions such as early stages of Paget's disease and others.

2. Technical: Injury for the soft tissues during extraction procedure, this may occur due to slipping of the surgical instruments specially the elevators during extraction. It may occur as well due to injury of one of the vital structure especially the inferior alveolar blood vessels.

• Reactionary Haemorrhage

This occur usually within first 24 hours after the Extraction some authors believe that any bleeding within the 48 hours from extraction considered as reactionary bleeding so they are believing that the time is not restricted to the first 24 hours after extraction time. The main cause of this kind of bleeding is a vaso-dilatation following metabolic degeneration of vaso-constrictive action of the epinephrine (or other vaso-constrictive substances) in the local anesthesia.

• Secondary Haemorrhage

This kind of bleeding occurs after 48 hours from the extraction procedure. The only cause of this bleeding is infection at the extraction site.

Root or Root Tip at the Maxillary Antrum

1. Good suction for the socket
2. If the root can be visualized, a blunt instrument should be used to retrieve it with great care not to injure the antrum mucosa, because it is usually intact in most cases.
3. If the above is not helpful the patient should be referred to Oral Surgeon for more specialized manipulation. The Caldwell-Luc procedures may be considered.

Oro-antral Communication

Oro-antral communication when occur at the time of extraction and when it is a fresh it is call Oro-antral sinus after 24 hours and when the epithelialization take place, it is called Oro-antral Fistula. In general this kind of communication should be repaired immediately at the time of extraction, it is always preferred to be done by an Oral Surgeon.

Generally, there are three main types of flaps can be used:

1. Buccal extended flap
2. Palatal rotational flap
3. Buccal fat bad for large defect

• Water tight suture is indicated, preferably horizontal mattress.

- After closure, the patient should be advised not to blow with a closing nose and avoid a sharp sneezing.
- Decongestant nasal drop may be prescribed as well.
- Broad spectrum antibiotic, many surgeon prefer Cephalexin since there is a wide believe that this antibiotic is the most effective one in maxillary sinus infection management.

Fracture Mandible

Fracture mandible is not a common complication. If this happened the patient should be referred to Oral & Maxillofacial Surgeon for definitive treatment.

Infective Endocarditis

Infective endocarditis is one of the most serious systemic complications may be associated with certain cardiac conditions. It is one of the most important post-operative systemic complications. It may occur in the following patients:

- 50% is on normal valves
- Abnormal -congenital, rheumatic fever, prosthetic.
- Caused by any bacteremia
- 60% no obvious cause
- 35-50% *S. Viridans*
- *S.faecalis*, *Staph aureus*, coxiella or chlamydia
- Vegetations can embolise
- Right heart endocarditis in IVDU
- High Risk Patients (List: 5.1). Patient with previous history for Infective Endocarditis. Patient with prosthetic valve replacement < 6 month.

Patients at highest risk for adverse outcome of infective endocarditis (IE):
- Prosthetic cardiac valve or prosthetic material used for cardiac valve repair
- Previous experience with infective endocarditis
- Congenital heart disease (CHD), including:
    1. Unrepaired cyanotic CHD, including palliative shunts and conduits
    2. Completely repaired congenital heart defect with prosthetic material or device, whether placed by surgery or by catheter intervention, during the first 6 months after the procedure
    3. Repaired CHD with residual defects at the site or adjacent to the site of a prosthetic patch or prosthetic device (which inhibits endothelialization)
- Cardiac transplantation recipients with cardiac valvulopathy

High risk dental procedures:
- Those involving manipulation of gingival tissue, periapical region of teeth, or perforation of the oral mucosa

Procedures not considered high risk:
- Routine anesthetic injections through noninfected tissue, taking dental radiographs, placement of removable prosthodontic or orthodontic appliances, adjustment of orthodontic appliances, placement of orthodontic brackets, shedding of deciduous teeth, and bleeding from trauma to the lips or oral mucosa

List 5.1. Dimension of dental hygiene, 2011.

Dental procedures requiring Prophylaxis in High Risk Patients:

- Exodontias
- placement of Dental implant or avulsed teeth reimplantation
- Periodontal treatment, including probing, scaling, root planing, and surgery
- Endodontic treatment or periapical surgery.

PROPHYLAXIS (Current Guideline):

For those operated under LA. , should be given one hour pre-operatively

- Current recommendation of AAC is 2g of amoxicillin
    Children<10: half the dose
    Children<5: quarter the dose
- Allergic to penicillin: Clindamycin 600mg
    Children<10: half the dose
    Children<5: quarter the dose
- OR
    Cephalexin….2 g, for children 50 mg/kg
- - OR
    Clindamycin…..600 mg. for children 20 mg/kg
- OR
    Azithromycinor clarithromycin….500 mg, for children 15 mg/kg
- - unable to take oral medication: Ampicillin….. 2 g IM or IV, for children 50 mg/kg IM or IV
- Allergic to penicillins group antibiotic including ampicillin and/or unable to take oral medication:
- Cefazolinor ceftriaxone…1 g IM or IV, for children 50 mg/kg IM or IV
- OR
    Clindamycin….600 mg IM or IV, for children 20 mg/kg IM or IV.

Antibiotic Prophylaxis Prior to Dental Procedures

The American Dental Association – (ADA) and the American Heart Association (AHA) released guidelines for the prevention of infective endocarditis in 2007, which were approved by the clinical skills assessment (CSA) as they relate to dentistry in 2008.8 In 2017, the AHA and American College of Cardiology (ACC) published a focused update to their 2014 guidelines on the management of valvular heart disease that reinforce the previous recommendations (list: 5.2-5.3).

Prevention of Prosthetic Joint Infection

The American Dental Association stated the following key points:

- Compared with previous recommendations, there are currently relatively few patient subpopulations for whom antibiotic prophylaxis may be indicated prior to certain dental procedures.
- In patients with prosthetic joint implants, a January 2015 ADA clinical practice guideline, based on a 2014 systematic review states, "In general, for patients with prosthetic joint implants, prophylactic antibiotics are not recommended prior to dental procedures to prevent prosthetic joint infection."
- According to the ADA Chairside Guide, for patients with a history of complications associated with their joint replacement surgery who are undergoing dental procedures that include gingival manipulation or mucosal incision, prophylactic antibiotics should only be considered after consultation with the patient and orthopedic surgeon; in cases where antibiotics are deemed necessary, it is most appropriate that the orthopedic surgeon recommend the appropriate antibiotic regimen and, when reasonable, write the prescription.
- For infective endocarditis prophylaxis, current guidelines support premedication for a relatively small subset of patients. This is based on a review of scientific evidence, which showed that the risk of adverse reactions to antibiotics generally outweigh the benefits of prophylaxis for many patients who would have been considered eligible for prophylaxis in previous versions of the guidelines. Concern about the development of drug-resistant bacteria also was a factor.
- Infective endocarditis prophylaxis for dental procedures should be recommended only for patients with underlying cardiac conditions associated with the highest risk of adverse outcome from infective endocarditis. For patients with these underlying cardiac conditions, prophylaxis is recommended for all dental procedures that involve manipulation of gingival tissue or the periapical region of teeth or perforation of the oral mucosa.[Key points (ADA: http://www.ada.org].

In 2014, the ADA Council on Scientific Affairs assembled an expert panel to update and clarify the clinical recommendations found in the 2012 evidence report and 2013 guideline, Prevention of Orthopaedic Implant Infection in Patients Undergoing Dental Procedures [1, 2].

As was found in 2012, the updated systematic review undertaken in 2014 and published in 2015 found no association between dental procedures and prosthetic joint infections.3 Based on this evidence review, the 2015 ADA clinical practice guideline states [3] "In general, for patients with prosthetic joint implants, prophylactic antibiotics are not recommended prior to dental procedures to prevent prosthetic joint infection."

"The new CSA guideline clearly states that for most patients, prophylactic antibiotics are not indicated before dental procedures to prevent [prosthetic joint infections]. The new guideline also takes into consideration that patients who have previous medical conditions or complications associated with their joint replacement surgery may have specific needs calling for premedication. In medically compromised patients who are undergoing dental procedures that include gingival manipulation or mucosal inclusion, prophylactic antibiotics should be considered only after consultation with the patient and orthopedic surgeon. For patients with serious health conditions, such as immunocompromising diseases, it may be appropriate for the orthopedic surgeon to recommend an antibiotic regimen when medically indicated, as footnoted in the new chair-side guide."

A 2017 commentary [3] published in the February 2017 issue of JADA written by ADA-appointed experts, offers guidance for using appropriate use criteria published by the American Academy of Orthopaedic Surgeons in January 2017 [4] that address managing care for patients with orthopedic implants undergoing dental procedures. The JADA editorial calls the appropriate use criteria "a decision-support tool to supplement clinicians in their judgment" and it emphasizes discussion of available treatment options between the patient, dentist and orthopedic surgeon, weighing the potential risks and benefits.The commentary encourages dentists to continue to use the 2015 guideline, consult the appropriate use criteria as needed, and respect the patient's specific needs and preferences when considering antibiotic prophylaxis before dental treatment. According to the ADA Chairside Guide, in cases where antibiotics are deemed necessary, it is most appropriate that the orthopedic surgeon recommend the appropriate antibiotic regimen and, when reasonable, write the prescription.

With input from the ADA, the American Heart Association (AHA) released guidelines for the prevention of infective endocarditis in 2007 [5], which were approved by the CSA as they relate to dentistry in 2008. In 2017, the AHA and American College of Cardiology (ACC) published a focused update [5] to their 2014 guidelines on the management of valvular heart disease that reinforce the previous recommendations.

These current guidelines support infective endocarditis premedication for a relatively small subset of patients. This is based on a review of scientific evidence, which showed that the risk of adverse reactions to antibiotics generally outweigh the benefits of prophylaxis for many patients who would have been considered eligible for prophylaxis in previous versions of the guidelines. Concern about the development of drug-resistant bacteria also was a factor.

Also, the data are mixed as to whether prophylactic antibiotics taken before a dental procedure prevent infective endocarditis. The guidelines note that people who are at risk for infective endocarditis are regularly exposed to oral bacteria during basic daily activities such as brushing or flossing. The valvular disease management guidelines [6] recommend that persons at risk of developing bacterial infective endocarditis (see "Patient Selection") establish and maintain the best possible oral health to reduce potential sources of bacterial seeding. They state, "Optimal oral health is maintained through regular professional dental care and the use of appropriate dental products, such as manual, powered, and ultrasonic toothbrushes; dental floss; and other plaque-removal devices."

Patient Selection

The current infective endocarditis/valvular heart disease guidelines state that use of preventive antibiotics before certain dental procedures is reasonable for patients with (List: 5.3):

- Prosthetic cardiac valves, including transcatheter-implanted prostheses and homografts;
- Prosthetic material used for cardiac valve repair, such as annuloplasty rings and chords;
- A history of infective endocarditis;
- A cardiac transplant with valve regurgitation due to a structurally abnormal valve;
- The following congenital (present from birth) heart disease:
- Unrepaired cyanotic congenital heart disease, including palliative shunts and conduits
- Any repaired congenital heart defect with residual shunts or valvular regurgitation at the site of or adjacent to the site of a prosthetic patch or a prosthetic device
  i. According to limited data, infective endocarditis appears to be more common in heart transplant recipients than in the general population; the risk of infective endocarditis is highest in the first 6 months after transplant because of endothelial disruption, high-intensity immunosuppressive therapy, frequent central venous catheter access, and frequent endomyocardial biopsies [7].
  ii. Except for the conditions listed above, antibiotic prophylaxis is no longer recommended for any other form of congenital heart disease.

List: 5.3 patient selections for prophylactic antibiotics ADA: http://www.ada.org.

Dental Procedures

Prophylaxis is recommended for the patients identified in the previous section for all dental procedures that involve manipulation of gingival tissue or the periapical region of the teeth, or perforation of the oral mucosa.

- Additional Considerations about Infective Endocarditis Antibiotic Prophylaxis (When Indicated) sometimes, patients forget to premedicate before their appointments. The recommendation is that for patients with an indication for antibiotic prophylaxis, the antibiotic be given before the procedure. This is important because it allows the antibiotic to reach adequate blood levels. However, the guidelines to prevent infective endocarditis state, "If the dosage of antibiotic is inadvertently not administered before the procedure, the dosage may be administered up to 2 hours after the procedure."
- Another concern that dentists have expressed involves patients who require prophylaxis but are already taking antibiotics for another condition. In these cases, the guidelines for infective endocarditis recommend that the dentist select an antibiotic from a different class than the one the patient is already taking. For example, if the patient is taking amoxicillin, the dentist should select clindamycin, azithromycin or clarithromycin for prophylaxis.

Other patient groups also may merit special consideration, which is discussed more fully in the guidelines.

In 2015, The Lancet published a study out of the United Kingdom that reported a correlation between institution of more limited antibiotic prophylaxis guidelines by the National Institute for Health and Clinical Evidence (NICE) in 2008 and an increase in cases of infective endocarditis.10 Because of the retrospective and observational nature of the study, the authors acknowledged that their "data do not establish a causal association." At this time, the ADA recommends that dentists continue to use the AHA guidelines discussed above. Dental professionals should periodically visit the ADA website for updates on this issue. ADA: http://www.ada.org.

Osteonecrosis

1. Osteoradionecrosis (Radio-osteo-necrosis)
2. Osteochemonecrosis   (chemo-osteo-necrosis)   Bisphosphonates   jaw osteonecrosis

Osteoradionecrosis

Osteoradionecrosis (ORN) is a condition of necrosis of bone in radiation site. ORN can be unconstrained, but in most cases results from tissue inflammation and injury such as ulcers, denture-related injury or tooth extraction. There are, three grades of disease (I, II, III) are recognized.

- Grade I: is the most common form, the necrotic alveolar bone is exposed.
- Grade II: is a category of ORN that does not respond positively to hyperbaric oxygen treatment (HBO) and requires sequestrectomy/saucerization.
- Grade III is used to describe a full-thickness involvement of bone and/or associated with pathologic fracture.
- The patients can present with grade I or grade III of ORN at initial presentation.

Patient who receive less than 60 gray (Gy) radiation therapy is unlikely to has ORN, but it has been reported in rare occasion. The incidence of ORN has decreased over the last 3 decades, as the incidence before 1970 was 5.4-11.8% but in recent studies it is less than 3.0%. Indeed there is no clear mechanism for reporting the disease, this make the exactly incidence not clear in recent studies. The Incidence is higher in patients who receive combined therapy (chemo-, radio-, therapy). The radiotherapist (RTOG - Radiation Therapy Oncology Group) members discuss report the possible radiation toxicity including ORN.

Osteoradionecrosis was first described by Marx in 1983 as local tissues hypoxia, hypocellularity and hypovascularity. Before Marx, there were many other theories described the etiology of ORN. Currently, there are huge clinical experiences, and subsequent studies support this widely accepted theory.

In the irradiated mandible, significant inflammation, hyperemia and endarteritis develop in the periosteum, and overlying soft tissue. These lead to massive thrombosis, progressive hypovascularity, cellular death and fibrosis.

The radiated bone becomes hypocellular, devoid of osteoblasts, fibroblasts and undifferentiated osteoid cells. Mandibular ORN usually develop after trauma like extraction or even spontaneously.

New Concept for Pathology of ORN

Recently, the "fibro-atrophic theory" has been widely accepted, it proposes that fibroblasts that undergo cellular depletion in response to radiation show a significant decrease in its ability to produce collagen into the surrounding tissue. This theory is based on the concept that osteoclasts damage occur earlier than the development of vascular alterations. Accordingly, the key factor in the development of ORN is the dysregulation of fibroblastic activity that initiate atrophic tissue changes within irradiated area. The histopathologic phases of the development of ORN include (List: 5.3) and (Table **5.1-5.3**):

- The prefibrotic phase:

In this phase, changes in endothelial cells predominate, along with the acute inflammatory response;

- The constitutive organized phase:

In this phase, abnormal fibroblastic activity predominates, and there is disorganization of the extracellular matrix.

- The late fibroatrophic phase.

In this phase, tissue remodeling occurs along with the formation of fragile healed tissues that carry a serious inherent risk of late reactivated inflammation in the event of local injury. [14, 15]

List 5.3. Staging of ORN.

Table 5.1. The histopathologic phases of the development of ORN.

	Score	Event
NCICTC [16]	0	None
	1	Asymptomatic and detected by imaging only
	2	Symptomatic and interfering with function, but not interfering with activities of daily living
	3	Symptomatic and interfering with activities of daily living
	4	Symptomatic, or disabling

Table 5.2. The histopathologic phases of the development of ORN.

	0	Mucosal defects only
Store & Boysen [17]	1	Radiological evidence of necrotic bone with intact mucosa
	2	Positive radiological findings with denuded bone intra-orally
	3	Clinically exposed radionecrotic bone, verified by imaging techniques, along with skin fistulas and infection

Table 5.3. The histopathologic phases of the development of ORN.

Glanzmann & Gratz [18]	1	**Bone exposure without signs of infection and persisting for at least three months**
	2	Bone exposure with signs of infection or sequester and without the signs of grade 3 ± 5
	3	Bone necrosis treated with mandibular resection with a satisfactory result
	4	Bone necrosis with persisting problems despite mandibular resection
	5	Death due to osteoradionecrosis

Management

- Dental evaluation and full mouth radiographs : before starting radiotherapy, all patients should be dentally examined (clinically and radiographically) and the prognosis for each tooth should be evaluated. A complete treatment plan and patient's motivation should be done before the radiotherapy. Patient education should inviscid on importance of meticulous oral hygiene and dental follow-up to avoid any intra-oral surgical procedure after radiotherapy.
- Definitive treatment protocol:
  1. Stage I: Perform 30 HBO dives for 90 minutes at 2.4 atmospheres pressure, 1 dive five days a week. the patient should be evaluated for decrease in bone exposure, granulation tissue, resorption of necrotic bone, and absence of inflammation. For patients who respond well, continue HBO treatment to a total of 40 dives. For patients who are not responding, advance to stage II.
  2. Stage II: Surgical sequestrectomy transoral should be done by transoral approach with primary wound closure followed by HBO for 40 dives over 8 weeks period.
  3. Stage III: Patients who show pathologic fracture, orocutaneous fistula or resorption to the inferior border of the mandible at time of presentation, should be categorized as Stage III. In these patient mandibular resection should be done *via* transcutaneous approach with tracking and excision of the fistula and wound closure, and mandibular fixation in case of fracture should be done with an external fixator or constructive plating system, followed by 10 postoperative HBO dives of period of 2 weeks.

Pentoxifylline and tocopherol are a new approach for the treatment of osteoradionecrosis

Pentoxifylline is:

- Anti-tumor necrosis factor (TNF)-α effect,
- Induce vasodilation,
- Increases erythrocyte flexibility,
- Anti-inflammatory,
- Enhance collagenase activity
- Inhibits human dermal fibroblast proliferation and extracellular matrix (ECM) production.

Pentoxifylline increases blood flow and enhances tissue oxygenation by decreasing the blood viscosity. The usual dosage of pentoxifylline is given in extended-release tablet form (400 mg), three times per day. The effect of pentoxifylline may be seen within 2 to 4 weeks, the treatment is recommended to be continued for at least 8 weeks.

Patients on oral anti-coagulant (warfarin) should be frequently monitoring for prothrombin times, while patients with other hemorrhagic risk factors (recent surgery and peptic ulceration) should be periodic examined for bleeding tendencies.

Vitamin E

Vitamin E exists in eight different forms, four tocopherols and four tocotrienols. Both the tocopherols and tocotrienols occur in α (alpha), β (beta), γ (gamma) and δ (delta) forms, determined by the number and position of methyl groups on the chromanol ring.

Tocopherols and tocotrienols are fat-soluble antioxidants, they have many functions in the body. They seem to:

- Protect cell membranes against lipid peroxidation,
- Inhibit TGF-ß1
- and Inhibit procollagen gene expression.

Recent reports of pentoxifylline and tocopherol combined therapy:

Combined pentoxifylline-tocopherol therapy has been proven effective in reducing chronic progressive septic ORN of the mandible. These two drugs act synergistically as potent anti-fibrotic agents and are available, inexpensive, well tolerated, and effective.

Pentoxifylline exerts an negative effect on TNF-α, increases erythrocyte flexibility, induce vasodilation, inhibits inflammation, increases collagenase activity, inhibits the human dermal fibroblasts proliferation and inhibit the production of extracellular matrix. When it is given with tocopherol, which reduces fibrosis by scavenging the free oxygen radical that were generated during oxidative stress, protecting cell membranes against the peroxidation of lipids, and partially inhibiting the expression of procollagen genes and TGF- β1. All these strongly contribute to effectiveness of this combination in cases of ORN.

Osteochemonecrosis - OCN

Osteochemonecrosis - OCN (Bisphosphonates jaw osteonecrosis - BJN, Medication related osteonecrosis of the jaw – MRONJ, Antiresorptive drug related osteonecrosis of the jaw – ARONJ, Bisphosphonates related osteonecrosis of the jaw - BRONJ):

Antiresorptive Medications

a. Bisphosphonates (BPs)
   ○ Intravenous (IV) bisphosphonates (BPs) are antiresorptive medications used in management of:
      - Cancer-related conditions including hypercalcemia of malignancy,
      - Lytic lesion such as multiple myeloma
      - Metastases in breast cancer, prostate cancer and lung cancers,
      - Skeletal-related events (SRE) associated with bone
   ○ Oral bisphosphonates are used for treatment of:
      - Osteoporosis
      - Osteopenia
      - Paget's disease of bone
      - Osteogenesis imperfecta.
b. RANK ligand inhibitor is a fully humanized antibody against RANK ligand (RANK-L)
   ○ Inhibits osteoclast activity
   ○ Reduce in the risk of fractures in osteoporotic patients, usually is administered subcutaneously every 6 months
   ○ Effective in reducing SRE related to metastatic bone disease from solid tumors when administered monthly. It is not indicated for the treatment of multiple myeloma.
      Interestingly, in contrast to bisphosphonates, RANK ligand inhibitors do not bind to bone and their effects on bone remodeling are mostly diminished within 6 months of treatment cessation. Antiangiogenic medications
c. Angiogenesis inhibitors interfere with the formation of new blood vessels by binding to various signaling molPAGE.
   ○ Disrupt the angiogenesis-signaling cascade. These medications have demonstrated efficacy in the treatment of
      - Neuroendocrine tumors,

- Gastrointestinal tumors,
- Renal cell carcinomas,
- and Others.

Bisphosphonates are used for treatment of bone metastatic disease such as Paget's disease and widely used in the treatment of osteoporosis. Bisphosphonates have a strong affinity to osteoclasts. These group of medicine inhibit the osteoclast,s activity and function. Bisphosphonates bind to bone mineral around osteoclasts and inhibit the osteoclastmediated bone resorption, and turnover.

At a cellular level, the drugs inhibit the differentiation of osteoclasts from marrow osteocomponent precursors and initiate apoptosis at the bone surface, which contribute to reducing of the life-span. Many studies reported that, the stimulation of osteoclast inhibitory factor, responsible for the prevention of osteoclast development from bone marrow precursors, and down regulation of matrix metalloproteinases. The bisphosphonates may modulate osteoclast function by interacting with an intracellular enzyme or cell surface receptor.

Bone resorption and remodeling are an essential function in maintaining normal bone homeostasis. Bisphosphonate inhibit the osteoclast function and decrease bone resorption. It inhibits the normal bone turnover. However, bisphosphonates may cause sufficient change in bone homeostasis that makes the bone ability to heal after minor difficult. The bone may also become secondarily infected and sequestrate after simple oral trauma like extraction, resulting in a lesion that appears clinically similar to osteoradionecrosis.

The localized vascular insufficiency is a constant pathology finding in the Osteochemonecrosis. However, osteocytes are not replaced if osteoclastic function is severely impaired, this resulting in loss of bone capillary network maintenance and avascular bone necrosis development.

Pathophysiology

The pathophysiology of MRONJ is not fully understood. Proposed hypotheses that attempt to explain the unique localization of MRONJ exclusively to the jaws include:

1. Inhibition of osteoclastic bone resorption and remodeling
2. Inhibition of angiogenesis
3. Constant microtrauma,
4. Vitamin D deficiency
5. Soft tissue BP toxicity
6. Suppression of immunity

7. Inflammation or infection

A. Inhibition of Osteoclastic Bone Resorption and Remodeling

Bisphosphonates (BP), and other antiresorptives, inhibit osteoclast differentiation and function, and increase apoptosis, all leading to decreased bone resorption and remodeling. Osteoclast differentiation and activity plays a vital role in bone remodeling and healing An increased remodeling rate in the jaws may explain the predisposition to MRONJ compared to other bones.

B. Inflammation/Infection

Both systemic and local oral risk factors have been implicated in MRONJ pathogenesis, where several human studies have implicated dental disease or bacterial infection. systemic antiresorptives are sufficient to induce MRONJ.

Inflammation or infection has long been considered an important component of MRONJ. Early studies identified bacteria, especially Actinomyces species, in biopsied of MRONJ. The presence of bacteria has prompted studies to evaluate the possibility of a complex biofilm on exposed bone.

C. Inhibition of Angiogenesis

Angiogenesis process involves:

• Growth,
• Migration
• and Differentiation of endothelial cells to form new blood vessels.

Angiogenesis influences tumor growth and invasion of vessels, resulting in minimize the tumor metastasis. Angiogenesis requires binding of signaling molecules (such as vascular endothelial growth factor - VEGF) to their receptors on the endothelial cells. These signals promote new blood vessel proliferation and growth.

Osteonecrosis is essentially considered as an interruption in vascular supply (avascular necrosis). These make the angiogenesis inhibition a strong possible hypothesis in MRONJ pathophysiology. Studies in cancer patients treated with angiogenesis inhibitors support these data as a decreased circulating VEGF levels have been reported.

Risk Factors for MRONJ

Medication-related risk factors. The MRONJ disease frequency estimates by two parameters:

- Therapeutic indications
- and Type of medications.

The therapeutic indications are grouped into two categories:

- Osteoporosis/osteopenia
- or Malignancy.

The Medications are grouped into two categories:

- BP (antiresorptive medications)
- and Non-BP (antiangiogenic medications).
- MRONJ risk among cancer patients

To measure the risk for MRONJ among patients exposed to a medication, the risk for MRONJ in patients not exposed to antiresorptive or antiangiogenic medications must be known. The risk for MRONJ among cancer patients enrolled in clinical trials and assigned to placebo groups ranges from 0% to 0.019% (0-1.9 cases per 10,000 cancer patients) [18 - 20].

Among cancer patients ex:

The cumulative incidence of MRONJ with low single digits of antiresorptive medications is (range = 0.7% - 6.7%). The risk of MRONJ in subjects exposed to BP approximates 1% (100 cases per 10,000 patients) [18 - 20, 22]. The risk of MRONJ among cancer patients exposed to antiresorptive medications ranges between 50-100 times higher than cancer patients treated with placebo.

Among cancer patients ex:

The cumulative incidence of MRONJ with (RANK-L) inhibitor ranges from 0.7% - 1.9% (70-90 cases per 10,000 patients) [18, 22]. The risk among cancer patient exposed to RANK-L is comparable to the risk of ONJ in patients exposed to antiresorptive medications.

The risk for MRONJ among cancer patients exposed to antiangiogenic agent is 0.2%. (20 cases per 10,000) [24]. The risk may be higher among patients exposed to both antiangiogenic agent and antiresorptive medications.

Many studies have highlighted the potential additive toxic effect of antiangiogenic drugs (TKIs and monoclonal antibody targeting VEGF) in patients having a history of bisphosphonate medication use [24, 29 - 35].

Many case reports underscore the potential for novel medications such as TKIs and VEGF inhibitors being implicated in the development of MRONJ in the absence of concomitant antiresorptive medication use [25 - 29].

- Risk for ONJ among osteoporotic patients exposed to oral BPs: In a survey study of over 13,000 Kaiser Permanente members, the prevalence of BRONJ in patients receiving long-term oral bisphosphonate therapy was reported at 0.1% (10 cases per 10,000) which increased to 0.21 (21 cases per 10,000) among patients with greater than 4 years of oral BP exposure [48].
  Many studies reported that the risk of MRONJ among osteoporotic patients exposed to IV BP or RANK-L inhibitors almost the same as exposed to oral BP. Studies analyzing patients with osteoporosis exposed to yearly BP therapy for 3 years reported a risk for MRONJ of 0.017% (1.7 cases per 10,000 subjects) [42].
- Duration of medication therapy as a risk factor for MRONJ: The duration of BP therapy continues to be a risk factor for developing ONJ. the incidence of developing MRONJ Among cancer patients exposed to BP or RANK-L inhibitors was respectively, 0.6 and 0.5% at 1 year, 0.9 and 1.1% at 2 years, and 1.3 and 1.1% at 3 years [23]. In a study by Saad *et al.*, the investigators combined three-blinded phase three trials and found similar results, including a plateau after 2-years for patients exposed to denosumab.108 Among cancer patients exposed to zolendronate or denosumab (n=5723), the incidence of developing ONJ was, respectively, 0.5 and 0.8% at 1 year, 1.0 and 1.8% at 2 years, and 1.3 and 1.8% at 3 years [45].
- Operative treatment: Dentoalveolar surgery is considered a major risk factor for developing MRONJ. Several studies reported MRONJ after tooth extraction. The extraction is a common predisposing factor; as up of 52 to 61% of patients reported with MRONJ have a history of tooth extraction [21, 45, 46]. The risk of developing MRONJ among patients who have been involved in other oral procedures such as endodontic, dental implant placement and periodontal surgery is unknown.
- Anatomic factors: The MRONJ is more likely to appear in the mandible (73%) than the maxilla (22.5%) but can appear in both jaws (4.5%) [45]. The lower blood supply for the mandible than the maxilla and osteoid cell viability can be considered as an explanation for that.
- Concomitant oral disease: Pre-existing dental inflammation such as periapical pathology or periodontal disease is considered as strongly relevant risk factor. Among cancer patients with MRONJ, pre-existing dental inflammation was a risk factor among 50% of the cases [45, 49].
- Demographic and systemic factors: Age and sex are variably reported as risk factors for MRONJ. Its risk is higher after the age of 55 and in female it is higher than male of equal age. The higher prevalence in the female is likely a reflection of the underlying disease for which the agents are being prescribed

(*i.e.* osteoporosis, breast cancer). [45, 47, 49, 52, 53]
• Medication factors
  The medications those are associated with an increased risk for MRONJ:
    ○ Corticosteroids are associated with an increased risk for MRONJ [45]
    ○ Immunosuppressive medication
    ○ Others
• Co-morbid conditions among cancer patients that are inconsistently reported to be associated with an increased risk for MRONJ include [45, 52]:
    ○ Anaemia (haemoglobin < 10g/dL)
    ○ and Diabetes.
• Tobacco use has been inconsistently reported as a risk factor for MRONJ. In a case-control study, tobacco use approached statistical significance as a risk factor for ONJ in cancer patients (OR=3.0; 95% CI= 0.8 - 10.4) [47]. In a more recent case-controlled study, tobacco use was not associated with MRONJ in a sample of cancer patients exposed to BP. Vahtsevanos did not report an association between tobacco use and MRONJ.
• Genetic factors: Genetic predisposition has been described in many studies. There are several reports describing relation between single nucleotide polymorphisms (SNPs, Note: 9.1) and the development of MRONJ. Most of these SNPs were located within regions of the gene responsible for bone metabolism, turnover, collagen formation, or certain metabolic bone diseases. An ONJ event of 57% rate has been reported when SNPs were present in 5 candidate genes that were responsible for bone turnover. [54, 55] In a genome wide study, Nicoletti reported that patients with an SNP in the RBMS3 gene (associated with bone density and collagen formation) were 5.8 times more likely to develop ONJ. In a study that analyzed polymorphisms related to farnesyl diphosphate synthase activity (the enzyme specifically inhibited by bisphosphonates) a positive correlation was established with the carrier status and ONJ [55]. Collectively, these studies suggest that a germ line sensitivity to bisphosphonates may exist.

Due to increased bioavailability when using IV bisphosphonates, the Osteochemonecrosis is more likely to develop in patients who are receiving intravenous compared with oral therapy (94.2% *vs.* 5.8% of patients).

Dental Risks

Poor dental health and lack of regular dental assessment may result in dental complications. A history of invasive dental procedures, dental extraction, and periodontal pathology, has been linked with the development of Osteochemonecrosis in approximately 70% to 80% of cases of patients using Bisphosphonates.

Note 5.1. Relation between single nucleotide polymorphisms and the development of MRONJ.

Single nucleotide polymorphisms, frequently called SNPs (pronounced "snips"), are the most common type of genetic variation among people. Each SNP represents a difference in a single DNA building block, called a nucleotide. For example, a SNP may replace the nucleotide cytosine (C) with the nucleotide thymine (T) in a certain stretch of DNA.

SNPs occur normally throughout a person's DNA. They occur once in every 300 nucleotides on average, which means there are roughly 10 million SNPs in the human genome. Most commonly, these variations are found in the DNA between genes. They can act as biological markers, helping scientists locate genes that are associated with disease. When SNPs occur within a gene or in a regulatory region near a gene, they may play a more direct role in disease by affecting the gene's function.

Most SNPs have no effect on health or development. Some of these genetic differences, however, have proven to be very important in the study of human health. Researchers have found SNPs that may help predict an individual's response to certain drugs, susceptibility to environmental factors such as toxins, and risk of developing particular diseases. SNPs can also be used to track the inheritance of disease genes within families. Future studies will work to identify SNPs associated with complex diseases such as heart disease, diabetes, and cancer

Diagnosis

Symptoms of Osteochemonecrosis include:

- Odontalgia,
- Deep dull pain in the jaw,
- Altered lip sensation and other neurosensory functions in facial area. any patient with these symptoms should be referred to an oral and maxillofacial surgeon for special assessment.

Stage 1: the patient at time of presentation show exposed or necrotic bone. These patients may be asymptomatic with no evidence of infection.
Stage 2: when the patient present with pain and infection in the exposed necrotic bone.
Stage 2: when the patient have one or more of the following:
  ○ Pathologic fracture,
  ○ Necrotic bone extending beyond the alveolar region,
  ○ An extra-oral fistula,
  ○ Oral antral/oral nasal communications,
  ○ Osteolysis extending to the lower mandible of the sinus floor.

For Further Reading

1. American Academy of Orthopaedic Surgeons/American Dental Association. Prevention of Orthopaedic Implant Infection in Patients Undergoing Dental Procedures: Evidence-based Guideline and Evidence Report. American Academy of Orthopaedic Surgeons 2012. http://www.aaos.org/ Research/ guidelines/ PUDP/PUDP_guideline.pdf. Accessed February 3, 2016.
2. Rethman MP, Watters W, 3rd, Abt E, *et al*. The American Academy of Orthopaedic Surgeons and the American Dental Association clinical practice guideline on the prevention of orthopaedic implant infection in patients undergoing dental procedures. J Bone Joint Surg Am 2013; 95(8): 745-7.
3. Sollecito TP, Abt E, Lockhart PB, *et al*. The use of prophylactic antibiotics prior to dental procedures in patients with prosthetic joints: Evidence-based clinical practice guideline for dental practitioners a report of the American Dental Association Council on Scientific Affairs. J Am Dent Assoc 2015; 146(1): 11-16 e8.
4. Meyer DM. Providing clarity on evidence-based prophylactic guidelines for prosthetic joint infections. J Am Dent Assoc 2015; 146(1): 3-5.
5. American Dental Association-Appointed Members of the Expert Writing and Voting Panels Contributing to the Development of American Academy of Orthopedic Surgeons Appropriate Use Criteria. American Dental Association guidance for utilizing appropriate use criteria in the management of the care of patients with orthopedic implants undergoing dental procedures. J Am Dent Assoc 2017; 148(2): 57-59.
6. Quinn RH, Murray JN, Pezold R, Sevarino KS. The American Academy of Orthopaedic Surgeons Appropriate Use Criteria for the Management of Patients with Orthopaedic Implants Undergoing Dental Procedures. J Bone Joint Surg Am 2017; 99(2): 161-63.
7. Wilson W, Taubert KA, Gewitz M, *et al*. Prevention of infective endocarditis: guidelines from the American Heart Association: a guideline from the American Heart Association Rheumatic Fever, Endocarditis, and Kawasaki Disease Committee, Council on Cardiovascular Disease in the Young, and the Council on Clinical Cardiology, Council on Cardiovascular Surgery and Anesthesia, and the Quality of Care and Outcomes Research Interdisciplinary Working Group. Circulation 2007; 116(15): 1736-54.
8. Wilson W, Taubert KA, Gewitz M, *et al*. Prevention of infective endocarditis: guidelines from the American Heart Association: a guideline from the American Heart Association Rheumatic Fever, Endocarditis and Kawasaki Disease Committee, Council on Cardiovascular Disease in the Young, and the Council on Clinical Cardiology, Council on Cardiovascular Surgery and Anesthesia, and the Quality of Care and Outcomes Research Interdisciplinary Working Group. J Am Dent Assoc 2008; 139 Suppl: 3S-24S.

9. Nishimura RA, Otto CM, Bonow RO, *et al.* 2017 AHA/ACC Focused Update of the 2014 AHA/ACC Guideline for the Management of Patients With Valvular Heart Disease: A Report of the American College of Cardiology/American Heart Association Task Force on Clinical Practice Guidelines. Circulation 2017.

10. Archer WH (1975) Oral and maxillofacial surgery, 5th edn. Saunders, Philadelphia, Pa.

11. Gans BJ (1972) Atlas of oral surgery. Mosby, St. Louis, Mo. Guralnick WC (1968) Text book of oral surgery. Little Brown, Boston, Mass.

12. Braid DP, Scott DB: The systemic absorption of local analgesic drugs. Br J Anaesth 1965; 37: 394-404.

13. Goebel WM, Allen G, Randall F: The effect of commercial vasoconstrictor preparations on the circulating venous serum level of mepivacaine and lidocaine. J Oral Med 1980; 35: 91-96.

14. Keesling GR, Hinds EC: Optimal concentration of epinephrine in lidocaine solutions. J Am Dent Assoc 1963; 66: 337-340.

15. Gangarosa LP, Halik FJ: A clinical evaluation of local anesthetic solutions containing graded epinephrine concentrations. Arch Oral Biol 1967; 12: 611-621.

16. Kennedy WF Jr, Bonica JJ, Ward RJ, Tolas AG, Martin WE, Grinstein A: Cardiorespiratory effects of epinephrine when used in regional anesthesia. Acta Anesthesiol Scand Suppl 1966; 23: 320-333.

17. Cowan A: Minimum dosage technique in the clinical comparison of representative modern local anesthetic techniques. J Dent Res 1964; 43: 1228-1249.

18. Tolas AG, Pflug AE, Halter JB: Arterial plasma epinephrine concentrations and hemodynamic responses after dental injection of local anesthetic with epinephrine. J Am Dent Assoc 1982; 104: 41-43.

19. Cioffi GA, Chernow B, Glahn RP, Terezhalmy GT, Lake CR: The hemodynamic and plasma catecholamine responses to routine restorative dental care. J Am Dent Assoc 1985; 111: 67-70.

20. Chernow B, Balestrieri F, Ferguson CD, Terezhalmy GT, Fletcher JR, Lake CR: Local dental anesthesia with epinephrine: minimal effects on the sympathetic nervous system or on hemodynamic variables. Arch Intern Med 1983; 143: 2141-2143.

21. Goldstein OS, Dionne RA, Sweet J, Gracely R, Brewer HB, Gregg R: Circulatory plasma catecholamine, cortisol, lipid and psychological responses to a real-life stress (third molar extractions): effects of diazepam sedation and of inclusion of epinephrine with the local anesthetic. Psychosom Med 1982; 44: 259-272.

22. Dionne RA, Goldstein OS, Wirdzek PR: Effects of diazepam premedication

and epinephrine containing local anesthetic on cardiovascular and plasma catecholamine responses to oral surgery. Anesth Analg 1984; 63: 640-646.

23. Knoll-Kohler E, Knoller M, Brandt K, Becker J: Cardiohemodynamic and serum catecholamine response to surgical removal of impacted mandibular third molars under local anesthesia: a randomized double-blind parallel group and crossover study. J Oral Maxillofac Surg 1991; 49: 957-962.

24. Clutter WB, Bier OM, Shah SD, Cryer PE: Epinephrine plasma metabolic clearance rates and physiologic thresholds for metabolic and hemodynamic actions in man. J Clin Invest 1980; 66: 94-101.

25. Fragiskos D.(2007) Oral surgery. Springer Berlin Heidelberg New York Hayward JR (1976) Oral surgery. Thomas, Springfield, Ill.

26. Hooley JR, Whitacre RA (1986) A self-instructional guide to oral surgery in general practice, vol 2, 5th edn. Stoma, Seattle, Wash.

27. Howe GL (1997) Minor oral surgery, 3rd edn. Wright, Oxford

28. Howe GL (1996) The extraction of teeth, 2nd edn. Wright, Oxford

29. Kruger GO (1984) Oral and maxillofacial surgery, 6th edn. Mosby, St. Louis, Mo.

30. Laskin DM (1980) Oral and maxillofacial surgery, vol 1. Mosby, St. Louis, Mo.

31. Peterson LJ, Ellis E III, Hupp JR,TuckerMR(1993)Contemporary oral and maxillofacial surgery, 2nd edn. Mosby, St. Louis, Mo.

32. Rounds CE (1962) Principles and technique of exodontia, 2nd edn. Mosby, St. Louis, Mo.

33. Sailer HF, Pajarola GF (1999) Oral surgery for the general dentist. Thieme, Stuttgart

34. Waite DE (1987) Textbook of practical oral and maxillofacial surgery, 3rd edn. Lea and Febiger, Philadelphia, Pa.

35. Wahl MJ. Osteoradionecrosis prevention myths. Int J Radiat Oncol Biol Phys. 2006 Mar 1. 64(3): 661-9.

36. Marx RE. Osteoradionecrosis: a new concept of its pathophysiology. J Oral Maxillofac Surg. 1983 May. 41(5): 283-8.

37. Marx RE. A new concept in the treatment of osteoradionecrosis. J Oral Maxillofac Surg. 1983 Jun. 41(6): 351-7.

38. Ruggiero SL, Mehrotra B, Rosenburg T J *et al*. Osteonecrosis of the jaws associated with the use of bisphosphonates: a review of 63 cases. J Oral Maxillofac Surg 2004; 62: 527-534.

39. Purcell P M, Boyd I W. Bisphosphonates and osteonecrosis of the jaw. Med J Australia 2005; 182: 417-418.

40. Melo M D, Obeid G. Osteonecrosis of the maxilla in a patient with a history of bisphosphonate therapy. J Canadian Dent Assoc 2005; 71: 111-113.

41. Marx R E. Pamidronate (Aredia) and Zoledronate (Zometa) induced avascular

necrosis of the jaws: a growing epidemic. J Oral Maxillofac Surg 2003; 61: 1115-1117.

42. Carter G, Goss A N, Doecke C. Bisphosphonates and avascular necrosis of the jaw: a possible association. Med J Australia 2005; 182: 413-415.

43. Durie B G, Katz M, Crowley J. Osteonecrosis of jaw and bisphosphonates. New Engl J Med 2005; 353: 99-102.

44. King AE, Umland EM. Osteonecrosis of the jaw in patients receiving intravenous or oral bisphosphonates. Pharmacotherapy. 2008 May; 28(5): 667-77.

45. Varun, BR *et al.* "Bisphosphonate Induced Osteonecrosis of Jaw in Breast Cancer Patients: A Systematic Review." Journal of Oral and Maxillofacial Pathology : JOMFP 16.2 (2012): 210-214. PMC. Web. 24 Apr. 2017.

46. Ruggiero SL, Dodson TB, Assael LA, Landesberg R, Marx RE, Mehrotra B; American Association of Oral and Maxillofacial Surgeons. American Association of Oral and Maxillofacial Surgeons position paper on bisphosphonate-related osteonecrosis of the jaws-2009 update. J Oral Maxillofac Surg. 2009 May; 67(5 Suppl): 2-12.

REFERENCES

[1]   Wahl MJ. Osteoradionecrosis prevention myths. Int J Radiat Oncol Biol Phys 2006; 64(3): 661-9.
        [http://dx.doi.org/10.1016/j.ijrobp.2005.10.021]

[2]   Marx RE. Osteoradionecrosis: a new concept of its pathophysiology. J Oral Maxillofac Surg 1983; 41(5): 283-8.
        [http://dx.doi.org/10.1016/0278-2391(83)90294-X]

[3]   Marx RE. A new concept in the treatment of osteoradionecrosis. J Oral Maxillofac Surg 1983; 41(6): 351-7.
        [http://dx.doi.org/10.1016/S0278-2391(83)80005-6]

[4]   Ruggiero SL, Mehrotra B, Rosenburg TJ, *et al.* Osteonecrosis of the jaws associated with the use of bisphosphonates: a review of 63 cases. J Oral Maxillofac Surg 2004; 62: 527-34.
        [http://dx.doi.org/10.1016/j.joms.2004.02.004]

[5]   Purcell PM, Boyd IW. Bisphosphonates and osteonecrosis of the jaw. Med J Aust 2005; 182: 417-8.

[6]   Melo MD, Obeid G. Osteonecrosis of the maxilla in a patient with a history of bisphosphonate therapy. J Can Dent Assoc 2005; 71: 111-3.

[7]   Marx RE. Pamidronate (Aredia) and Zoledronate (Zometa) induced avascular necrosis of the jaws: a growing epidemic. J Oral Maxillofac Surg 2003; 61: 1115-7.
        [http://dx.doi.org/10.1016/S0278-2391(03)00720-1]

[8]   Carter G, Goss AN, Doecke C. Bisphosphonates and avascular necrosis of the jaw: a possible association. Med J Aust 2005; 182: 413-5.

[9]   Durie BG, Katz M, Crowley J. Osteonecrosis of jaw and bisphosphonates. N Engl J Med 2005; 353: 99-102.
        [http://dx.doi.org/10.1056/NEJM200507073530120]

[10]   King AE, Umland EM. Osteonecrosis of the jaw in patients receiving intravenous or oral bisphosphonates. Pharmacotherapy 2008; 28(5): 667-77.
        [http://dx.doi.org/10.1592/phco.28.5.667]

[11]   Varun BR, *et al.* Bisphosphonate Induced Osteonecrosis of Jaw in Breast Cancer Patients: A Systematic Review. Journal of Oral and Maxillofacial Pathology: JOMFP 162 2017; 210-4.

[12]   Ruggiero SL, Dodson TB, Assael LA, Landesberg R, Marx RE, Mehrotra B. American Association of Oral and Maxillofacial Surgeons. American Association of Oral and Maxillofacial Surgeons position paper on bisphosphonate-related osteonecrosis of the jaws--2009 update. J Oral Maxillofac Surg 2009; 67(5) (Suppl.): 2-12.
[http://dx.doi.org/10.1016/j.joms.2009.01.009]

[13]   Lyons A, Ghazali N. Osteoradionecrosis of the jaws: current understanding of its pathophysiology and treatment. Br J Oral Maxillofac Surg 2008; 46: 653-60.
[http://dx.doi.org/10.1016/j.bjoms.2008.04.006]

[14]   Jacobson AS, Buchbinder D, Hu K, Urken ML. Paradigm shifts in the management of osteoradionecrosis of the mandible. Oral Oncol 2010; 46: 795-801.
[http://dx.doi.org/10.1016/j.oraloncology.2010.08.007]

[15]   Delanian S, Lefaix JL. The radiation-induced fibroatrophic process: therapeutic perspective *via* the antioxidant pathway. Radiother Oncol 2004; 73: 119-31.
[http://dx.doi.org/10.1016/j.radonc.2004.08.021]

[16]   Bennett MH, Feldmeier J, Hampson N, Smee R, Milross C. Hyperbaric oxygen therapy for late radiation tissue injury. Cochrane Database Syst Rev 2012; 16(5): CD005005.

[17]   Epstein JB, Hatcher DC, Graham M. Bone scintigraphy of fibro-osseous lesions of the jaw. Oral Surg Oral Med Oral Pathol 1981; 51: 346-50.
[http://dx.doi.org/10.1016/0030-4220(81)90140-7]

[18]   Ubios AM, Piloni MJ, Cabrini RL. Mandibular growth and tooth eruption after localized x-radiation. J Oral Maxillofac Surg 1992; 50: 153-6.
[http://dx.doi.org/10.1016/0278-2391(92)90361-3]

[19]   Qi WX, Tang LN, He AN, *et al.* Risk of osteonecrosis of the jaw in cancer patients receiving denosumab: a meta-analysis of seven randomized controlled trials. Int J Clin Oncol 2013.

[20]   Coleman R, Woodward E, Brown J, *et al.* Safety of zoledronic acid and incidence of osteonecrosis of the jaw (ONJ) during adjuvant therapy in a randomised phase III trial (AZURE: BIG 01-04) for women with stage II/III breast cancer. Breast Cancer Res Treat 2011; 127: 429.
[http://dx.doi.org/10.1007/s10549-011-1429-y]

[21]   Mauri D, Valachis A, Polyzos IP, *et al.* Osteonecrosis of the jaw and use of bisphosphonates in adjuvant breast cancer treatment: a meta-analysis. Breast Cancer Res Treat 2009; 116: 433.
[http://dx.doi.org/10.1007/s10549-009-0432-z]

[22]   Vahtsevanos K, Kyrgidis A, Verrou E, *et al.* Longitudinal cohort study of risk factors in cancer patients of bisphosphonate-related osteonecrosis of the jaw. J Clin Oncol 2009; 27: 5356.
[http://dx.doi.org/10.1200/JCO.2009.21.9584]

[23]   Scagliotti GV, Hirsh V, Siena S, *et al.* Overall survival improvement in patients with lung cancer and bone metastases treated with denosumab *versus* zoledronic acid: subgroup analysis from a randomized phase 3 study. J Thorac Oncol 2012; 7: 1823.
[http://dx.doi.org/10.1097/JTO.0b013e31826aec2b]

[24]   Henry DH, Costa L, Goldwasser F, *et al.* Randomized, double-blind study of denosumab *versus* zoledronic acid in the treatment of bone metastases in patients with advanced cancer (excluding breast and prostate cancer) or multiple myeloma. J Clin Oncol 2011; 29: 1125.
[http://dx.doi.org/10.1200/JCO.2010.31.3304]

[25]   Guarneri V, Miles D, Robert N, *et al.* Bevacizumab and osteonecrosis of the jaw: incidence and association with bisphosphonate therapy in three large prospective trials in advanced breast cancer. Breast Cancer Res Treat 2010; 122: 181.
[http://dx.doi.org/10.1007/s10549-010-0866-3]

[26] Koch FP, Walter C, Hansen T, *et al.* Osteonecrosis of the jaw related to sunitinib. Oral Maxillofac Surg 2011; 15: 63.
[http://dx.doi.org/10.1007/s10006-010-0224-y]

[27] Nicolatou-Galitis O, Migkou M, Psyrri A, *et al.* Gingival bleeding and jaw bone necrosis in patients with metastatic renal cell carcinoma receiving sunitinib: report of 2 cases with clinical implications. Oral Surg Oral Med Oral Pathol Oral Radiol 2012; 113: 234.
[http://dx.doi.org/10.1016/j.tripleo.2011.08.024]

[28] Fleissig Y, Regev E, Lehman H. Sunitinib related osteonecrosis of jaw: a case report. Oral Surg Oral Med Oral Pathol Oral Radiol 2012; 113
[http://dx.doi.org/10.1016/j.tripleo.2011.06.023]

[29] Brunello A, Saia G, Bedogni A, *et al.* Worsening of osteonecrosis of the jaw during treatment with sunitinib in a patient with metastatic renal cell carcinoma. Bone 2009; 44: 173.
[http://dx.doi.org/10.1016/j.bone.2008.08.132]

[30] Ayllon J, Launay-Vacher V, Medioni J, *et al.* Osteonecrosis of the jaw under bisphosphonate and antiangiogenic therapies: cumulative toxicity profile? Ann Oncol 2009; 20: 600.
[http://dx.doi.org/10.1093/annonc/mdn788]

[31] Christodoulou C, Pervena A, Klouvas G, *et al.* Combination of bisphosphonates and antiangiogenic factors induces osteonecrosis of the jaw more frequently than bisphosphonates alone. Oncology 2009; 76: 209.
[http://dx.doi.org/10.1159/000201931]

[32] Balmor GR, Yarom N, Weitzen R. Drug-induced palate osteonecrosis following nasal surgery. Isr Med Assoc J 2012; 14: 193.

[33] Hoefert S, Eufinger H. Sunitinib may raise the risk of bisphosphonate-related osteonecrosis of the jaw: presentation of three cases. Oral Surg Oral Med Oral Pathol Oral Radiol Endod 2010; 110: 463.
[http://dx.doi.org/10.1016/j.tripleo.2010.04.049]

[34] Bozas G, Roy A, Ramasamy V, *et al.* Osteonecrosis of the jaw after a single bisphosphonate infusion in a patient with metastatic renal cancer treated with sunitinib. Onkologie 2010; 33: 321.
[http://dx.doi.org/10.1159/000313680]

[35] Beuselinck B, Wolter P, Karadimou A, *et al.* Concomitant oral tyrosine kinase inhibitors and bisphosphonates in advanced renal cell carcinoma with bone metastases. Br J Cancer 2012; 107: 1665.
[http://dx.doi.org/10.1038/bjc.2012.385]

[36] Smidt-Hansen T, Folkmar TB, Fode K, *et al.* Combination of zoledronic acid and targeted therapy is active but may induce osteonecrosis of the jaw in patients with metastatic renal cell carcinoma. J Oral Maxillofac Surg 2013; 71: 1532.
[http://dx.doi.org/10.1016/j.joms.2013.03.019]

[37] United States. Food and Drug Administration http://www.fda.gov/Safety/MedWatch/ Safety Information/ ucm275758.htm

[38] United States. Food and Drug Administration http://www.fda.gov/safety/medwatch/ safetyinformation/ ucm224050.htm

[39] Background Document for Meeting of Advisory Committee for Reproductive Health Drugs and Drug Safety and Risk Management Advisory Committee. United States 2011. http://www.fda.gov/ downloads/ Advisory Committees/ Committees Meeting Materials/ drugs/ Drug Safetyand RiskManagementAdvisoryCommittee/ ucm270958.pdf

[40] Lo JC, O'Ryan FS, Gordon NP, *et al.* Prevalence of osteonecrosis of the jaw in patients with oral bisphosphonate exposure. J Oral Maxillofac Surg 2010; 68: 243.
[http://dx.doi.org/10.1016/j.joms.2009.03.050]

[41] Malden N, Lopes V. An epidemiological study of alendronate-related osteonecrosis of the jaws. A

case series from the south-east of Scotland with attention given to case definition and prevalence. J Bone Miner Metab 2012; 30: 171.
[http://dx.doi.org/10.1007/s00774-011-0299-z]

[42] Grbic JT, Black DM, Lyles KW, *et al.* The incidence of osteonecrosis of the jaw in patients receiving 5 milligrams of zoledronic acid: data from the health outcomes and reduced incidence with zoledronic acid once yearly clinical trials program. J Am Dent Assoc 2010; 141: 1365.

[43] Black DM, Reid IR, Boonen S, *et al.* The effect of 3 *versus* 6 years of zoledronic acid treatment of osteoporosis: a randomized extension to the HORIZON-Pivotal Fracture Trial (PFT). J Bone Miner Res 2012; 27: 243.
[http://dx.doi.org/10.1002/jbmr.1494]

[44] Briefing Information for the September 9, 2011 Joint Meeting of the Reproductive Health Drugs Advisory Committee and the Drug Safety and Risk Management Advisory Committee. 2011.http://www.fda.gov/AdvisoryCommittees/CommitteesMeetingMaterials/Drugs/DrugSafetyand RiskManagementAdvisoryCommittee/ucm270957.htm

[45] Saad F, Brown JE, Van Poznak C, *et al.* Incidence, risk factors, and outcomes of osteonecrosis of the jaw: integrated analysis from three blinded active-controlled phase III trials in cancer patients with bone metastases. Ann Oncol 2012; 23: 1341.
[http://dx.doi.org/10.1093/annonc/mdr435]

[46] Fehm T, Beck V, Banys M, *et al.* Bisphosphonate-induced osteonecrosis of the jaw (ONJ): Incidence and risk factors in patients with breast cancer and gynecological malignancies. Gynecol Oncol 2009; 112: 605.
[http://dx.doi.org/10.1016/j.ygyno.2008.11.029]

[47] Kyrgidis A, Vahtsevanos K, Koloutsos G, *et al.* Bisphosphonate-related osteonecrosis of the jaws: a case-control study of risk factors in breast cancer patients. J Clin Oncol 2008; 26: 4634.
[http://dx.doi.org/10.1200/JCO.2008.16.2768]

[48] Kunchur R, Need A, Hughes T, *et al.* Clinical investigation of C-terminal cross-linking telopeptide test in prevention and management of bisphosphonate-associated osteonecrosis of the jaws. J Oral Maxillofac Surg 2009; 67: 1167.
[http://dx.doi.org/10.1016/j.joms.2009.02.004]

[49] Yamazaki T, Yamori M, Ishizaki T, *et al.* Increased incidence of osteonecrosis of the jaw after tooth extraction in patients treated with bisphosphonates: a cohort study. Int J Oral Maxillofac Surg 2012; 41: 1397.

[50] Mozzati M, Arata V, Gallesio G. Tooth extraction in patients on zoledronic acid therapy. Oral Oncol 2012; 48: 817.
[http://dx.doi.org/10.1016/j.oraloncology.2012.03.009]

[51] Scoletta M, Arata V, Arduino PG, *et al.* Tooth extractions in intravenous bisphosphonate-treated patients: a refined protocol. J Oral Maxillofac Surg 2013; 71: 994.
[http://dx.doi.org/10.1016/j.joms.2013.01.006]

[52] Tsao C, Darby I, Ebeling PR, *et al.* Oral health risk factors for bisphosphonate-associated jaw osteonecrosis. J Oral Maxillofac Surg 2013; 71: 1360.
[http://dx.doi.org/10.1016/j.joms.2013.02.016]

[53] Brown JJ, Ramalingam L, Zacharin MR. Bisphosphonate-associated osteonecrosis of the jaw: does it occur in children? Clin Endocrinol (Oxf) 2008; 68: 863.

[54] Katz J, Gong Y, Salmasinia D, *et al.* Genetic polymorphisms and other risk factors associated with bisphosphonate induced osteonecrosis of the jaw. Int J Oral Maxillofac Surg 2011; 40: 605.

CHAPTER 6

Wisdom Teeth & Maxillary Canine Impaction

Wamiq Musheer Fareed[*]

Department of Oral & Maxillofacial Surgery, College of Dentistry, Taibah University, Madinah, Saudi Arabia

Abstract: Any tooth that fails to erupt to its normal anatomic position in the jaw, by the end of its eruption time; despite of having eruptive forces, due to a specific physical (bone/soft tissue) barrier or ectopic position is said to be impacted. The removal of impacted mandibular third molars is the most common procedure in the specialty of oral and maxillofacial surgery. The third molars are the last teeth to erupt therefore by far the most frequently impacted teeth. This chapter includes the Impaction of maxillary mandibular wisdom teeth and maxillary mandibular canine impactions. Association of clinical, radiology clinical variables which combined level of difficulties:

1. Age,
2. Radiological variables to the combined level of difficulty are
   a. Angulation
   b. Relation to second molar
   c. Depth from point of elevation.

With the above topics classifications and surgeries of wisdom teeth are also illustrated with figures, tables and diagrams.

Mandibular and maxillary canine impactions are also discussed with diagrams .All the Pre, Intra and post-surgical aspects are covered in details.

The chapter also deals with different types of incisions, radiographs, surgical anatomy and surgical procedures.

Keywords: Canine Impaction, Causes Impactions, Classification, Maxillary Third Molar, Radiological Interpretation, Surgical Management.

DEFINITION OF IMPACTION

Archer (1975) quoted "A tooth which is completely or partially unerupted and

---
[*] **Corresponding author Esam Ahmad Z Omar:** Department of Oral & Maxillofacial Surgery, College of Dentistry, Taibah University, Madinah, Saudi Arabia; Tel: 009660550152401; Fax: 00966148494710; E-mail: wmfareed@gmail.com

positioned against another tooth, bone or soft tissue so that its further eruption is unlikely".

Mac Gregor (1985) stated Impaction is present if the occlusal surface of the tooth does not conform to the curves of Manson and Spee, when the third molar is fully formed and the growth of the jaws is complete.

- According to Scottish intercollegiate guidelines (1999) An unerupted tooth is a tooth lying within the jaws, entirely covered by soft tissue, and partially or completely covered by bone.
- A partially erupted tooth is a tooth that has failed to erupt fully into a normal position. The term implies that the tooth is partly visible or in communication with the oral cavity.
- An impacted tooth is a tooth, which is prevented from completely erupting into a normal functional position. This may be due to lack of space, obstruction by another tooth, or an abnormal eruption path.
- Fonseca *et al.* (2000) defined impaction as a cessation of the eruption of a tooth caused by a clinically or radiographically detectable physical barrier in the eruption path such as teeth, odontomas, cysts, crowded tooth germs or erupted teeth or by an ectopic position of the tooth.

ETIOLOGY OF THIRD MANDIBULAR MOLAR IMPACTION

Hunter (1771) is one of the early authors who noted 'want of room in the jaws for these late teeth'.

Henry and Ivlorant (1936) were of the opinion that impaction of third molars was related to their mesiodistal crown width. Small third molars appeared to be less at risk of impaction than large ones.

Late mineralization of the mandibular third molar crown is associated with a higher incidence of impaction in boys (Bjork, Jensis, Palling, 1956).

Individuals with wide alveolar shelves and deep buccinator grooves run less risk of third molar impaction than individuals with a different morphology (Willis Tha 1966).

Initial extreme mesial inclination of the third molar germs has been found to enhance the risk of impaction (Tait, Williams 1978).

MacGregor (1985) noted that in the course of primate evolution, an increase of brain size at the expense of jaw size has not always been accompanied by a commensurate reduction in tooth size or number. An alteration of diet/ food habits has followed in the last 2000 years has resulted in the teeth being underused and not worn down.

Svendsen, Maertens (1997) indicated that causal factors for lack of space in the third molar region include insufficient growth in length of the mandible, vertical condylar growth direction, posteriorly directed eruption of the dentition, size of dental arch perimeter and resorption of the anterior border of the ramus.

INCIDENCE OF THIRD MANDIBULAR MOLAR

Classification

Winter (1926) classified the impacted tooth in relation to the long axis of the second molar as:

1. Vertical
2. Mesiooblique
3. Horizontal
4. Distoangular

Pell, Gregory (1933) classified mandibular third molars impacted as:

(I). Relation of the Tooth to the Ramus of the Mandible (Fig. 6.1)

Class I: Sufficient/Adequate space or distance exists among the distal aspect of second molar and the anterior border of ramus, for accommodation of the mesiodistal diameter of the crown of third molar.

Class II: The distance between the distal aspect of second molar and the anterior border of ramus is less than the mesiodistal diameter of the crown of wisdom molar.

Class III: Entire third mandibular molar tooth is within the ramus.

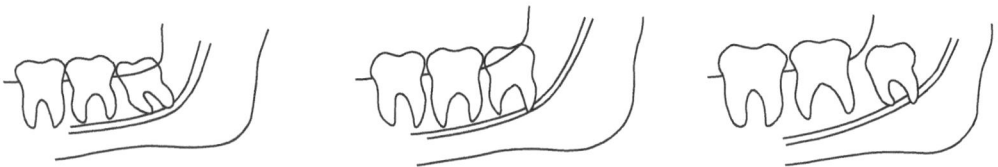

Fig. (6.1). Relation of the tooth to the ramus of the Mandible.

(II). Mandibular Third Molars Relative Depth in Bone (Fig. 6.2)

Position A: The highest or uppermost portion of the impacted tooth is in level with or above the occlusal plane.

Position B: The highest or uppermost portion of the tooth (impacted) is lower than the occlusal plane, but above the cervical line of the second molar.

Position C: The highest/uppermost portion of the impacted tooth is below the cervical line of the second molar.

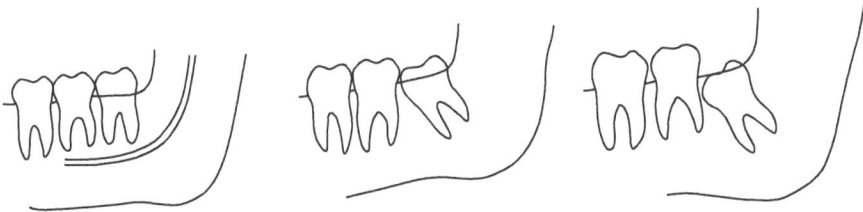

Fig. (6.2). Mandibular third molars relative depth in Bone.

(III). Position of the Tooth in Relation to the Long Axis of the Second Molar

1. Vertical
2. Horizontal
3. Inverted
4. Mesioangular
5. Distoangular

These possibly will occur in:

1. Buccal deflection
2. Lingual deflection
3. Torsion

(IV). Complications

1. Abnormal/unusual root curvature
2. Hypercementosis
3. Proximity or closeness to the mandibular canal
4. Bone density
5. Adipose tissue
6. Lack of accessibility
7. Inflexibility of the muscle of the mouth

Killey, Kay (1965) classified the wisdom mandibular third molars according to:

A. **Angulation and position**
    a. Vertical
    b. Mesio-angular
    c. Disto-angluar

    d. Horizontal
    e. Transverse displacement
    f. Aberrant positions
B. **State of Eruption**
    a. Erupted
    b. Partially erupted
    c. Unerupted
C. **Number of roots**
    a. Fused roots
    b. Two roots
    c. Multiple roots

The roots may be surgically favourable or unfavourable. Macgregor (1985) proposed the WHARF Assessment:

1. Winter's Classification

Horizontal	2
Distoangular	2
Mesioangular	1
Vertical	0

2. Height of the Mandible

1-30 mm	0
31-34 mm	1
35-39 mm	2

3. Angulation of Third Molar

1-50	0
60-69	1
70-79	2
80-89	3
90°+	4

4. Root shape

Complex	1
Favorable curvature	2
Unfavorable curvature	3

5. Follicles

Normal	0
Possibly enlarged	1
Enlarged	2

6. Exit Path

Space	0
Distal cusp covered	1
Mesial cusp also covered	2
Both covered	3

Third Molar Difficulty Index: Mandibular Impactions (Pederson 1988).

Spatial relationship

Mesioangular	1
Horizontal/Transverse	2
Vertical	3
Distoangular	4

Depth

Level A	1
Level B	2
Level C	3

Ramus relationship/space available

Class I	1
Class II	2
Class III	3

Age

Young (roots nearly formed)	1
Young (no root formation)	2
Young (roots recently formed, *i.e.*, 18-24)	3
Mid-age range (25-35)	4
Older age (over 35)	5

Facial form

Tapering	1
Mid-range, tapering to compact	2
Compact	3

Difficulty Index

Very Difficult	7 - 10
Moderately Difficult	5 - 6 (5 - 7 in original index)
Minimally Difficult	3 - 4

Yuasa *et al.* (2002) stated that Proximity/vicinity to the mandibular canal were classified by Pederson as close or distant. Abnormal or unusual root curvature was classified as straight, incomplete or curved root. Width of the root is defined as: thin, where the width of the middle root is thinner than the width of the neck, bulbous, the width of the middle root is thicker than the width of the neck and the roots do not separate; or thick (multiple roots), the width of the middle root is thicker than the width of the neck and the roots separately. The quantity of roots was categorized as singular, multiple, or incomplete.

RADIOLOGICAL INTERPRETATION

According to Killey, Kay (1965) basic radiographic views required are:

a. Accurate periapical view
b. Occlusal view
c. Lateral oblique view Abramovich *et al.* Despite the relative ease in imaging impacted teeth, any acceptable diagnostic radiograph or set of diagnostic radiographs must demonstrate the following:
   ○ Entire outline of the impacted tooth
   ○ Outline of the follicular sac
   ○ More than 2.0 mm of healthy cancellous bone around the follicular sac and impacted root outline.
   The first two points are necessary to properly evaluate the position of the impacted tooth and assist in the development of a treatment plan. The last point is particularly significant of diagnose pathological conditions associated with the impacted tooth that may affect the treatment plan.
d. **Orthopantomogram**
   Venta *et al.* (2001) quoted Panoramic radiographs bite wings, frontal cephalometric radiographs and lateral head films have predominantly been used. The study carried out by Sewerin and Wowern is one of the first to report on following up on third molars using periapical radiographs.

INFORMATION OBTAINED FROM STANDARD RADIOGRAPHS

Kruger *et al.* (1980), Peterson (1999) stated anatomically accurate and clear radiographs will define the morphology of each impacted tooth. Any anomalies that may alter the probable surgical management can be identified. Examples of such conditions include sclerotic cancellous bone; unusual coronal shapes; dilacerated roots; and the number, length, shape, and curvature of the roots of an impacted tooth. Improper radiographic evaluation that fails to detect this anomaly could lead to various types of complications, including root fracture, jaw fracture, and aspiration of a tooth fragment.

Radiographs can also yield information about the density of the surrounding bone. Sclerotic cancellous bone may require that the surgeons remove more bone to facilitate moving a tooth, whereas bone with sparse trabeculation would require less force and less bone removal.

Similar predictions about the surgical access and degree of difficulty need to be made regarding the position of an impacted mandibular third molar as it relates to the position of the inferior border, angle, and ramus of the mandible. Also of major importance is the position of the impaction relative to the neurovascular bundle in the mandible, *i.e.*, the inferior alveolar (mandibular) canal. A review of Miller and associates reported that the incidence of inferior alveolar nerve dysesthesia following surgery of impacted third molars was 0.57 to 5.30%.

Access

Howe (1966) stated that the radio-opaque line casted by external oblique ridge concludes the easiness of access to the surgical site. If this line is inclining or tending to be vertical this leads to poor access, but if it is horizontal, excellent access is gained.

Position and Depth

Winter (1926) describes by drawing three imaginary lines on the radiographic film, by this method the position and depth of the tooth is assessed. These lines have been designated as:

- **White line** - represents the occlusal plane. The line is drawn touching the occlusal surfaces of first mandibular, second mandibular molar and is extended posteriorly over the third molar region. It indicates the axial inclination of the impacted mandibular third molar in relation to the long axis or elongation of the second mandibular molar.
- **Amber line** - represents the bone level. The line is drawn from the crest of the

interdental septum between the molars and extended posteriorly to the ascending ramus. This line signifies covering of the alveolar bone on the impacted tooth. This will indicate the amount of the bone taken out for the extraction of the impacted tooth.

- **Red line** - The line is drawn perpendicular *i.e.* 90 degree from the amber line to an imaginary point of application of the elevator. It indicates the depth of the tooth in bone.

Howe (1966) stated that any tooth/teeth with a red line 5 mm or more in length is better removed under an endotracheal anesthesia or sedation. Increase in the length of the red line of every surplus millimeter renders the surgical removal of the impacted tooth three times more challenging and difficult.

Relationship to the Inferior Dental Canal (Fig. 6.3)

The relation radiographically between the wisdom third molar tooth and the inferior alveolar nerve was superimposition in 37% teeth, the root apex just touched the upper border of the outline of the neurovascular bundle in 32% teeth and in 18% teeth a separation of more than 1mm between the roots and the neurovascular bundle was found (Bell 2003).

Bell (2003) listed each mandibular wisdom tooth was categorized according to its relation to the inferior alveolar neurovascular bundle.

These were:

- Darkening of the root (Howe and Poyton, Main).
- Deflecting of the roots (Stockdale, Waggener)
- Narrowing of the root (Seward)
- Dark and bifid apex of the root (Seward)
- Interruption of white lines of the canal (Howe and Poyton, Seward)
- Diversion of the inferior alveolar canal (Seward, MacGregor)
- Narrowing of the inferior alveolar canal (Seward, Macgregor, Killey and Kay)
- Root of tooth more than 1 mm distant from the neurovascular bundle.
- Root of tooth just touching the upper outline of the neurovascular bundle.
- Root of toot superimposed on the neurovascular bundle.

Intraoral Periapical Radiographs

Intraoral radiography is the most commonly used imaging method in general dentistry; however, for evaluating impacted teeth panoramic and occlusal radiographic techniques are usually indicated. Minimally geometric and vertical distortion of the objects occurs when a paralleling technique is used.

Paralleling procedures require that the film be positioned medial to the target toot but parallel to long axis/alignment of the teeth. In the mandible, the film can be positioned close to the alveolar ridge and remain parallel to the mandibular teeth. In the maxilla, however, the curvature of the palatal vault and the buccal inclination of the crowns make it necessary to increase the tooth film distance. A properly positioned maxillary film usually deviates in alignment with the sagittal plane by approximately 6 to 22 degrees.

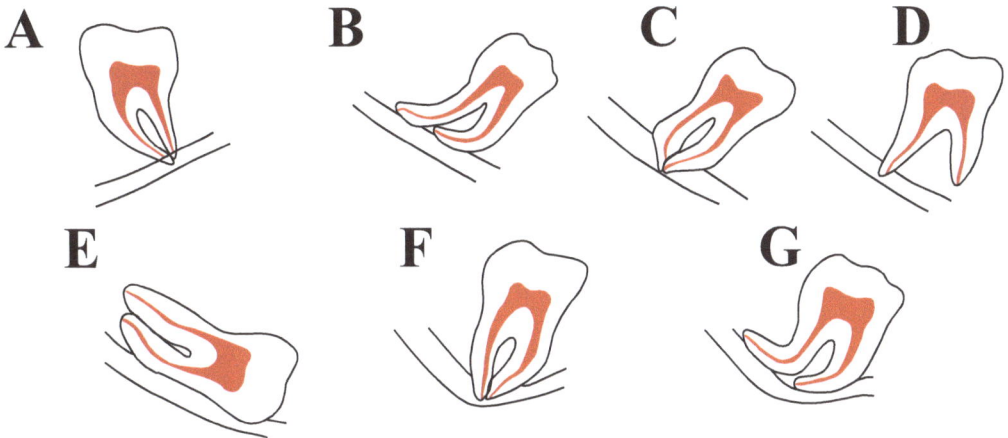

Fig. (6.3). Relationship to the inferior dental canal.

Occlusal Radiography

Occlusal radiography represents an excellent imaging method when the image field extends more apically than the coverage of standard intraoral radiographs. It is also helpful on patients with a limited opening that restricts access for intraoral film placement. Occlusal techniques use either standard size intraoral film (1¾ x 1¼") or the larger size occlusal film (3.0 x 2¼"). Film stabilization is accomplished by placing the film on the occlusal plane and having the patient close lightly on the film.

Lateral Oblique Mandibular Radiography

Lateral oblique projections of the mandible are extraoral projections. Prior to panoramic radiography, these views were the only option for viewing mandibular impactions that could not be imaged on intraoral film.

The film is placed on the lateral aspect of the jaw with the impaction. The beam is directed from the opposite side of the mandible at a negative oblique angle. The central rays of the X-ray beam are focused and directed approximately 1 inch inferior to the contralateral (opposite) mandible toward the side with the impacted teeth. This projection provides greater periapical coverage than is available on standard periapical views. Given figure shows the horizontal impaction of a second premolar in an otherwise edentulous mandible.

Computed tomography (CT) is an imaging modality that uses x-radiation to scan the patient from multiple angles. This technology uses sensitive X-ray receptors that reduce patient exposure by 80 to 90%, as compared with standard oral and dental exposures, and produces a visual image on a monitor within seconds following the radiographic exposure.

The X-ray generator for digital radiography is similar to standard dental X-ray generators except that it requires a microprocessor except that it requires a microprocessor timer to more precisely control the very short exposure times.

The exposure times are dramatically reduced because a charge-coupling device (CCD) is used as the image receptor instead of film. The radiographic CCD is similar to the CCDs used in video camera technology.

Aside from the advantages of time and decreased radiation, the major advantage of this technology is the ability to digitize the information from the CCD and store the images electronically.

The film must also parallel the teeth in the horizontal dimensions; this is accomplished by paralleling the film with a line that joins the tangents of the buccal and/or lingual crests of curvature. With the film position parallel to the long axis of the teeth, the x-radiation central beam must be projected perpendicular to both of these paralleled planes. This is also achieved by aligning the end of the cone, *i.e.*, the beam-indicating device (BID), parallel to the film packet. The center of the X-ray beam should then be directed toward the center of the film to avoid "cone-cutting". Several commercial instruments are available to facilitate the paralleling technique.

Indications for Extraction/Removal of Wisdom Teeth

Westcott *et al.* (2002) listed Indications for extraction/removal of wisdom teeth by Royal College of Surgeons of England, (1997):

Overt or previous history of infection including pericoronitis
Unrestorable caries
Non-treatable pulpal or periapical disease or both
Cellulitis, abscess and osteomyelitis

Cellulitis, abscess and osteomyelitis
Periodontal disease
Orthodontic abnormalities
Prophylactic removal in the presence of specific medical and surgical conditions
Facilitation of restorative treatment including provision of prosthesis
Internal external resorption of tooth or adjacent teeth
Pain directly related to third molar
Tooth in the line of bony fracture or impeding trauma management
Fracture of tooth
Disease of follicle including cyst tumor
Tooth teeth impeding orthognathic surgery or reconstructive jaw surgery
Tooth involved in within field of tumor resection
Satisfactory tooth for use as donor for transplantation
Hamasha *et al.* (2006) studied the reasons for third molar tooth extraction

Category	Reason
Dental caries and its consequences	Badly carious tooth
	Remaining root
	Periapical lesion
	Failure of restoration
	Deep root caries
Eruption problems	Impacted tooth
	Pericoronitis
	Cheek bite
	No opposing tooth
	Pressure on the adjacent teeth
	Impinging on opposing soft tissues
	Food impaction in wisdom area
	Eruption buccally or lingually
	Periocoronal abscess
Periodontal diseases	Periodontitis
	Mobility
Dentists choice	Prosthodontist request
	Prophylactic removal
	Investigating facial pain
	Orthodontists request
Miscellaneous	Fractured teeth due to trauma

Contd.....

Category	Reason
	Patient's choice
	Root resorption
	Attempt extraction elsewhere

CHOICE OF ANAESTHESIA

The removal of impacted or displaced mandibular third molars may be carried out under local analgesia or general anaesthesia (Kay, Killey 1965).

Technically there is no contra-indication to the removal of any impaction under local analgesia. But, surgery involving the removal of deeply buried impacted tooth may be prolonged, and it is more suitable for both patient and operator if such cases are performed under general anaesthesia. Another important factor is the nervous state of the patient. If there is no general medical reason which dictate the type of anesthesia to be used, then patients can decide by themselves, which anaesthesia they prefer (Kay, Killey 1965).

SURGICAL MANAGEMENT

(Kay, Killey 1965) divided the operation for the removal of impacted lower third molars into the following stages:

- The incision to obtain access to the area
- Removal of an adequate amount of bone
- Elevation of the tooth from its socket
- Preparation of the wound before closure
- Closure of the incision

Types of Incision

I. **Ward's Incision (Fig. 6.4)**: According to Kay, Killey (1965) the incision should begin from a point above 1/4 inch down in buccal sulcus approximately at the junction of the posterior and middle thirds of the second molar. The anterior line of the incision with the scalpel blade, pressed firmly down to bone passes upwards to the disto-buccal angle of the second molar at the gingival margin. Here the course of the incision passes cervically behind the tooth to the middle of the posterior surface if the third molar is unerupted. From this point on the distal aspect of the second molar, the cut is taken backwards and buccally, but not directed straight up the ramus. The lateral extension avoids the small vessels emerging from the retromolar triangle or fossa.

II. **Modified Ward's Incision (Fig. 6.5)**: Incision differs from ward`s incision only in that the anterior incision starts from the distobuccal angle of first molar at the gingival margin. This is advocated to obtain better access. (Howe 1966).

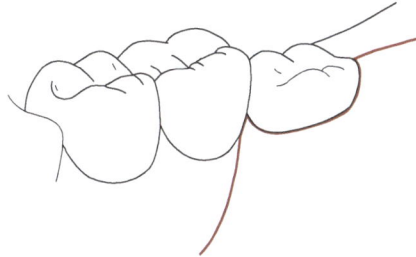

Fig. (6.4). Ward's Incision.

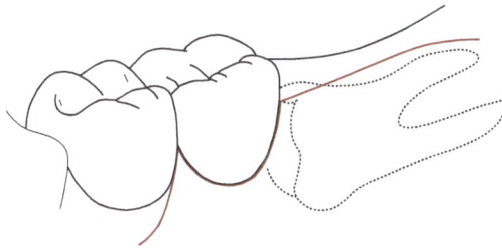

Fig. (6.5). Modified Ward's Incision.

III. **Envelope Type (Fig. 6.6)**: The incision starts on the ascending ramus, following the center of the third molar shelf to the distobuccal surface of the second molar, and then extends as a sulcular incision to the mesiobuccal corner of the second molar. This flap is adequate for most mesially inclined and superficial impactions Szmyd (1971), Kay-Killey, Flap can be extended to the mesiobuccal corner of the first molar to allow better visibility.

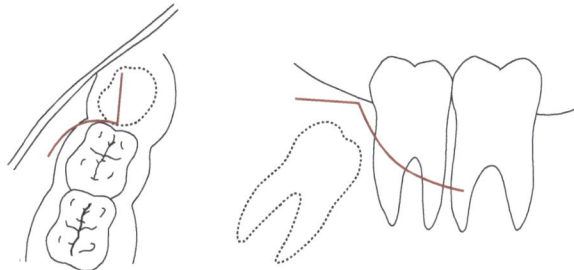

Fig. (6.6). Envelope type.

IV. **L-shaped (Fig. 6.7)**: Another variant of the previously mentioned flap is to place the incision a couple of millimeters away from the marginal gingiva. This procedure optimizes marginal attachment healing next to the second molar (Groves, Moore 1970) but requires that the main surgical approach to the third molar is at a distance from the second molar.

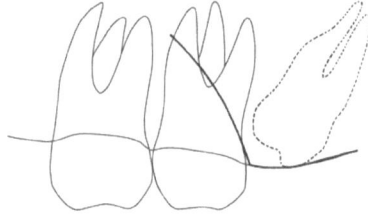

Fig. (6.7). L-shaped.

V. **Bayonet Shaped:** This flap uses an incision similar to the envelope flap incision. However, an oblique vestibular extension is made in the sulcus region (MacGregor 1985). This extension should be angled forward to facilitate suturing and to optimize blood supply to the anterior part of the flap. This type of incision gives excellent buccal visibility.

Removal of an Adequate Amount of Bone

Bone removal from around the impacted or displaced tooth is carried out by a mallet and chisel or by a bur, sometimes a combination of both methods may be a appropriate, provided that sufficient bone is removed to free the tooth from obstruction and provide a point of application for an elevator, it does not matter which technique is chosen (Kay, Killey 1965).

Thermal necrosis due to drilling has been reported by Anderson *et al.* (1943), Peterson (1952).

Gregory (1933) in which they advocated occlusal, buccal and distal bone removal to facilitate removal of mandibular third molars and whenever required a modified tooth splitting technique to split off distal portion of crown. They noted need for less extensive incision and bone removal and lesser surrounding tissue injury with less operating time required.

Split-bone technique for the removal of mandibular third molars was proposed by Kelsey Fry, and described by Ward in 1956. The wedge-shaped lingual piece of bone is fractured inwards to facilitate removal of impacted tooth. The advantages of this technique are its quick atraumatic nature and elimination of the distolingual bone allowing the lingual tissues to fall in and eliminate much of the dead space. The bone is clean, fresh cut and there is little or no late sequestration (Ward 1956).

Simplified split bone technique was described by Yeh (1995) in which an osteomucoperiosteal flap was created by making a cut with the chisel superiorly, distally and lingually to expose the crown and root as much as possible. Chisel in this technique is used as an osseous elevator to reflect the bone, periosteum and mucosa simultaneously and to displace the lingual nerve.

Buccal corticotomy is an alternative approach that offers access to deeply impacted mandibular teeth (Miloro 1995).

Tooth Sectioning

The tooth sectioning is done to create an easy bath of removal. It decease the amount of bone need to be removed. There are different types of sectioning (Fig. **6.8**-**6.11**), selection of the proper one depend on pre-operative assessment of:

- Root curvature,
- Path of removal,
- Amount of bone and relation of the tooth to ramus,
- Relation of the tooth to second molar

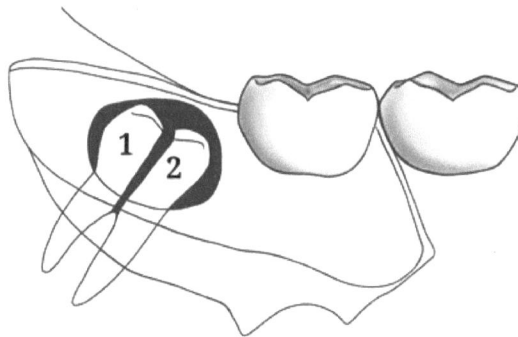

Fig. (6.8). Tooth sectioning.

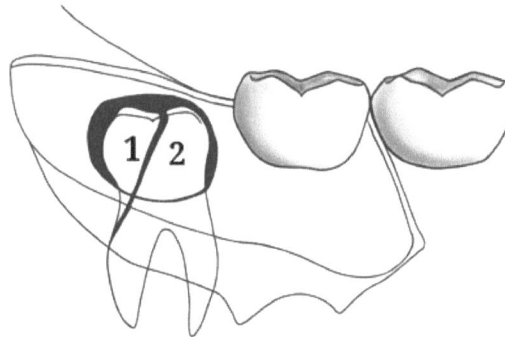

Fig. (6.9). Tooth sectioning.

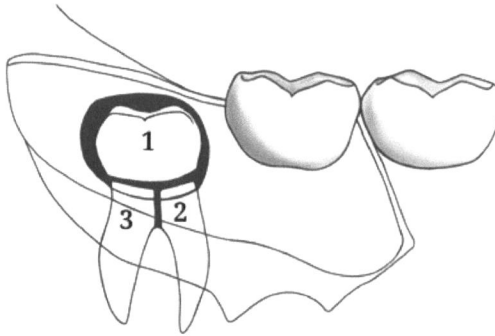

Fig. (6.10). Tooth sectioning.

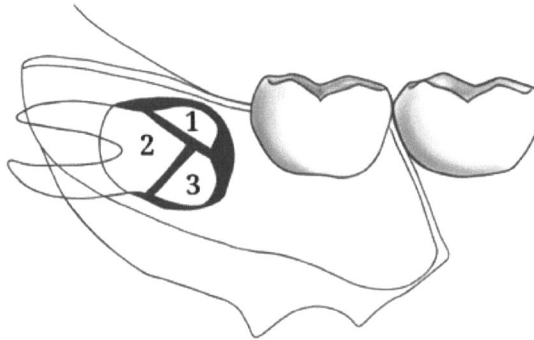

Fig. (6.11). Tooth sectioning.

Elevation of the Tooth From its Socket

After adequate removal of surrounding bone, the impacted lower third molar should be elevated from its socket with the help of elevators such as Warwick-James patterns which are not of great mechanical efficiency. Excessive force should never be applied during elevation of the impacted tooth otherwise tooth or jaw may fracture. This is also the reason why forceps should not be used in removal of impacted third molar. (Kay, Killey 1965).

Elevators are applied at a point of access which is cut after removing the impeding bone. This depends upon the position of the tooth and configuration of the roots (Kay, Killey 1965).

Preparation of the Wound for Closure

The wound should be gently irrigated with sterile warm saline solution with a chi p syringe to remove minute tooth and bone debris after removal of the impacted mandibular wisdom molar (Kay, Killey 1965).

Loose tags of mucosa, any granulation tissue and also the tooth follicle should be removed gently with a pair of curved Halstead's mosquito forceps. Irregular bony margins should be trimmed to a smooth surface with a pair of Jansen-Middleton bone nibblers. Bleeding points are controlled by pressure with swabs and finally the wound is again irrigated thoroughly prior to closure (Kay, Killey 1965).

Well designed flaps fall back easily into place aided by pressure from the fold of the cheek. If the impacted wisdom tooth was unerupted, then the wound can be closed merely by returning the muco-periosteal flap to its original position. With a partially erupted tooth an essential preliminary is to trim the flap with a pair of long curved scissors before suturing (Kay, Killey 1965).

The curved Denis-Browne needle is inserted into the lingual gingiva just distal to the second molar and then through the buccal flap in such a position that the flap will be in its correct position when the suture is tied loosely (Kay, Killey 1965).

Usually a single suture will suffice to close the wound, but occasionally a second suture is required to approximate the tissues either at the anterior buccal part of the incision line or along the distal extension into the cheek (Kay, Killey 1965).

The ends of the sutures after knotting should be cut so that approximately 1/4 inch in length remains. Larger ends tend to be irritating to the patient. (Kay, Killey 1965).A primary closure is preferred by Howe (1971), Archer (1975), Kruger (1974), and Killey-Kay (1975). Blair-Ivy (1923) prefers the wound to heal by secondary intention. However, Clark (1965), Winter (1947) indicated that the wound may be treated by either method. Woodward (1976) advocated the use of a small V-opening posterior to the second molar to facilitate postoperative irrigation of the wound.

Maxillary Third Molar

The first evidence of calcification of maxillary third molars usually is seen on X-ray films from patients ages 8 to 10. The enamel covering the coronal portion is completed in the middle of the second decade, from 11 to 17 years, and the root is completed from 15 to 25 years. Normal eruption is expected from the 17th to the 21st year of life. The maxillary third molar may have a wide variety of appearances.

Wheeler observed: The maxillary third molar often appears as a developmental anomaly. It can vary considerably in size, contour and relative position to other teeth .All third molars, mandibular and maxillary, show more variation in development than any other teeth in the mouth. Occasionally they appear as anomalies bearing little to no resemblance to neighboring teeth.

Third Molar and Second Molar Relationships

The position of a maxillary third molar is often described, as with a mandibular third molar, by a statement of its relationship to the second molar. The maxillary third molar, compared with the long axis of the second molar, may be in positions described as mesioangular, vertical, and distoangular, horizontal, transverse, and unusual, such as inverted or displaced to distant locations in the mid facial skeleton.

The level of impaction may be described, from inferior to superior in association with the second molar, as being crown of the third molar to crown of the second molar, crown to cervix, crown to root, and displaced. These positions may be modified by direction of the entire axis of the third molar from the apex to the crown in relation to the midline of the dental arch, palatal (medial), directly posterior, or buccal (lateral) to the second molar.

One of the challenging relationships of the maxillary third molar to second molar is coalescing of the root surfaces. This coalescence poses a treatment problem if there is a need to perform endodontic treatment or to remove one tooth or the other.

Classification of Impacted Maxillary Third Molars (Fonseca *et al.* 2000)

The classification of impacted maxillary teeth is similar to mandibular teeth but variations do exist. The following are the classifications which are commonly used.

Classification of maxillary third molar impactions, based on anatomic position

Relative depth of the impacted maxillary third molar in bone (Pell and Gregory)
> **Class A:** The lowest portion of the crown of the impacted maxillary third molar is on a line with the occlusal plane of the second molar.
> **Class B:** The lowest portion of the crown of the impacted maxillary third molar is between the occlusal plane of the second molar and the cervical line.
> **Class C:** The lowest portion of the crown of the impacted maxillary third molar is at or above the cervical line of the second molar.

The position of the long axis of the impacted maxillary third molar in relation to the long axis of the second molar (Fonseca *et al.* 2000)
1. Vertical
2. Horizontal
3. Mesioangular
4. Distoangular
5. Inverted

    6. Buccoangular

    7. Linguoangular

These may also occur simultaneously as

    a. Buccal version

    b. Lingual version

    c. Torsoversion

Relationship of the impacted maxillary third molar to the maxillary sinus (Fonseca *et al.* 2000) (Fig. 6.12)

1. Sinus approximation (SA): No bone or a thin partition/ wall of bone between the impacted maxillary third molar and the maxillary sinus is known as 'maxillary sinus approximation'.

2. No sinus approximation (NSA): 2 mm or more of bone sandwiched between the impacted maxillary third molar and the maxillary sinus is known as 'no maxillary sinus approximation'.

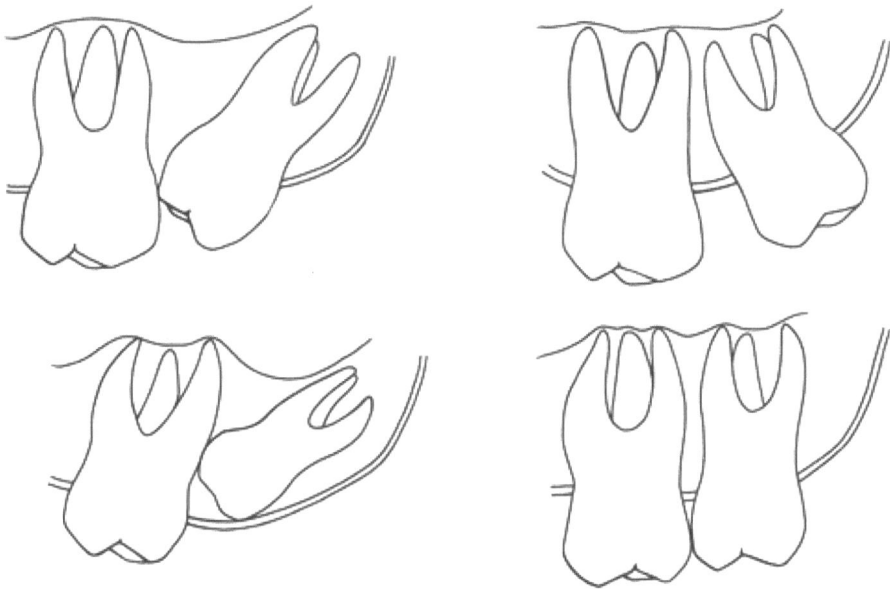

Fig. (6.12). Relationship of the impacted maxillary third molar to the maxillary sinus (Fonseca *et al.* 2000).

Third Molar Skeletal Relationships

Contiguous, non dental structures are important in assessing the status and the prognosis of impacted maxillary third molars .The structures that are always present as surgical hazards are the tuberosity and the maxillary sinus of the maxilla, the infratemporal fossa, and the pterygopalatine fossa. Other structures that may present problems are the buccal part of the masticatory fat pad, the posterior superior alveolar artery, the descending palatine nerve and the mandibular retromolar triangle.

Tuberosity

On the lateral aspect, the tuberosity, as a continuation of the alveolar process, is covered with the gingival mucoperiosteum extending from the gingival crest to the free mucosa of the vestibule. Just superior to the vestibule is the horizontal linear superior origin of the buccinator muscle. The buccinator muscle will tend to direct inflammatory products either from the normal postoperative edema or from a dissecting purulent exudate arising from pericoronal, parietal, and periapical areas toward the oral cavity, into the facial tissues, or into the infratemporal space.

Therefore, the surgeon could consider that placement of an incision for surgery involving a maxillary third molar will have two objectives regarding the buccinator muscle: to elevate it in the flap and to return it to its normal anatomical location. These two objectives would be served by a subperiosteal elevation of the muscle in the soft tissue flap.

Although the osseous height of the alveolar process that constitutes the tuberosity does not decrease in the second and third molar region, the apparent height, when inspected from the medial side, does. This apparent height decrease is due to soft tissue covering of the anterior and posterior palatine foramina through which pass the anterior (greater) and the posterior (lesser) palatine nerves and vessels. The soft tissue also covers, immediately posterior and medial to the third molar region, the tensor veli palatini muscle as it passes through the hamular notch and then medial to the soft palate.

The posterior curve of the tuberosity of the maxilla joins the medial and lateral sides and contains the maxillary third molar. The medial posterior curve of the tuberosity has no clinical height that may be observed by inspection because it is draped with the lateral soft palate mucosa that blends posterior and lateral, with buccal mucosa. Beneath the mucosa is the pterygomandibular raphe, passing from the hamular process inferiorly to the mandibular retromolar trigone area. This raphe is at the union between the buccinator muscle and the superior constrictor muscle of the pharyngeal tissues. Penetrating the buccinator muscle leads to the space beneath the zygomatic arch. Penetrating the superior constrictor muscle leads posteriorly to the lateral pharyngeal space. Both of these routes represent surgical hazards if a maxillary tooth or portions of a tooth were displaced.

Aside from the presence of the third molar in the tuberosity, the substance of the tuberosity will vary from containing the sparse trabeculations of cancellous bone to being a virtually hollow receptacle for an alveolar extension of the maxillary sinus. The maxillary sinus may extend down and around an impacted third molar.

Mandibular Retromolar Triangle Area: The mandibular retromolar trigone area is frequently afflicted with an inflammatory response from Uvaula by malposed by palatally impacted maxillary third molars, This trauma often manifests as a pericoronitis of a mandibular third molar and the trauma may be superimposed on an existing pericoronitis or may be the etiology. In these situations, the removal of the maxillary third molar usually is the first step in managing the mandibular third molar pericoronitis.

Radiographs

Periapical X-ray views that demonstrate the entire tooth will overcome the possibility that a panoramic X-ray tomographic view may exclude the plane of the impacted tooth. Periapical views may be supplemented with a bitewing X-ray view. The bitewing views will provide the information, described above, of the posterior dental occlusion relationships between the mandible and the maxilla, and the periapical films will supply the doctor with the information needed for evaluating the status of the impacted tooth. Periapical and bitewing views may demonstrate, more clearly than panoramic views, localized destruction of second molars by impacted third molars.

Occlusal radiographs have some application in imagery for maxillary third molars in exceptional circumstances. The indications are for localizing maxillary third molars that have been displaced. The tooth may be displaced into the maxillary sinus, into the spaces lateral to the maxilla and superior to the buccinator muscles, or through the superior constrictor muscle into the lateral pharyngeal space.

INDICATIONS OF REMOVAL/EXTRACTION OF MAXILLARY THIRD MOLAR

A unique indication for removal of an impacted maxillary wisdom molar is noted in the· origins of the pterygoid muscles. The internal pterygoid muscle arises from the pterygoid fossa and from the medial surface of the pterygoid plate; a few fibers, which are lateral to the lateral pterygoid muscle, arise from the palatine bone and the maxillary tuberosity. A distoangular position and eruption of an impacted maxillary third molar may be into, or near enough to affect, the medial pterygoid muscle fibers. As a result, there may be local musculofascial pain, referred pain, or a deleterious effect on the temporomandibular (TM) joint.

Other indications for removal/extraction of impacted maxillary wisdom molars are similar to those for other teeth: removal of local inflammation associated. with abortive attempts to erupt; protection of the second molar from the abortive attempts of the third molar to erupt; treatment of periodontal defect or disease between the second and third molars; removal of noxious stimulus to the mandibular retromolar triangle, and preservation of the alignment of the dental arch.

Complications of Maxillary Third Molar Removal

- The most common complicating factor of the maxillary third molar removal is thin non-fused roots with curvature.
- Structure and position of the maxillary sinus play an important role in determination of the difficulty of maxillary third molar removal.
- Possibility of maxillary tuberosity fracture is also another complicating factor.
- Small orbicularis oris muscle or small mouth interferes with a clear access.
- As in case of mandibular molars, the presence of thin periodontal ligament covering the impacted maxillary tooth makes the removal of the tooth more difficult. As the age advances, the periodontal ligament becomes progressively thinner.
- Relationship of the impacted tooth with the maxillary second molar:
- Roots of the impacted tooth in close approximation with roots of the maxillary second molar
- Fusion of the roots of the second and third maxillary molar.
- Hypercementosis or abnormal curvature of the root of the impacted tooth.
- Extreme density of the bone/follicular space filled with bone (commonly seen in elderly patients)
- In close proximity with the zygomatic process of the maxillary bone.

Incisions: Balaji *et al.* (2007) quoted "following are the different types of incisions made to expose the site of operation for the removal of maxillary third molar":

- Buccal sulcular incision
- Sulcular incision with vestibular extension
- Palatal incision flap.

According to one of the questions asked in a survey of oral and maxillofacial surgeons, who were Diplomates of the American Board of Oral and Maxillofacial Surgery (ABOMS) and members of committees of the American Society of Oral and Maxillofacial Surgeons, pertained to the design of the incision for removal of impacted maxillary third molars. The situation given in the survey was of a 20-year-old male patient with a mesioangular positioned third molar, slightly buccal to the second molar, and in a crown to cervix relationship.

All of the surgeons except one had the incision line beginning over the tuberosity, usually lateral to the midline, and extending anteriorly in the crest of the gingival tissues, with some variations as to the inclusion or not of the papillae. The exception was one surgeon who removes impacted third molars with incisions that extend only for the length of the tuberosity; for mandibular third molars, the incision line is, similarly, just the length of the retromolar triangle.

The usual incision (Fig. **6.13**), which is described from posterior to anterior, is routinely placed over the mid portion of the tuberosity or slightly to the buccal to intersect the distobuccal aspect of the second molar. As the incision passes anteriorly, in the gingival crest, it passes into the embrasure between the second and first molars and usually terminates lateral to the first molar. However, the terminating point depends on the required access and the surgical preference of the doctor, and the termination may be any place from the second molar to the bicuspid areas.

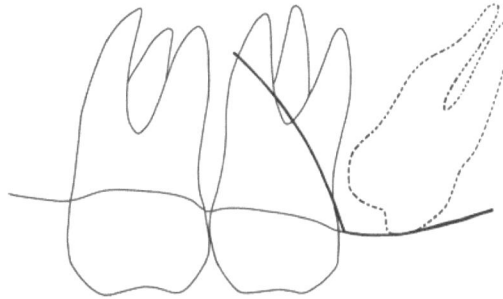

Fig. (6.13). Incisions: Balaji *et al.* (2007).

Incision Posterior to the Second Molar

Following the placement of the incision in the gingival crevice, and the possible use of an oblique extension for access, a submucous elevator or the scalpel is used to incise immediately posterior to the maxillary second molar. This incision intersects the tuberosity incision and passes from the distobuccal to the distopalatal margin of the second molar; this incision is made to bone or to the impacted tooth. This technique permits the elevation of the medial soft tissues from the tuberosity without tearing and provides a clean incision through which repair may take place posterior to the second molar.

Oblique Extension Arms

The higher the impacted third molar is positioned, the more difficult the surgical access, and the more important it is to increase the length of the incision and/or place an oblique releasing incision. If additional access is needed, a reasonable option would be to extend the incision in the gingival crevice or place an oblique incision superiorly toward the vestibule of the maxilla.

If the extension of the incision past the papilla between the ·first and second molar is used, the incision continues in the gingival crevice, around the second molar and into the embrasure between the first molar and second bicuspid. Alternatively, an oblique incision is made just anterior to the papilla between the first and second molars so that the papilla is in the flap that will be raised. By including the papilla in the flap, the surgeon can accurately replace the flap and immobilize it with sutures.

The surgeon may place the incision lines slightly buccal to the crest of the tuberosity and then obliquely toward the vestibule after either leaving a collar of gingival crest mucosa untouched adjacent to the second molar or just touching, for a few millimeters, the distobuccal surface of the second molar cervical region.

Incisions for Palatally Positioned Third Molars

For maxillary third molars with limited lateral access or for palatally positioned maxillary third molars, the incision may begin on the palatal aspect of the tuberosity and pass to the distopalatal corner of the second molar, and then pass first laterally through the posterior gingival attachments of the second molar and then laterally to the second molar.

Operations on Osseous Tissues

The objectives of the osseous operations are (1) to permit easy removal of the impacted maxillary third molar in one piece, without sectioning; (2) to expose a tooth to assist in eruption; and (3) to transplant a suitable donor tooth.

Preparation for Removal

The contiguous bone is prepared to permit removal of the tooth without the need to exert pressures that would fracture roots, fracture the tuberosity, or displace the tooth into the sinus or into the infrazygomatic arch area. The procedures on osseous tissues are performed with unibevel chisels, periosteal elevators, submucous elevators, or similar instruments, or the equivalent of a No. 8 or No.6 round bur operating under a lavage of sterile normal saline and suctioning. If chisels are used, they must be sharp to avoid slipping and producing inaccurate cuts; the chisels may be powered with hand pressure or with taps from a mallet. The use of powered sprays on bur tips is avoided to prevent inducing emphysema of the facial tissues and the spaces.

For the usual impacted maxillary third molar, the surgeon removes the bone that may be accessed from a lateral approach and overlays the crown and the coronal one fourth of the root system. The same is true if a palatal approach is used.

The bone posterior to the impacted maxillary third molar may be removed with lateral to medial to lateral horizontal sweeps of a bur operating at a low speed. This technique will tend to prevent an impacted maxillary third molar from being-displaced into the infratemporal or pterygopalatine fossas during a subsequent elevation maneuver on the tooth. This maneuver may be performed, without direct vision, using a round bur to diminish the possibility of entangling the overlying soft tissue flap in the serrations of the bur, as may occur if a fissure bur was used. The surgeon will know, through digital sensations, when the bur is operating in the bone that is being removed and when it is touching the tooth. The bur is simply inserted under the soft tissue flap, and the posterior bone is painted away by action of the bur. This will provide posterior relief of bone and probably assure ease of delivery of the tooth.

The posterior relief of bone imprisoning an impacted maxillary third molar may be performed with a tooth-elevating instrument or with a periosteal or submucous elevator. The instrument is placed between the tooth and the posterior curve of bone, and the bone is wedged in a posterior direction. This maneuver will provide space for elevation of the tooth inferiorly and slightly posterior without fracturing the thin bony margin of the tuberosity. One must take extreme care to avoid anterior or superior displacement of the impacted third molar during this tech-nique. The purpose is to create a space on the posterior of the impacted tooth by forcing an instrument between the tooth and the bone.

Preparation to Permit Eruption

For a tooth to be exposed to· promote its eruption, bone is removed, using a round bur operating at a low speed, from the occlusal surface to the greatest width of the crown. A fenestration is made in the overlying flap, and the surgical site may be covered with a periodontal pack for 1 week postoperatively. Similarly, in most patients, the bone may be removed with hand instrumentation chisels, or periosteal, submucous, or tooth elevators.

Operations on Tooth Structures

Impacted maxillary third molars destined to be removed rarely are sectioned; the teeth are usually removed intact following preparation of the osseous structures. After the bone has been relieved from the lateral and posterior aspects of the crown and coronal surfaces of the roots, elevators are placed at angles to ensure that the vector of forces is downward and lateral, not superior and posterior. As the recipients of referrals from dentist colleagues for several decades, the authors have received patients in whom posterior pressure from elevators was applied to impacted maxillary third molars and the teeth suddenly departed from view. The referring doctor usually suspects that the teeth are in the maxillary sinus; however, in many cases the teeth have passed posteriorly into the area lateral to the zygomatic process of the maxilla, below the anterior aspect of the zygomatic arch. Removal of a rim of bone from the posterior of the tooth, as described above, will prevent the dislodging of a tooth because less force is required to move the tooth, and it may be guided into the oral cavity with the dental structure elevating instruments.

After the tooth has been luxated and is ready for removal, it may be delivered from the alveolus with a dental forceps, an end cutting rongeur, hemostat, or fingers depending on the situation and the surgeon's preference. The universal maxillary forceps is useful for deciduous teeth. The beaks are small and curved enough to fit around crown shapes of maxillary third molars without obscuring vision of the crown as should be the situation with a forceps with thicker beaks. However, selection of the instrument depends on the surgeon's preference.

Following removal of an impacted maxillary third molar, the surgical area is molded with finger pressure in a pinching manner, and the bony margins of the surgical site are smoothed with hand files or by the light passage of a bur. The alveolus undergoes debridement with a lavage of saline and suctioning; we suggest that the surgeon use the suction device to inspect the site for signs of wayward rootlets and splinters of bone.

It is important to palpate the bony surgical area, through the overlying soft tissue flaps, to detect any rough or sharp areas. The anterior bony margin is particularly likely to give the patient a sharp, uncomfortable sensation in the postoperative course. The margins are corrected, as indicated, with burs or hand files. Intraoral medicaments are placed in the maxillary third molar surgical sites. Dry socket occurrence is very rare owing to the surgical drainage from the surgical site and the soft medullary quality of the bone as compared with the mandible.

Closure of the surgical site is accomplished with a non-absorbable suture, usually 000 or 0000 black silk, or with our preference of an absorbable suture, 000 plain gut. During the seventh day postoperative visit, the gut suture may have disappeared or may be so loose that it can be removed with a suction tip.

Moistened 10 cm x 10 cm gauze is folded so that the side next to the tongue is smooth, and the gauze is placed between the maxillary and the mandibular surgical sites, with the free ends of the gauze being packed against the lateral flaps of mucosal tissues. The gauze is left in place for 1 to 2 hours without changing.

Following the initial period, gauze may be placed by the patient or the sponsor, if necessary, owing to oozing hemorrhage. Usually, however, only the initial gauze pack is necessary.

Maxillary third molars, as with all teeth, may be displaced from the normal anatomical location either by an abnormal eruption phenomenon or by a tumor or a cyst.

The developmental factors that produce impaction of mandibular impacted third molars are retention of a full arch of teeth owing to modern soft diets as well as decreased skeletal space-are also responsible for the impaction of maxillary third molars. Additionally, owing to the aborted attempts to erupt, extended opportunities arise for the development of cysts and tumors originating from various phases of the eruptive process.

To prevent and to correct problems produced by impacted maxillary third molars, one must assess these problems as a part of the patient's total oral and general health care. Impacted maxillary third molars should not be regarded as isolated targets, unassociated with the patient's total health.

The evaluation of impacted maxillary third molars requires the appropriate basic science knowledge to which is added accurate clinical and imagery examinations of the impacted teeth as well as knowledge of the relationship to contiguous teeth and the relationship to the maxillary sinus.

The surgical anatomy the maxillary third molar region is the result of normal growth However, roots are introduced by the presence either an embedded or an impacted third molar that has no normal anatomical route for eruption, by extensions of the maxillary sinus, and by molding of the maxilla by the internal pterygoid muscle attached to the tuberosity area.

The first evidence of calcification of maxillary third molars usually is seen on X-ray films from patients ages 8 to 10. The enamel covering the coronal portion is completed in the middle of the second decade, from 11 to 17 years, and the root is completed from 15 to 25 years. Normal eruption is expected from the 17th to the 21st year of life. The maxillary third molar may have a wide variety of appearances. Wheeler[3] observed: The maxillary third molar often appears as a developmental anomaly. It can vary considerably in size, contour and relative position to other teeth. All third molars, mandibular and maxillary, show more variation in development than any other teeth in the mouth. Occasionally they appear as anomalies bearing little to no resemblance to neighboring teeth.

Third Molar and Second Molar Relationships

The position of a maxillary third molar is often described, as with a mandibular third molar, by a statement of its relationship to the second molar. The maxillary third molar, compared with the long axis of the second molar, may be in positions described as mesioangular, vertical, distoangular, horizontal, transverse, and unusual, such as inverted or displaced to distant locations in the mid facial skeleton.

The level of impaction may be described, from inferior to superior in association with the second molar, as being crown of the third molar to crown of the second molar, crown to cervix, crown to root, and displaced. These positions may be modified by direction of the entire axis of the third molar from the apex to the crown in relation to the midline of the dental arch, palatal (medial), directly posterior, or buccal (lateral) to the second molar.

One of the challenging relationships of the maxillary third molar to second molar is coalescing of the root surfaces. This coalescence poses a treatment problem if there is a need to perform endodontic treatment or to remove one tooth or the other. One may visualize the formative radicular activities of the teeth occurring in the same tight anatomical area, especially with the propensity for the third molar to be displaced owing to the lack of anatomical space, and the formation of the roots producing a physical unity. If removal or endodontic treatment is necessary for one of the involved teeth, a sharp surgical division of the union may be made and endodontic procedures initiated for the tooth to be salvaged.

Third Molar Skeletal Relationships

Contiguous, non-dental structures are important in assessing the status and the prognosis of impacted maxillary third molars. The structures that are always present as surgical hazards are the tuberosity and the maxillary sinus of the maxilla, the infratemporal fossa, and the pterygopalatine fossa. Other structures that may present problems are the buccal part of the masticatory fat pad, the posterior superior artery, the descending palatine nerve, and the mandibular retromolar triangle.

Infratemporal Fossa

The anterior wall of the infratemporal fossa is bounded by the thin cortex of the maxilla, which is the posterior border of the maxillary sinus. Displacement of a tooth or a fragment of a tooth is possible through the weak maxillary bone. The superior boundary of the infratemporal fossa is a portion of the greater wing of the sphenoid and a small area of the temporal bones; the superior boundary extends from the foramen ovale to the infratemporal crest and is perforated by the foramen ovale, the foramen spinosum, and, when present, the foramen of Vesalius. The lateral wall of the fossa is the ramus of the mandible, the medial wall is the lateral pterygoid plate, and there is no osseous posterior wall.

Pterygopalatine Fossa

The pterygopalatine fossa is a narrow, cylindrical area bounded on the anterior by the medial portion of the maxillary tuberosity. The other boundaries are on the superior, the greater wing of the sphenoid bone and foramen rotundum: on the posterior, the anterior surface of the pterygoid process of the sphenoid bone; on the medial, the vertical plate of the palatine bone; and on the lateral, the communication with the infratemporal fossa.

Buccal Fat Pad

The buccal part of the masticatory fat pad is located between the buccinator and the masseter muscles and is part of a larger mass of fat. The entire mass of the masticatory fat pad includes compartments in the pterygomandibular space, the zygomaticotemporal space, and the buccal space; the pterygomandibular compartment communicates with the lateral pharyngeal space. When a lateral mucoperiosteal flap is raised, it usually carries the origins of the superior portion of the buccinator muscle. Care is exercised to keep the periosteum intact for several reasons. One very practical reason is to avoid an encounter with the bothersome buccal compartment of the masticatory fat pad. If the buccinator muscle is pierced during maxillary third molar surgery and if a large buccal fat pad is present, copious amounts of fat may ooze into the surgical field. Attempts to remove the fat, because it is an impediment to vision, by drawing the fat pad through the buccinator muscle and out of its anatomical space are frustrated by the amount of fat emerging into a constricted surgical field, especially if the fat pad had extensions superiorly and inferiorly from the temporal fossa arid the pterygomandibular space. We suggest sharply excising the fat that is in the surgical field and then arranging retractors to keep the remaining fat pad in place during the surgery for management of a maxillary third molar.

Posterior Superior Alveolar Artery

The posterior superior alveolar artery may be bound to the maxilla by periosteum in an area just lateral to the maxillary third molar on paranasal sinus X-ray views, the radiolucency indicative of the presence of the artery when it makes a groove in the maxilla is termed an arterial niche. If the artery is present, it may be opened (because it cannot escape by rolling in the soft tissues) by the point of a local anesthetic injection needle; the immediate hemorrhage will be contained by the intact tissues and will be manifested by an infraorbital swelling. The hemorrhage ceases when the extravascular accumulation of fluids produces sufficient pressures to stem the hemorrhage.

If effective analgesic has been produced by the local anesthetic agent, a simple surgical' procedure could proceed, However, in most cases, one may wish to defer surgery until the coagulum has been resolved. If the artery is encountered during the elevation of a soft tissue flap, there will be a dramatic moment of hemorrhage that is contained by application of pressure from hemostats or crushing of a minute amount of the contiguous bone.

Descending Palatine Artery and Nerve

The descending palatine artery and nerve emerge from the greater (major) palatine foramen after descending through the pterygopalatine canal. After emerging from the greater palatine foramen, the artery is termed the anterior (greater) palatine artery and courses anteriorly, at the junction of the alveolar process and the horizontal plate of the maxilla, to enter the nasopalatine foramen; from there it passes superiorly into the nasal cavity to anastomose with the sphenopalatine artery on the nasal septum. If the artery is encountered in the greater palatine foramen area, a vigorous hemorrhage may ensue. Injecting a local anesthetic agent containing epinephrine into the pterygopalatine canal will stanch the flow. The greater palatine nerve emerges from the greater palatine foramen and then passes anteriorly to carry sensory fibers to the mucosa, postganglionic parasympathetic fibers to the accessory salivary glands, and afferent taste fibers to the palatal mucosa as far anteriorly as the premaxillary area. The unlikely loss of the nerve incidental to maxillary third molar surgery is usually not discernible to the patient. Mandibular Retromolar Triangle Area : The mandibular retromolar trigone area is frequently afflicted with an inflammatory response from by malposed or by partially impacted maxillary third molars , This trauma often manifests as a pericoronitis of a mandibular third molar and the trauma may be superimposed on an existing pericoronitis or may be the etiology. In these situations, the removal of the maxillary third molar usually is the first step in man-aging the mandibular third molar pericoronitis. The surgical spaces associated with impacted maxillary third molars include the intraoral vestibular spaces, the buccal space, and the temporal spaces or compartments. Normal postoperative inflammatory processes as well as inflammations secondary to infections may be limited to the oral cavity by the buccinator and superior constrictor muscles or may be spread to the adjacent spaces by passing through the barrier of these muscles. If the normal postoperative inflammatory process is limited by the buccinator muscle, the manifestations will be limited to the vestibular area of the maxilla. Lateral to the buccinator muscle is the buccal facial space, which contains portions of the buccal fat pad and loose areolar connective tissue. The boundaries of the space define the postoperative edema that may be a side effect of third molar surgery: superiorly, the anterior-most part of the zygomatic arch; posteriorly, the anterior border of the masseter muscle; inferiorly, the body of the mandible; and anteriorly, two of the muscles of facial expression, the depressor anguli oris and the zygomaticus major muscles. The temporal spaces are filled with loose areolar connective tissue and communicate with the infratemporal region and the pterygopalatine fossa. The superficial space is between the temporalis muscle and the cutaneous tissues; the deep space is between the temporalis muscle and the skull. Passage of an inflammatory process or an object through the buccinator muscle and into the temporalis spaces will be manifested by trismus of the temporalis muscle; if the superficial space is involved, there may be a swelling noted above and below the zygomatic arch, with the area of the arch clearly viewed. A deep temporal space inflammation will be more difficult to identify by inspection but may be suspected based on the case history and the physical findings of temporalis muscle trismus. In unusual circumstances, it would be possible for inflammations associated with either needle tract infection or maxillary third molar surgery to involve the pterygomandibular, the masticator, or the lateral pharyngeal spaces. However, these spaces are usually associated with mandibular third molar surgery. The position of an impacted maxillary third molar must be defined before formulating a definitive treatment plan. However, anatomical features associated with the medial sweep of the maxilla toward the tuberosity area, the origins of insertions of the soft palate musculature, the presence of the hamular process, and the confluence of the maxillary sinus with the location of maxillary third molars tend to obfuscate clinical and imagery evaluations. For example, if an impacted maxillary third molar is located in the midline or to the medial of the dental arch, as compared with the second molar, or is in a very superior position in the maxilla, it will not be detected by the physical evaluations of inspection and palpation; radiographic views may also be somewhat obfuscated, especially if there is an alveolar extension of them maxillary sinus. The medial sweep of the lateral aspect of the posterior maxilla toward the tuberosity and, on the medial, the confluence of the soft palate and the hamular process, just medial to the posterior maxilla, limit effective' inspection. Furthermore, the anterior border of the mandibular ramus will tend to overlap the area as the mandible is moved to open positions.

Inspection is aided by having the patient open the mandible only 25 or 30 mm and then gently move or swing it laterally away from the maxillary third molar site being inspected. A mouth mirror is used to inspect the third molar site. Findings may include partial eruption of the crown of the third molar; the possible presence of a pericoronitis; periodontal disease or defect posterior to the second molar owing to the presence of the third molar; and the character of the soft tissue overlying the tuberosity.

With the mandible in the same position as described for inspection, a palpating finger may note the likely presence of an impacted maxillary third molar. Usually, an impacted maxillary third molar will be positioned to the buccal side, as related to the second molar, owing to the cross-sectional configuration of the maxillary tuberosity. The presence of an impacted maxillary third molar may be noted as a rounded bulge, or sharp cusps of the crown may be sensed by palpation. The absence of these findings may indicate the impacted maxillary third molar is directly posterior, is posterior and medial, or is extremely superior to the second molar.

The usual extraoral imagery technique for evaluating maxillary third molars is a panoramic X-ray view. A panoramic view is a single tomographic plane, and it is possible that a maxillary third molar may be eclipsed by the plane if the tooth is displaced markedly to the medial of the usual location.

We recommend that the panoramic X-ray view be made without a device in the oral cavity that properly locates the· head and provides a slightly mouth-opened view. The mouth-opened view will display the dentition without overlap, but there is no normal relationship displayed between the mandible and maxilla. If the view is made with the dentition in full occlusion, a normal dosed occlusion relationship is visualized between the mandible and the maxilla. The normal relationship displayed in a closed occlusion view is useful as a training aid for informing patients of the role that maxillary third molars may play in some cases of mandibular third molar pericoronitis. By viewing the X-ray film, patients will have an informed understanding of the traumatic relations that may occur, for example, between partially impacted, malposed, or supraerupted maxillary third molars and the structures in the mandibular retromolar triangle area.

Periapical X-ray views that demonstrate the entire tooth will overcome the possibility that a panoramic X-ray tomographic view may exclude the plane of the impacted tooth. Periapical views may be supplemented with a bitewing X-ray view. The bitewing views will provide the information, described above, of the posterior dental occlusion relationships between the mandible and the maxilla, and the periapical films will supply the doctor with the information needed for evaluating the status of the impacted tooth. Periapical and bitewing views may demonstrate, more clearly than panoramic views, localized destruction of second molars by impacted third molars.

Occlusal radiographs have some application in imagery for maxillary third molars in exceptional circumstances. The indications are for localizing maxillary third molars that have been displaced. The tooth may be displaced it into the maxillary sinus, into the spaces lateral to the maxilla and superior to the buccinator muscles, or through the superior constrictor muscle into the lateral pharyngeal space.

In some cases in the maxillary third molar region, as with the displacements described above and for teeth displaced by pathological lesions, indications exist for selected cephalometric, paranasal sinus, and cross-sectional radiography using CT scans or standard tomographic techniques.

SURGICAL MANAGEMENT

The surgical management of an impacted maxillary third molar includes assessing the options and alternatives to treatment and informing the patient. If a surgical solution is selected, the management consists of satisfying the surgical principle of access, taking the logical steps of incision, elevation of soft tissues, retraction of soft tissues, operations on osseous tissues, and operations on tooth structures, and applying the indicated direct postoperative regional care.

The options for care of an impacted maxillary third molar are exposure of the tooth to permit eruption, transplantation, removal, and long-term observation.

Exposure

In some patients, a maxillary third molar with appropriate anatomy and potential for participating in useful occlusion will have eruption impeded by overlying mucosa, follicle, bone, or a supernumerary tooth. Removal of the overlying impediment and exposure of the crown from the height of contour of the crown to the occlusal surface may permit the eruption to proceed. These instances are extremely rare because the third molar crowns are usually malformed and would not be useful for occlusion, and the roots are usually too short to supply support for the tooth as an abutment. The posterior maxilla, in individuals who have maintained a full dental arch, usually directs the eruption of a maxillary third molar into an untenable position.

However, the possibility of salvage of a maxillary third molar does exist in a few patients if the second molar is absent. As with all teeth, an eruption potential for maxillary third molars exists throughout life, though it is more pronounced in the first three decades.

Transplantation

The transplantation of maxillary third molars, as with other autogenous donor transplanted teeth, may be to any suitable location in either the maxillary or mandibular arch. The transplantation of a maxillary third molar often takes advantage of its frequently malformed molar crown, which may be of similar dimensions to a bicuspid or cuspid, and consideration may be given to using an impacted maxillary third molar as a donor transplant to replace a bicuspid or cuspid, in either arch. A unique indication for removal of an impacted maxillary third molar is noted in the· origins of the pterygoid muscles. The internal pterygoid muscle arises from the pterygoid fossa and from the medial surface of the pterygoid plate; a few fibers,' which are lateral to the lateral pterygoid muscle; arise from the palatine bone and the maxillary tuberosity. A distoangular position and eruption of an impacted maxillary third molar may be into, or near enough to affect, the medial pterygoid muscle fibers. As a result, there may be local musculofascial pain, referred pain, or a deleterious effect on the temporomandibular (TM) joint.

Other indications for removal of impacted maxillary third molars are similar to those for other teeth: removal of local inflammation associated with abortive attempts to erupt; protection of the second molar from the abortive attempts of the third molar to erupt; treatment of periodontal defect or disease between the second and third molars; removal of noxious stimulus to the mandibular retromolar triangle; and preservation of the alignment of the dental arch. Of course, control of associated pathology, is an indication for removal of a maxillary third molar.

If an impacted maxillary third molar is not a clear present or pending challenge to a patient's health, long-term observation may be in order. In this instance, the periodic recall of a patient for preventive dentistry should include specific evaluation, with at least biennial radiographic views, of the status of the impacted maxillary third molar.

The fusion of maxillary third and second molar root systems is an indication for long term observation. An attempt to remove the impacted third molar may lead to the loss of the second molar. The probable loss of a maxillary second molar may be a reason to retain an impacted maxillary third molar. If the maxillary third molar is in a slight mesioangular position, is in the midline of the dental arch posterior to the second molar, and has appropriate crown and root forms, it may erupt into useful occlusion. However, the plan of routinely and electively removing sound and useful second molars to permit third molars to erupt into the position of the second molars is not totally logical. It is an assumption that the third molar will follow a correct eruption plan from both the medial-lateral and anterior posterior viewpoints; it is an assumption that the third molar will indeed drift anteriorly to accurately land against the first molar; on the other hand, it is a fact that maxillary third molar surgery produces very little morbidity for the patients and is not daunting to surgeons; and it is a fact that anatomists have correctly described the maxillary third molars as often being so malformed that they appear as anomalies. There are instances where the removal of second molars is necessary and the useful eruption of third molars is indicated; these instances should be carefully considered with the referring doctor, often an orthodontist. The concept of a maxillary third molar subsequently erupting into the site of an extracted maxillary second molar is used, in many practices, as a method of controlling the length of dental arches. To pursue the concept when there is a healthy second molar in useful occlusion, one must be assured that the third molar has an appropriate crown and root form and is in a position to erupt into useful occlusion.

Access for surgical management of an impacted maxillary third molar is enhanced by having the patient open the mandible a comfortable distance, perhaps moving it laterally toward the affected side. The lips and buccal tissues are controlled with retracting instruments or finger retraction.

The site of an impacted maxillary third molar may be relatively inaccessible if the mandibular ramus has a long anterior-posterior dimension and, owing to the osseous anatomy of either the maxilla or the ramus, very little clearance from the maxilla. A confluence of the above, a tight oral orifice, a high posterior curve of the dental arch, and restricted lateral access to the third molar site will reduce surgical access and visibility for the usual lateral approach to the third molar region. In these cases, the patient may be more comfortable under a full general anesthetic owing to possibly increased operating time needed to manage an impacted maxillary third molar. Depending on the intraosseous location of the third molar and the contiguous anatomy, the surgeon may elect to utilize a combination occlusal and palatal approach with the usual buccal surgical avenue.

Incision Designs

One of the questions asked in a survey of oral and maxillofacial surgeons, who were Diplomates of the American Board of Oral and Maxillofacial Surgery (ABOMS) and members of committees of the American Society of Oral and Maxillofacial Surgeons, pertained to the design of the incision for removal of impacted maxillary third molars. The situation given in the survey was of a 20-year-old male patient with a mesioangular positioned third molar, slightly buccal to the second molar, and in a crown to cervix relationship.

All of the surgeons except one had the incision line beginning over the tuberosity, usually lateral to the midline, and extending anteriorly in the crest of the gingival tissues, with some variations as to the inclusion or not of the papillae . The exception was one surgeon who removes impacted third molars with incisions that extend only for the length of the tuberosity; for mandibular third molars, the incision line is, similarly, just the length of the retromolar triangle. The length of the incisions and the routine use of an oblique incision.

The usual incision, which is described from posterior to anterior, is routinely placed over the mid portion of the tuberosity or slightly to the buccal to intersect the distobuccal aspect of the second molar. As the incision passes anteriorly, in the gingival crest, it passes into the embrasure between the second and first molars and usually terminates lateral to the first molar. However, the terminating point depends on the required access and the surgical preference of the doctor, and the termination may be any place from the second molar to the bicuspid areas.

Incision Posterior to the Second Molar

Following the placement of the incision in the gingival crevice, and the possible use of an oblique extension for access, a submucous elevator or the scalpel is used to incise immediately posterior to the maxillary second molar. This incision intersects the tuberosity incision and passes from the distobuccal to the distopalatal margin of the second molar; this incision is made to bone or to the impacted tooth. This technique permits the elevation of the medial soft tissues from the tuberosity without tearing and provides a clean incision through which repair may take place posterior to the second molar.

Oblique Extension Arms

The higher the impacted third molar is positioned, the more difficult the surgical access, and the more important it is to increase the length of the incision and/or place an oblique releasing incision. If additional access is needed, a reasonable option would be to extend the incision in the gingival crevice or place an oblique incision superiorly toward the vestibule of the maxilla.

If the extension of the incision past the papilla between the ·first and second molar is used, the incision continues in the gingival crevice, around the second molar and into the embrasure between the first molar and second bicuspid. Alternatively, an oblique incision is made just anterior to the papilla between the first and second molars so that the papilla is in the flap that will be raised. By including the papilla in the flap, the surgeon can accurately replace the flap and immobilize it with sutures.

The surgeon may place the incision lines slightly buccal to the crest of the tuberosity and then obliquely toward the vestibule after either leaving a collar of gingival crest mucosa untouched adjacent to the second molar or just touching, for a few millimeters, the distobuccal surface of the second molar cervical region.

Incisions for Palatally Positioned Third Molars

For maxillary third molars with limited lateral access or for palatally positioned maxillary third molars, the incision may begin on the palatal aspect of the tuberosity and pass to the distopalatal corner of the second molar, and then pass first laterally through the posterior gingival attachments of the second molar and then laterally to the second molar The lateral portion of the incision may be either in the gingival crevice or in the mucosa lateral to the second molar. An incision may be indicated that begins on the tuberosity area and then passes anteriorly to the palatal gingival sulci of the first and second molars and passes, with the elevating instrument in firm contact with bone, superior and posterior to the impacted tooth. If one tries to elevate the flap directly from an impacted tooth, the presentation of the follicular sac and crown through the overlying bone may cause the flap to tear; by freeing the soft tissues around the sac and crown, one can readily dissect these structures free and obtain generous exposure.

The elevating instrument is then used to lift the mucoperiosteal tissues off of the tuberosity in one block. The submucous elevator is passed, in a sweeping anterior-to-posterior motion, medially beneath the soft tissues of the tuberosity with the tip either in firm contact with bone overlying the impacted tooth or in firm contact with the crown that may have erupted through the bone. As the elevator moves past the height of contour of the midline of the tuberosity, the surgeon elevates the soft tissue in one block by using the elevator as a Class I lever with the tips of the elevator serving as the fulcrum. This elevation is facilitated by the incision made posterior to the second molar. The space provided by the elevation of the tuberosity tissues will prevent lacerations of the tissues during the surgery on osseous and tooth structures. It is not necessary to retract the tuberosity soft tissues medial from the incision line.These tissues will passively remain out of the surgical field. The surgeon usually retracts the lateral soft tissue flap, although different techniques are used by various surgeons. An example of a retraction instrument would be a design that features a broad flat blade that is placed on bone, superior to the surgical site, and is left in place, as much as possible, throughout the remaining surgery. Many surgeons use a curved instrument with a broad handle that will provide retraction of the buccal and lip tissues as well as the lateral soft tissue flap.

The principle of retraction is to perform as little manipulation of the operated tissues, the flap, as possible. The more the tissues are handled, the greater the inflammatory response; therefore, the tissues should be handled in a deft, delicate, accurate manner. As a surgical technique discipline, it is interesting to place the retracting instrument and then complete all the surgical steps to the point of soft tissue closure before moving the retracting instrument; the steps to be completed would be operations on bone and on tooth, and debridement.

Operations on Osseous Tissues

The objectives of the osseous operations are (1) to permit easy removal of the impacted maxillary third molar in one piece, without sectioning; (2) to expose a tooth to assist in eruption; and (3) to transplant a suitable donor tooth.

Preparation for Removal

The contiguous bone is prepared to permit removal of the tooth without the need to exert pressures that would fracture roots, fracture the tuberosity, or displace the tooth into the sinus or into the infrazygomatic arch area. The procedures on osseous tissues are performed with unibevel chisels, periosteal elevators, submucous elevators, or similar instruments, or the equivalent of a No. 8 or No. 6 round bur operating under a lavage of sterile normal saline and suctioning. If chisels are used, they must be sharp to avoid slipping and producing inaccurate cuts; the chisels may be powered with hand pressure or with taps from a mallet. The use of powered sprays on bur tips is avoided to prevent inducing emphysema of the facial tissues and the spaces.

For the usual impacted maxillary third molar, the surgeon removes the bone that may be accessed from a lateral approach and overlays the crown and the coronal one fourth of the root system. The same is true if a palatal approach is used. The bone posterior to the impacted maxillary third molar may be removed with lateral to medial to lateral horizontal sweeps of a bur operating at a low speed. This technique will tend to prevent an impacted maxillary third molar from being-displaced into the infratemporal or pterygopalatine fossa's during a subsequent elevation maneuver on the tooth. This maneuver may be performed, without direct vision, using a round bur to diminish the possibility of entangling the overlying soft tissue flap in the serrations of the bur, as may occur if a fissure bur was used. The surgeon will know, through digital sensations, when the bur is operating in the bone that is being removed and when it is touching the tooth. The bur is simply inserted under the soft tissue flap, and the posterior bone is painted away by action of the bur. This will provide posterior relief of bone and probably assure ease of delivery of the tooth. The posterior relief of bone imprisoning an impacted maxillary third molar may be performed with a tooth-elevating instrument or with a periosteal or submucous elevator. The instrument is placed between the tooth and the posterior curve of bone, and the bone is wedged in a posterior direction. This maneuver will provide space for elevation of the tooth inferiorly and slightly posterior without fracturing the thin bony margin of the tuberosity. One must take extreme care to avoid anterior or superior displacement of the impacted third molar during this technique. The purpose is to create a space on the posterior of the impacted tooth by forcing an instrument between the tooth and the bone.

Preparation to Permit Eruption

For a tooth -to be exposed to· promote its eruption, bone is removed, using a round bur operating at a low speed, from the occlusal surface to the greatest width of the crown. A fenestration is made in the overlying flap, and the surgical site may be covered with a periodontal pack for 1 week postoperatively. Similarly, in most patients, the bone may be removed with hand instrumentation-chisels, or periosteal, submucous, or tooth elevators.

Preparation to Permit Transplantation

If a tooth is to be transplanted, bone is removed from the entire coronal surface with great care not to touch the root surfaces with a bur or chisel. The tooth has to be luxated and removed gently to preserve the soft tissue cap over the apical region. If the soft tissue cap covering an immature apical opening is damaged, the transplanted tooth will fail.

Operations on Tooth Structures

Impacted maxillary third molars destined to be removed rarely are sectioned; the teeth are usually removed intact following preparation of the osseous structures. After the bone has been relieved from the lateral and posterior aspects of the crown and coronal surfaces of the roots, elevators are placed at angles to ensure that the vector of forces is downward and lateral, not superior and posterior.

As the recipients of referrals from dentist colleagues for several decades, the authors have received patients in whom posterior pressure from elevators was applied to impacted maxillary third molars and the teeth suddenly departed from view. The referring doctor usually suspects that the teeth are in the maxillary sinus; however, in many cases the teeth have passed posteriorly into the area lateral to the zygomatic process of the maxilla, below the anterior aspect of the zygomatic arch. Removal of a rim of bone from the posterior of the tooth, as described above, will prevent the dislodging of a tooth because less force is required to move the tooth, and it may be guided into the oral cavity with the dental structure elevating instruments.

After the tooth has been luxated and is ready for removal, it may be delivered from the alveolus with a dental forceps, an end cutting rongeur, hemostat, or fingers depending on the situation and the surgeon's preference. The universal maxillary forceps is useful for deciduous teeth. The beaks are small and curved enough to fit around the variety of crown shapes of maxillary third molars without obscuring vision of the crown as should be the situation with a forceps with thicker beaks. However, selection of the instrument depends on the surgeon's preference.

Following removal of an impacted maxillary third molar, the surgical area is molded with finger pressure in a pinching manner, and the bony margins of the surgical site are smoothed with hand files or by the light passage of a bur. The alveolus undergoes debridement with a lavage of saline and suctioning; we suggest that the surgeon use the suction device to inspect the site for signs of wayward rootlets and splinters of bone.

It is important to palpate the bony surgical area, through the overlying soft tissue flaps, to detect any rough or sharp areas. The anterior bony margin is particularly likely to give the patient a sharp, uncomfortable sensation in the postoperative course. The margins are corrected, as indicated, with burs or hand files. Or intraoral medicaments are placed in the maxillary third molar surgical sites. Dry socket occurrence is very rare owing to the surgical drainage from the surgical site and the soft medullar quality of the bone as compared with the mandible.

Closure of the surgical site is accomplished with a nonabsorbable suture, usually 000 or 0000 black silk, or with our preference of an absorbable suture, 000 plain gut. During the seventh day postoperative visit, the gut suture may have disappeared or may be so loose that it can be removed with a suction tip. In the surveys conducted among oral and maxillofacial surgeons, 30% reported that the surgical site as not sutured closed in the maxilla following removal of an impacted maxillary third molar.

A moistened 10 cm x 10 cm gauze is folded so that the side next to the tongue is smooth, and the gauze is placed between the maxillary and the mandibular surgical sites, with the free ends of the gauze being packed against the lateral flaps of mucosal tissues· The gauze is left in place for I to 2 hours without changing. Following the initial period, gauze may be placed by the patient or the sponsor, if necessary, owing to oozing hemorrhage. Usually, however, only the initial gauze pack is necessary.

Maxillary third molars, as with all teeth, may be displaced from the normal anatomical location either by an abnormal eruption phenomenon or by a tumor or a cyst.

Abnormal Eruption Phenomenon

Maxillary third molars may be carried to various locations in the mid facial skeleton and reside in the walls of the maxillary sinus, the floor or lateral walls of the nose, or the infraorbital area. Removal may require Trans nasal or one of several variations of Le Fort midfacial osteotomies for access and removal. If the infraorbital nerve is transected, it should be: repaired, intraoperatively, with perineural sutures. Microsurgical techniques or the use of Loupes by the surgeon may assist in visualizing the repair.

Displacement by a Tumor or Cyst

Obviously, if a lesion caused the displacement of a maxillary third molar, the tooth is just an incident in the scenario. Attention is directed to managing the pathology.

In the case of a cyst, the ideal surgical plan would be to enucleate the lesion and to remove the associated tooth. An alternative approach would be to obtain a biopsy specimen of the lining, and, if not contraindicated, a marsupialization procedure could then be performed. Performing the biopsy usually provides the opening that will lead to decompression and decreasing the size of the cyst. After the cyst is small enough, it may be enucleated *via* a transoral operation. A tumor should be removed, and the advent of mid facial skeletal surgery has provided routine down fracturing operations to gain surgical access, if applicable, depending on the type of tumor and the associated anatomy.

SIDE EFFECTS AND COMPLICATIONS

The normal physiological responses to surgery include edema that will be macroscopically apparent for most patients. The majority of unplanned problems associated with maxillary third molar surgery center around inadequate surgical access and surgical visibility. Performing blind procedures in the posterior maxilla leads to inadvertent challenges by producing displacements of the tooth or segments of the tooth into the maxillary sinus and into the infratemporal fossa; fracture of the tuberosity is more likely if the preparation for delivery of the tooth was incomplete and without maximal visibility.

The posterior superior alveolar artery may be embraced by the overlying periosteum and held immobile on the lateral surface of the posterior tuberosity. If this is the case, it may be lacerated by the tip of a local anesthetic injection needle or during the elevation of a mucoperioseal flap. The arterial hemorrhage will be vigorous, and, if it was produced by an anesthetic needle, the intact overlying tissues will balloon and stem the hemorrhage by pressure against the artery. If the hemorrhage is produced during the raising of a flap, it is initially stanched by pressure from a metal instrument followed by either crushing of the contiguous bone onto the small vessel or by electrode or by cautery.

Hemorrhage from the abundant and widespread pterygoid plexus of veins may follow laceration by the tip of a needle. No specific immediate treatment is necessary. The small local hemorrhages will, in time, produce extravascular pressures to collapse the affected venous, In the case of the arterial hemorrhage from the posterior superior alveolar artery or pterygoid plexus of veins, a hematoma may be produced. Hematomas, as a coagulum of blood, have no self-defense system and may be the repository of circulating microorganisms: Therefore, systemic antibiosis may be indicated because of the possibility that both oral and circulating microorganisms may reside in the hematoma. An initial antibiotic coverage of penicillin is suggested, *e.g.*, for adults, penicillin V potassium, 500 mg immediately and 500 mg four times a day (before meals and at bedtime) for 7 days.

The raising of the intraoral flaps may produce a normal postoperative ecchymosis, creating subcutaneous discolorations in the facial tissues. Although this ecchymosis are usually limited to the buccal facial space, in very young patients, without well-defined muscles of facial expression, and in elderly patients, with a normal diminution of subcutaneous fibrous connective tissue demarcations, the ecchymosis may dissect to distant sites.

Trismus is not often associated with impacted third molar postoperative inflammatory conditions or with secondary hemorrhage; nor is it often a finding attributed to surgery. However, inflammations and hemorrhages that arise in the facial buccal and in the infratemporal fossa areas owing to the surgery may secondarily afflict the masticator space and produce a trismus. Prudent treatment would require effective use of antibiotics (*e.g.*, for adults, clindamycin, 150 mg four times a day) and a possible incision and drainage.

Tooth displacement or Segment into the Maxillary Sinus

A maxillary third molar or the root portion may be displaced during surgery, lodging in or near the maxillary sinus. The alveolar extensions of the maxillary sinus, sometimes seen in both normal dentate and edentate areas, are potential surgical hazards in terms of displacing a tooth fragment or tooth into the sinus.

If a tooth or a root should disappear from the surgical field, the team must realize that the event, though unusual, is not an acute emergency and is not indicative of negligent care. The surgeon may elect to complete other planned procedures before identifying the location of the root or tooth and planning for its management. For a patient who has incurred the displacement of a tooth or fragment of a tooth into the maxillary antrum, the surgeon may elect to include, in the first 7 days of initial supportive care, antibiotics, antihistamines, and nasal decongestants (*e.g.*, for adults, cefaclor, 250 mg, three times daily; pseudo-ephedrine hydrochloride, 60 mg, three to four times daily; oxymetazoline hydrochloride 0.05% nasal spray, twice daily). The fragment must be accurately localized.

The displacement of a maxillary third molar root segment or tooth may be in one of four different areas. It may pass through the sinus membrane and be in the sinus; it may pass between the sinus membrane and the osseous wall of the sinus; it may be lodged under the mucoperiosteum lateral to the alveolar process; or it may pass posteriorly in the infratemporal fossa. The use of shift-shot X-ray studies, often with periapical films, may identify the exact location of the structure.

The localization of a root or tooth in the sinus may include both cross-fire localization X-ray studies and X-ray studies taken with the patient's head in various positions to ascertain if the fragment is free within the sinus. The positional X-ray films are taken with the patient's head in an upright position, forward in the prone position, and posteriorly in the supine position.

If a non-infected root is in the sinus of a patient who is historically and clinically free of inflammations, there is no need to surgically remove the root. The antral cilia should be given an opportunity to carry the root to the ostium of the antrum. If this occurs, within 10 days or less of the time of the displacement of the root into the sinus, it will be expelled through the nose. The patient may recover the root by sneezing, or by blowing the nose, or by having the root drop over the soft palate and into the oral pharynx.

If the root remains in the antrum, the patient should be monitored to determine whether it will cause an inflammatory response. If the root is a psychological problem to the patient, or if the doctor believes it is in the best interests of prudent prophylactic management, the root should be removed. Roots that have resided in the maxillary sinus for months or years are usually bound to the normal sinus membrane by mature fibrotic tissues.

An empty alveolus should never be enlarged to recover a root or tooth from the maxillary sinus. This approach will not provide surgical access and may produce an oral antral fistula.

Recovery of a root may be accomplished by one of two approaches. If the root is trapped in a convolution or under the sinus, an opening may be made through the posterior lateral wall of the sinus, perhaps in the lower aspect of the zygomatic recess of the maxilla. A second surgical approach is through an opening in the canine fossa of the anterior surface of the maxilla.

If the sinus is acutely inflamed, there may be an indication for establishing a nasal antral drainage window following the removal of a root or tooth. Usually, however, neither antral packing nor nasal antrostorpy is necessary when removing an uninfected root or tooth.

Displacement to the Infratemporal or Pterygopalatine Fossa

Entire maxillary third molars have been displaced posteriorly and superiorly to be lodged in the soft tissues behind the maxilla and superiorly under the anterior aspect of the zygomatic arch. In some cases, dental extraction forceps beaks were placed on the occlusal third of the crown, thereby launching the tooth in a superior direction when the beaks were squeezed together. In other cases, the use of dental elevators has culminated in a sharp release of the bone posterior to the impacted tooth, causing the tooth to move out of the surgical field and into a position beneath the zygomatic process of the maxilla at the anterior-most location of the zygomatic arch.

As with tooth fragments and teeth displaced into the maxillary sinus, there is no immediate emergency. Localization by imagery is necessary; sometimes fortunate occlusal radiography will identify the tooth, or a CT scan may be necessary. Recovery is carried at under general anesthesia from a transoral approach. Teeth displaced posterior to the maxilla have tended to be fibrosed in position after 3 or 4 days and have been identified and removed following sharp and blunt dissection through an enlarged initial incision. It is possible that a patient will require sectioning of the coronoid process to obtain surgical access.

The maxillary tuberosity may be weakened by an alveolar extension of the maxillary sinus anterior to the maxillary third molar. This may occur idiopathically, or it may be secondary to the loss of a first or second molar. The stage may be set for a fracture of the tuberosity by an impacted tooth's being in dense sclerotic bone and/or by the tooth's having bulbous, ankylosed, or widespread roots. The fracture may be produced by an impacted tooth in any position.

In the preceding instances, exerting pressures on a tooth with an elevator or through an extraction forceps may produce a fracture of the tuberosity. The fracture will be immediately sensed by the surgeon by sound, by sudden ease of movement of the tooth, and often by an oozing hemorrhage.

The objective, following fracture of the tuberosity, is to preserve as much of the osseous tissue as possible and to avoid producing an oral-antral fistula. If the fracture is small, the impacted tooth should be removed, and the alveolus closed with a mattress suture to ensure primary repair. If the fracture is large, the tooth may be replaced and stabilized with either a palatal splint or a buccal orthodontic arch wire to produce bone of repair; the tooth is removed 2 or 3 months later following elevation of appropriate Raps, removal of lateral and posterior bone, sectioning, and removal of the tooth segments.

The area of potential or actual oral sinus opening should never be probed, explored, or packed with medicaments. There is no point to making the defect larger and possibly to introducing a secondary infection.

Air and powered sprays used to cool burs in high-speed hand pieces may dissect into the soft tissues contiguous to the oral cavity. The dissection may be surprisingly rapid and extend throughout the mid-face facial soft tissues on the affected side if the dissection was incurred during maxillary third molar surgery. The subcutaneous emphysema will produce an enlargement of the tissues that is usually non-painful and is characterized by a diagnostic crackling or crepitus on palpation.

Treatment is preventive antibiosis (*e.g.*, for adults, cephalexin, 500 mg, four times daily) and observation. Absorption of the gases occurs rapidly, and resolution of a non-infected case requires less than 7 days.

The incision is made similar to that in case of lingual split technique. A mucoperiosteal flap is elevated on the buccal side to expose the bone enclosing the impacted tooth. A vertical stop cut is made in the anterior end of the impacted tooth using a chisel.

Now the chisel is placed horizontally with the bevel facing downwards just below the vertical stop cut, and a horizontal cut is made extending backwards.

A point of application for an elevator is made with a chisel by excising the triangular piece of bone bounded anteriorly by the lower end of the stop cut and above by the anterior end of the horizontal cut. The distolingual bone is now fractured inward by placing the chisel on the line. The chisel is held at an angle of 45° to the bone surface and pointing in the direction of second premolar on the contralateral side. The cutting edge of the chisel is kept parallel to the external oblique ridge and a few light taps are given with the mallet which separates the lingual plate from the alveolar bone and hinges it inward on the soft tissue attached to it. At this point care must be taken that the cutting edge of the chisel is not held parallel to the internal oblique ridge as this may lead to the extension of the lingual split to the coronoid process.

- The "peninsula" of bone which then remains distal to the tooth and between the buccal and lingual cuts is excised.
- A sharp, pointed, fine-bladed straight elevator is then applied to the mesial surface of the tooth and minimum of force is used to displace the tooth upward and backward out of its socket.

- As the tooth moves backward, the fractured lingual plate is displaced from its path of withdrawal, thus facilitating delivery of the tooth. After the tooth has been removed from its socket, the lingual plate is grasped in fine hemostats, and the soft tissues are freed from it by blunt dissection.
- The fractured lingual plate is then lifted from the wound, thus completing the saucerization of the bony cavity.
- The bone edges are smoothened with bone files; the wound is irrigated with saline and closed with sutures.
- A transient lingual anesthesia may be experienced by the patient in the postoperative period.

Maxillary Canine Impaction

Stewart et al. **(2001)** quoted the canine is the second most commonly impacted tooth(after the third molar),with the rate of maxillary canine impaction ranging from approximately 1% to 3%.Palatal displacement of the maxillary canine is more common than labial displacement; studies shows a highly variable ratio of 2:1 to 9:1 for palatal :labial canine impactions.

Ronald L. Otto et al. **(2003)** quoted Canine impaction is not a new phenomenon. A case has recently been reported in an excavated skull dated at 2700 to 2724 BC.

Incidence of Canine Impaction

Bishara et al. **(1998)** reviewed that *Dachi and Howell* reported that the incidence of maxillary canine impaction is 0.92% where as *Thilander and Myrberg* estimated the cumulative prevalence of canine impaction in 7- to- 13- year old children to be 2.2%. The incidence in the Swedish population at 1.7% was quoted by *Ericson and Kurol* Impactions are twice as common in females (1.17%) than in males (0.51%).Of all individuals with maxillary impacted canines, it is estimated that 8% have bilateral impactions. The incidence of mandibular canine impaction is 0.35%.According to *Yamaoka et al.* there was no difference in the prevalence of completely impacted canines in the edentulous as compared with the dentate maxillae.

According to *Dewel* maxillary canines have the longest period of development, as well as the longest and most tortuous course to travel from their point of formation, lateral to the piriform fossa , until they reach their final destination in full occlusion.During their course of development, the crowns of the permanent canines are intimately related to the roots of the lateral incisor The removal of impacted maxillary cuspids is one of the most difficult procedures encountered in the oral cavity. The frequency of impaction of maxillary cuspids is 20 times greater than that in the mandibular cuspid. Impaction of maxillary cuspids on the palatal aspect is 3 times more than that on the buccal or labial side. The tooth may be embedded deeply close to the maxillary sinus, in close approximation with the nasal cavity, present in the orbit, in the lower lip, or in the floor of the mouth (mandibular impacted cuspids). It may be impacted horizontally or palatally. The maxillary cuspids are mostly impacted in a horizontal position on the palatal aspect, whereas mandibular canine is usually impacted on the labial or buccal aspect.

Classification Usually Followed for Impacted Maxillary Cuspids:

Class I: Impacted cuspids located in the palate
  1. Horizontal
  2. Vertical
  3. Semi vertical.
Class II: Impacted cuspids located in the labial or buccal surface of the maxilla
  1. Horizontal
  2. Vertical
  3. Semi vertical.
Class III: Impacted cuspids located in both the palatal process and labial or buccal maxillary bone, *e.g.* the crown is on the palate and the root passes between the roots of the adjacent teeth in alveolar process, ending in a sharp angle on the labial or buccal surface of the maxilla.
Class IV: Impacted cuspids located in the alveolar process, usually vertically between the incisor and first bicuspid.
Class V: Impacted cuspids located in an edentulous maxilla.

Etiological Factors Affecting the Impaction of the Maxillary Cuspids

- In case of palatally impacted cuspids, the hard palate offers greater resistance to the eruption of the cuspids.
- Prolonged retention or delayed resorption of the roots of the deciduous canine affects the eruption of the canine.
- The canine passes through a greater distance before reaching its normal occlusal position. In this course, there is every possibility for the canine to get deflected from its normal path resulting in impaction.
- Presence of dilacerated roots of the canine increases its chances of impaction.
- Ankylosed cupid's fail to erupt.
- Presence of canine in relation to clefts of the alveolus or the palate leads to its impaction.
- Lack of space also leads to impaction of canine. The canine erupts between already existing teeth and at about the same time when the second molars are erupting which compete with the canine for space.
- Sometimes the thick mucoperiosteum covering the palate offers considerable

resistance to the eruption of the canine.
• The mesiodistal width of the primary canine is less when compared to the mesiodistal width of the permanent canine which also accounts for lack of space for eruption of the permanent canine.
• Certain endocrinal changes also lead to impaction of the maxillary canine.

The generalized evaluation is similar to that for any other minor oral surgical procedure. Clinically a bulge can be noticed in the region of the palate or the alveolus depending upon the position of the impacted canine. The movements of the lateral incisor are also indicative of the type of maxillary canine impaction. However, this movement can only be used as a guide after carrying out all other diagnostic investigations:

• When lateral incisor is deflected distally, impacted canine might be present in close approximation with the mesial aspect root apex of the lateral incisor.
• When lateral incisor is tipped labially, it implies that impacted canine is present on the buccal or labial aspect of the root of lateral incisor.
• When lateral incisor is inclined lingually, canine is impacted on the palatal aspect of the root of lateral incisor. Though periapical and panoramic radiographs are available for localizing the impacted canine, the exact location of the impacted cuspids cannot be determined merely in one plane. Two radiographs taken in two lanes horizontal and vertical are necessary for accurate positioning of the impacted tooth.

CAUSES OF CANINE IMPACTIONS

Harry Jacoby (1983) studied the:

1. Primary Cause
   ○ Rate of root resorption of deciduous teeth
   ○ Trauma of the deciduous teeth bud
   ○ Disturbances in tooth eruption sequence
   ○ Availability of space in the arch
   ○ Rotation of tooth buds
   ○ Premature root closure

Canine eruption into cleft area in a person with cleft palate.

2. Secondary causes:
   ○ Abnormal muscle pressure
   ○ Febrile diseases
   ○ Endocrine disturbances
   ○ Vitamin D deficiency

According to Shafer *et al.* (1997) Sequelae might be associated with canine impaction:

1. Labial or lingual malpositioning of the impacted tooth.
2. Migration of the neighboring teeth and resultant loss of arch length
3. Internal resorption
4. Dentigerous cyst formation
5. External root resorption of the impacted as well as the neighboring teeth
6. Infections particularly associated with partial eruption
7. Referred pain
8. Various combinations of above sequelae.

It is estimated that 0.7% of children in the 10-13 age group have resorbed permanent incisor roots because of the ectopic eruption of maxillary canines.

Radiographs

One radiograph is taken in the horizontal plane which can either be a posterior or anterior and occlusal radiograph shows the position of the impacted canine. Another radiograph is taken in the vertical plane which reveals the height of the tooth in the maxilla.

Tube Shift Method: In this method, two periapical radiographs are taken in the same position. The first radiograph is taken in usual manner, but while taking the second radiograph, film is positioned in the same place but the tube or cone of the X-ray is moved horizontally in anyone direction (either to right or left).

Principle

Due to changes in horizontal direction while taking the second radiograph, unerupted tooth seems to be moving in a mesial or distal direction with respect to the adjacent teeth the surrounding anatomical structures.

SLOB (Same side - lingual, opposite side - buccal) rule. Applying the above mentioned principle, the SLOB rule can be used to determine the exact location of the impacted tooth.

If the impacted tooth seems to be moving towards the same side in which the tube is shifted, it is located on the lingual side.

If the impacted tooth seems to be moving in the opposite direction to which the tube is shifted, it is located on the buccal or labial side.

Complications of the Removal of Impacted Maxillary Cuspids

- Most of the time the impacted maxillary cuspid is situated in close proximity with the maxillary sinus; inadvertent instrumentation may displace the tooth into the sinus.
- The roots of the impacted canines may be extensively curved or hooked rendering the delivery of these teeth difficult.
- The tooth may be present in close approximation with the adjacent teeth. • After securing adequate local anaesthesia, an incision made starting from palatal aspect of neck of the maxillary canine involved side, and extending around the neck of the partially impacted crown of canine or around the expected position of the crown of the canine of the second bicuspid.
- Another incision is made midline starting from the of the interdental papilla, between the central incisors on the palatal aspect extending posteriorly for bleeding from the nasopalatine vessel maybe encountered which can be controlled using pressure packs.
- The mucoperiosteum is elevated to expose the impaction site adequately.
- Now the bulge of the crown of the impacted canine can be seen. Sufficient bone is removed by means of bur or chisel. However, most of the surgeons prefer burs to chisels. Holes are drilled around the crown of the impacted canine, appropriate elevator is applied and the tooth delivered out of the socket. If the curvature of the root resists the normal delivery or when the crown is present in close proximity with the adjacent tooth, sectioning should be considered. The crown should be sectioned first and removed followed by the root which can be pushed into the space created by removal of the crown.

Impaction on the Labial or Buccal Side

- The crown of the impacted teeth should be exposed with appropriately designed flap.
- The bone overlying the impacted tooth should be removed with bur or chisel.
- The tooth is elevated from the socket using elevators.
- If there is any resistance, the tooth should be sectioned and the root and crown removed separately.
- On the buccal side a semicircular incision is made and the root sectioned to remove it.
- On the palatal aspect, a palatal flap is reflected as previously mentioned and the crown of the impacted tooth is exposed by removing the overlying bone using bur or chisel. An appropriate instrument is inserted in the root end of the crown through the buccal crypt and the instrument is now tapped with mallet to remove it through the palatal exposure.

Removal of impacted canine in the edentulous jaw is essentially the same except for the incision which is made on the crest of the alveolar ridges due to lack of teeth.

Removal of bilaterally impacted maxillary canine differs in the type of incision and elevation of the flap. The incision is made around the necks of the teeth extending from one bicuspid region to the other, and a full thickness mucoperiosteal flap is elevated incising the nasopalatine nerve bundle and vessels (which re-establishes in a few weeks).

Placement of a palatal pack is important here. As mentioned earlier, mandibular cuspids are mostly impacted in a vertical position either buccally or lingual.

Removal of Vertically Impacted Cuspid on the Buccal Aspect

An incision is made and a mucoperiosteal flap is reflected adequately on the buccal side to expose the site of operation. The bone covering the crown of the tooth is removed using bur or chisel. Using the labial cortical plate as fulcrum, the tooth is luxated out of the socket. If there is any resistance to the normal delivery of the tooth out of the socket, segmentation of the crown and root should be considered. After removing the impacted tooth, the sharp bony edges are trimmed and smoothened. The socket is irrigated profusely using sterile saline solution and the flap sutured back.

Postoperative Management

- The socket should be thoroughly debrided with a surgical curette to remove pieces of bone chips, any granulation tissue and the dental follicle (to prevent the formation of cyst).
- The sharp bony edges should be smoothened with a blunt bur or bone file. Irrigation should be done profusely with sterile solution before approximating the flaps and suturing them.
- Medication prescribed by the surgeon should be taken by the patient regularly.
- Primary haemorrhage occurs immediately after removal of the tooth. Firm pressure should be applied at least for a period of 2 minutes with gauze over the socket. This would control most of the bleeding.
- Secondary haemorrhage, usually results due to incomplete or ineffective arrest of primary haemorrhage. This is often a result of increased blood pressure, alcoholic stimulation or indulgence in exercise.
- To treat secondary haemorrhage, coagulative properties of blood should be investigated to rule out any blood dyscrasia. Next a gauze sponge should be held firmly between the jaws and operative site for half an hour after the procedure. The patient should not rinse his/her mouth for 6 hours postoperatively since this

would disrupt the clot formation.

- Swelling of the face after impaction occurs over the outer surface of the jaws. Swelling on the lingual side is very rare. Cause of immediate swelling following surgery is usually mechanical trauma whereas cause of late swelling is generally infection.
- To treat immediate swelling ice cap should be applied over the area briefly and intermittently for the first day only, following which heat can be applied for at least four hours a day for the next four days. To prevent stiffness of the jaws, jaw exercise can be given like chewing gum as often as possible.
- Mastication of hard food substances should be avoided for a few days. The patient should take nutritious food rich in vitamins and minerals along with plenty of water.
- Strict oral hygiene instructions should be given.

Complications Arising from Retained Impacted Teeth

- Infections: The infections which can arise from retained impacted teeth are pericoronitis, abscess, cellulitis, osteitis and osteomyelitis
- Fractures: Impacted teeth cause weakening of the bone.
- Pain: It might be restricted to one area or may be referred to the ear, postauricular area or any part supplied by the trigeminal nerve.
- Cystic or neoplastic changes.
- Malocclusion and crowding of anterior teeth due to pressure effects of impacted third molar on the distal end of the arch.

Complications Arising During and After Removal of Impacted Third Molar

- Neurosensory injuries include injury to inferior alveoli nerve, lingual nerve, buccal nerve, mylohyoid nerve, all the resultant numbness of the area supplied by these nerve
- Infections
- Injury to the surrounding soft tissues
- Disturbance of the normal blood supply due to injury to the local blood vessels resulting in necrosis of the sur· rounding soft tissue or flap
- Acute trismus.
- Fracture of the root or accidental displacement of the fractured root into the maxillary sinus or other spaces
- Oroantral fistula
- Displacement of adjacent teeth out of the socket thus rendering it non-vital
- TMJ problem
- Alveolar osteitis
- Fracture of maxilla or mandible
- Excessive hemorrhage

- Adjacent teeth rendered non-vital
- Subcutaneous emphysema as a result of frequent use of air driven hand pieces
- Postoperative sequelae like excessive swelling, severe dysphagia, severe pain, and trismus
- Teeth may get displaced into maxillary sinus, submandibular space or may be accidentally swallowed or aspirated by the patient.

BIBLIOGRAPHY

[1]   Rafetto LK. Contemporary management of third molars. Philadelphia: Saunders 2012.

[2]   MacGregor AJ. The impacted lower wisdom tooth. Oxford: Oxford University Press 1985.

[3]   Killey HC, Kay LW. The impacted wisdom tooth. Edinburgh: Churchill Livingstone 1975.

[4]   Fragiskos FD. Oral surgery. Berlin: Springer 2007.
        [http://dx.doi.org/10.1007/978-3-540-49975-6]

[5]   Hooley JR, Whitacre RJ. A Self-instructional guide to oral surgery in general dentistry. Seattle, Wa.: Stoma Press 1979.

[6]   Howe GL. Minor oral surgery. 3rd ed., Oxford: Wright 1997.

[7]   Dimitroulis G. A synopsis of minor oral surgery. Oxford: Wright 1996.

[8]   Kruger GO. Textbook of oral and maxillofacial surgery. St. Louis: Mosby 1984.

[9]   Laskin DM. Oral and maxillofacial surgery. St. Louis: C.V. Mosby 1992.

[10]   Laskin DM, Abubaker AO. Decision making in oral and maxillofacial surgery. Chicago: Quintessence Pub. Co. 2007.

[11]   Kwon PH, Laskin DM. Clinician's manual of oral and maxillofacial surgery. Chicago: Quintessence Pub. Co. 1991.

[12]   Rounds CE, Rounds FW. Principles and technique of exodontia. St. Louis: Mosby 1962.

[13]   Peterson LJ. Contemporary oral and maxillofacial surgery. St. Louis: Mosby 1998.

[14]   Contemporary H. Oral and Maxillofacial Surgery. Elsevier 2014.

[15]   Sailer HF, Pajarola GF. Oral surgery for the general dentist. Stuttgart: Thieme 1998.

[16]   Dym H, Ogle OE. Oral surgery for the general dentist. Philadelphia: Saunders 2012.

[17]   Waite DE. Textbook of practical oral and maxillofacial surgery. Philadelphia: Lea & Febiger 1987.

[18]   Pell GJ, Gregory GT. Report on a ten-year study of a tooth division technique for the removal of impacted teeth. American Journal of Orthodontics and Oral Surgery 1942; 28(11): B660-6.

[19]   Read by Dr. Gregory before American Society of Oral Surgeons and Exodontists at the Houston meeting. From the Indiana University School of Dentistry Dental Digest. 1933

[20]   Yalcin S, Aktas I, Emes Y, Atalay B. Accidental displacement of a high-speed handpiece bur during mandibular third molar surgery: a case report. Oral Surgery, Oral Medicine, Oral Pathology, Oral Radiology, and Endodontology 2008; 105(3): e29-31.
        [http://dx.doi.org/10.1016/j.tripleo.2007.09.017]

[21]   Yeh CJ. Simplified split-bone technique for removal of impacted mandibular third molars. Int J Oral Maxillofac Surg 1995; 24(5): 348-50.
        [http://dx.doi.org/10.1016/S0901-5027(05)80489-8] [PMID: 8627100]

[22]   Veh. Clinic of Oral and Maxillofacial Surgery, Mackay Memorial Hospital. Int J Oral Maxillofac Surg 1995; 24: 148-350.

[PMID: 7608579]

[23]   Current clinical practice and parameters of care.The management of patients with third molar (syn: wisdom) teeth.American Association of Oral and Maxillofacial Surgeons in March 2007.

[24]   Siegel SC, von Fraunhofer JA. Irrigating solution and pressure effects on tooth sectioning with surgical burs. Oral Surg Oral Med Oral Pathol Oral Radiol Endod 1999; 87(5): 552-6.
[http://dx.doi.org/10.1016/S1079-2104(99)70132-0] [PMID: 10348511]

[25]   Edwards DJ, Brickley MR, Horton J, Edwards MJ, Shepherd JP. Choice of anaesthetic and healthcare facility for third molar surgery. Br J Oral Maxillofac Surg 1998; 36(5): 333-40.
[http://dx.doi.org/10.1016/S0266-4356(98)90643-X] [PMID: 9831052]

[26]   Ahmed N, Speculand B. Removal of ectopic mandibular third molar teeth: literature review and a report of three cases. Oral Surgery 2011; 5(1): 39-44.
[http://dx.doi.org/10.1111/j.1752-248X.2011.01145.x]

[27]   Holland IS, Stassen LF. Bilateral block: is it safe and more efficient during removal of third molars? Br J Oral Maxillofac Surg 1996; 34(3): 243-7.
[http://dx.doi.org/10.1016/S0266-4356(96)90278-8] [PMID: 8818259]

[28]   Meechan JG, Seymour RA. The use of third molar surgery in clinical pharmacology. Br J Oral Maxillofac Surg 1993; 31(6): 360-5.
[http://dx.doi.org/10.1016/0266-4356(93)90191-X] [PMID: 8286289]

[29]   Godfrey K, Dent KK. Prophylactic removal of asymptomatic third molars: a review. Aust Dent J 1999; 44(4): 233-7.
[http://dx.doi.org/10.1111/j.1834-7819.1999.tb00225.x] [PMID: 10687230]

[30]   Prophylactic removal of third molars. Dent Abstr 2008; 53(4): 201-2.
[http://dx.doi.org/10.1016/j.denabs.2008.02.030]

[31]   Bell GW. Use of dental panoramic tomographs to predict the relation between mandibular third molar teeth and the inferior alveolar nerve. Radiological and surgical findings, and clinical outcome. Br J Oral Maxillofac Surg 2004; 42(1): 21-7.
[http://dx.doi.org/10.1016/S0266-4356(03)00186-4] [PMID: 14706294]

[32]   Atieh MA. Diagnostic accuracy of panoramic radiography in determining relationship between inferior alveolar nerve and mandibular third molar. J Oral Maxillofac Surg 2010; 68(1): 74-82.
[http://dx.doi.org/10.1016/j.joms.2009.04.074] [PMID: 20006158]

[33]   Bishara SE, Andreasen G. Third molars: A review American Journal of Orthodontics 1983; 83(2): 131-7.

[34]   Jamileh Y, Pedlar J. Effect of clinical guidelines on practice for extraction of lower third molars: study of referrals in 1997 and 2000. Br J Oral Maxillofac Surg 2003; 41(6): 371-5.
[http://dx.doi.org/10.1016/S0266-4356(03)00172-4] [PMID: 14614863]

[35]   Yuasa H, Kawai T, Sugiura M. Classification of surgical difficulty in extracting impacted third molars. Br J Oral Maxillofac Surg 2002; 40(1): 26-31.
[http://dx.doi.org/10.1054/bjom.2001.0684] [PMID: 11883966]

[36]   Wang C-C, Kok S-H, Hou L-T, *et al.* Ectopic mandibular third molar in the ramus region: report of a case and literature review. Oral Surg Oral Med Oral Pathol Oral Radiol Endod 2008; 105(2): 155-61.
[http://dx.doi.org/10.1016/j.tripleo.2007.04.009] [PMID: 17764987]

[37]   Ventä IL, Turlola L, Murtomaa H, Ylipaavalniemi P. Assessing the eruption of lower third molars on the basis of radiographic features. Br J Oral Maxillofac Surg 1991; 29: 274-6.
[PMID: 1911678]

[38]   Ventä I, Schou S. Application of the Third Molar Eruption Predictor to periapical radiographs. Clin Oral Investig 2001; 5(2): 129-32.
[http://dx.doi.org/10.1007/s007840100103] [PMID: 11480811]

[39]   Westcott K, Irvine GH. Appropriateness of referrals for removal of wisdom teeth. Br J Oral Maxillofac
       Surg 2002; 40(4): 304-6.
       [http://dx.doi.org/10.1016/S0266-4356(02)00120-1] [PMID: 12175830]

[40]   Oral surgery: Distal cervical caries in the mandibular second molar: an indication for the prophylactic
       removal of the third molar? Br Dent J 2006; 200(8): 441.
       [http://dx.doi.org/10.1038/sj.bdj.4813470]

[41]   While KA. Jaw trabecular pattern varies with location, gender, age, and weight. Oral Surg Oral Med
       Oral Pathol 2003; 91-104.

[42]   Walters H. Lower third molar treatment. Br Dent J 1997; 182(6): 207.
       [http://dx.doi.org/10.1038/sj.bdj.4809347] [PMID: 9115836]

[43]   Friedman JW. The prophylactic extraction of third molars: a public health hazard. Am J Public Health
       2007; 97(9): 1554-9.
       [http://dx.doi.org/10.2105/AJPH.2006.100271] [PMID: 17666691]

[44]   Hamasha AA, Al Qudah MA, Bataineh AB, Safadi RA. Reasons for third molar teeth extraction in
       Jordanian adults. J Contemp Dent Pract 2006; 7(5): 88-95.
       [PMID: 17091144]

[45]   Alantar A, Roisin-Chausson M-H, Commissionat Y, *et al.* Retention of third molar roots to prevent
       damage to the inferior alveolar nerve. Oral Surg Oral Med Oral Pathol Oral Radiol Endod 1995; 80(2):
       126.
       [http://dx.doi.org/10.1016/S1079-2104(05)80190-8] [PMID: 7552873]

[46]   Alantar A, Roisin-Chausson M-H, Commissionat Y, *et al.* Retention of third molar roots to prevent
       damage to the inferior alveolar nerve. Oral Surg Oral Med Oral Pathol Oral Radiol Endod 1995; 80(2):
       126.
       [http://dx.doi.org/10.1016/S1079-2104(05)80190-8] [PMID: 7552873]

[47]   Husain J, Burden D, McSherry P, Morris D, Allen M. Clinical Standards Committee of the Faculty of
       Dental Surgery, Royal College of Surgeons of England. National clinical guidelines for management
       of the palatally ectopic maxillary canine. Br Dent J 2012; 213(4): 171-6.
       [http://dx.doi.org/10.1038/sj.bdj.2012.726] [PMID: 22918345]

[48]   Zuhal HK, Bahattin BC. Value of Computed Tomography (CT) in Imaging the Morbidity of
       Submerged Molars: A Case Report Journal List. Eur J Dent 2007; 1(4)

[49]   Ylikontiola L, Kinnunen J, Oikarinen K. Factors affecting neurosensory disturbance after mandibular
       bilateral sagittal split osteotomy. J Oral Maxillofac Surg 2000; 58(11): 1234-9.
       [http://dx.doi.org/10.1053/joms.2000.16621] [PMID: 11078134]

[50]   Roychoudhury S, Nagori SA, Roychoudhury A. Neurosensory disturbance after bilateral sagittal split
       osteotomy: A retrospective study. J Oral Biol Craniofac Res 2015; 5(2): 65-8.
       [http://dx.doi.org/10.1016/j.jobcr.2015.04.006] [PMID: 26258016]

[51]   Rood JP. Degrees of injury to the inferior alveolar nerve sustained during the removal of impacted
       mandibular third molars by the lingual split technique. Br J Oral Surg 1983; 21(2): 103-16.
       [http://dx.doi.org/10.1016/0007-117X(83)90054-9] [PMID: 6575812]

[52]   Benediktsdóttir IS, Wenzel A, Petersen JK, Hintze H. Mandibular third molar removal: risk indicators
       for extended operation time, postoperative pain, and complications. Oral Surg Oral Med Oral Pathol
       Oral Radiol Endod 2004; 97(4): 438-46.
       [http://dx.doi.org/10.1016/j.tripleo.2003.10.018] [PMID: 15088029]

[53]   Rakprasitkul S, Pairuchvej V. Mandibular third molar surgery with primary closure and tube drain. Int
       J Oral Maxillofac Surg 1997; 26(3): 187-90.
       [http://dx.doi.org/10.1016/S0901-5027(97)80817-X] [PMID: 9180228]

[54]   Yuasa H, Sugiura M. Clinical postoperative findings after removal of impacted mandibular third

molars: prediction of postoperative facial swelling and pain based on preoperative variables. Br J Oral Maxillofac Surg 2004; 42(3): 209-14.
[http://dx.doi.org/10.1016/j.bjoms.2004.02.005] [PMID: 15121265]

[55]   Benediktsdóttir IS, Wenzel A, Petersen JK, Hintze H. Mandibular third molar removal: risk indicators for extended operation time, postoperative pain, and complications. Oral Surg Oral Med Oral Pathol Oral Radiol Endod 2004; 97(4): 438-46.
[http://dx.doi.org/10.1016/j.tripleo.2003.10.018] [PMID: 15088029]

[56]   Scharff EU. Importance of early diagnosis and removal of mandibular third molar. Am J Orthod Oral Surg 1938; 24(4): 369-72.
[http://dx.doi.org/10.1016/S0096-6347(38)90144-9]

[57]   Oral surgery: Incidence and evolution of inferior alveolar nerve lesions following lower third molar extraction. Br Dent J 2005; 199(4): 209.
[http://dx.doi.org/10.1038/sj.bdj.4812618] [PMID: 15731796]

[58]   Valmaseda-Castellón E, Berini-Aytés L, Gay-Escoda C. Lingual nerve damage after third lower molar surgical extraction. Oral Surg Oral Med Oral Pathol Oral Radiol Endod 2000; 90(5): 567-73.
[http://dx.doi.org/10.1067/moe.2000.110034] [PMID: 11077378]

[59]   Shahana R. Lingual Nerve Damage during Third Molar Extraction – A Review. Research Journal of Pharmacy and Technology 2015; 8(6): 796.
[http://dx.doi.org/10.5958/0974-360X.2015.00128.6]

[60]   Robinson PP, Smith KG. Lingual nerve damage during lower third molar removal: a comparison of two surgical methods. Br Dent J 1996; 180(12): 456-61.
[http://dx.doi.org/10.1038/sj.bdj.4809126] [PMID: 8703598]

[61]   Park K-L. Which factors are associated with difficult surgical extraction of impacted lower third molars? J Korean Assoc Oral Maxillofac Surg 2016; 42(5): 251-8.
[http://dx.doi.org/10.5125/jkaoms.2016.42.5.251] [PMID: 27847732]

[62]   van der Linden W, Cleaton-Jones P, Lownie M. Diseases and lesions associated with third molars. Review of 1001 cases. Oral Surg Oral Med Oral Pathol Oral Radiol Endod 1995; 79(2): 142-5.
[PMID: 7614173]

[63]   Jerjes W, Swinson B, Moles D, *et al.* Permanent sensory nerve impairment following third molar surgery: a prospective study. Oral Surgery, Oral Medicine, Oral Pathology, Oral Radiology, and Endodontology 2006; 102(4): e1-7.
[http://dx.doi.org/10.1016/j.tripleo.2006.01.016]

[64]   Gargallo-Albiol J, Buenechea-Imaz R, Gay-Escoda C. Lingual nerve protection during surgical removal of lower third molars. a prospective randomised study. Int J Oral Maxillofac Surg 2000; 29(4): 268-71.
[http://dx.doi.org/10.1016/S0901-5027(00)80026-0] [PMID: 11030397]

[65]   Stivaros N, Mandall NA. Radiographic factors affecting the management of impacted upper permanent canines. J Orthod 2000; 27(2): 169-73.
[http://dx.doi.org/10.1093/ortho/27.2.169] [PMID: 10867073]

[66]   Stivaros N, Mandall NA. Radiographic factors affecting the management of impacted upper permanent canines. J Orthod 2000; 27(2): 169-73.
[http://dx.doi.org/10.1093/ortho/27.2.169] [PMID: 10867073]

[67]   Fleming C, Evans M. Re-exposure of impacted maxillary canines: the North Bristol experience. Oral Surgery 2009; 2(2): 71-6.
[http://dx.doi.org/10.1111/j.1752-248X.2009.01045.x]

[68]   Otto RL. Early and unusual incisor resorption due to impacted maxillary canines. Am J Orthod Dentofacial Orthop 2003; 124(4): 446-9.
[http://dx.doi.org/10.1016/S0889-5406(03)00563-8] [PMID: 14560276]

[69]   Jacoby H. The etiology of maxillary canine impactions. Am J Orthod 1983; 84(2): 125-32.
       [http://dx.doi.org/10.1016/0002-9416(83)90176-8] [PMID: 6576636]

[70]   Stewart JA, Heo G, Glover KE, Williamson PC, Lam EW, Major PW. Factors that relate to treatment
       duration for patients with palatally impacted maxillary canines. Am J Orthod Dentofacial Orthop
       2001; 119(3): 216-25.
       [http://dx.doi.org/10.1067/mod.2001.110989] [PMID: 11244415]

[71]   Milberg DJ. Labially impacted maxillary canines causing severe root resorption of maxillary central
       incisors. Angle Orthod 2006; 76(1): 173-6.
       [PMID: 16448288]

[72]   Strbac GD, Foltin A, Gahleitner A, Bantleon H-P, Watzek G, Bernhart T. The prevalence of root
       resorption of maxillary incisors caused by impacted maxillary canines. Clin Oral Investig 2013; 17(2):
       553-64.
       [http://dx.doi.org/10.1007/s00784-012-0738-9] [PMID: 22543896]

[73]   Barnard D. Surgical access to a complex composite odontome by sagittal splitting of the mandible. Br
       J Oral Surg 1983; 21(1): 44-8.
       [http://dx.doi.org/10.1016/0007-117X(83)90030-6] [PMID: 6573188]

[74]   Jr Fonseca. Textbook of Oral and Maxillofacial surgery. 2010.

[75]   Pye AD, Lockhart DE, Dawson MP, Murray CA, Smith AJ. A review of dental implants and infection.
       J Hosp Infect 2009; 72(2): 104-10.
       [http://dx.doi.org/10.1016/j.jhin.2009.02.010] [PMID: 19329223]

[76]   Ataoğlu H, Öz GY, Çandirli C, Kiziloğlu D. Routine antibiotic prophylaxis is not necessary during
       operations to remove third molars. Br J Oral Maxillofac Surg 2008; 46(2): 133-5.
       [http://dx.doi.org/10.1016/j.bjoms.2006.11.005] [PMID: 17188409]

[77]   Osaki T, Nomura Y, Hirota J, Yoneda K. Infections in elderly patients associated with impacted third
       molars. Oral Surg Oral Med Oral Pathol Oral Radiol Endod 1995; 79(2): 137-41.
       [http://dx.doi.org/10.1016/S1079-2104(05)80269-0] [PMID: 7614172]

[78]   Berge TI. Complications requiring hospitalization after third-molar surgery. Acta Odontol Scand 1996;
       54(1): 24-8.
       [http://dx.doi.org/10.3109/00016359609003505] [PMID: 8669237]

[79]   Yamalik K, Bozkaya S. The predictivity of mandibular third molar position as a risk indicator for
       pericoronitis. Clin Oral Investig 2008; 12(1): 9-14.
       [http://dx.doi.org/10.1007/s00784-007-0131-2] [PMID: 17619915]

[80]   Kirk DG, Liston PN, Tong DC, Love RM. Influence of two different flap designs on incidence of pain,
       swelling, trismus, and alveolar osteitis in the week following third molar surgery. Oral Surgery, Oral
       Medicine, Oral Pathology, Oral Radiology, and Endodontology 2007; 104(1): e1-6.
       [http://dx.doi.org/10.1016/j.tripleo.2007.01.032]

[81]   Pasqualini D, Cocero N, Castella A, Mela L, Bracco P. Primary and secondary closure of the surgical
       wound after removal of impacted mandibular third molars: a comparative study. Int J Oral Maxillofac
       Surg 2005; 34(1): 52-7.
       [http://dx.doi.org/10.1016/j.ijom.2004.01.023] [PMID: 15617967]

[82]   Santamaria J, Arteagoitia I. Radiologic variables of clinical significance in the extraction of impacted
       mandibular third molars. Oral Surg Oral Med Oral Pathol Oral Radiol Endod 1997; 84(5): 469-73.
       [http://dx.doi.org/10.1016/S1079-2104(97)90259-6] [PMID: 9394375]

[83]   Eliav E, Gracely RH. Sensory changes in the territory of the lingual and inferior alveolar nerves
       following lower third molar extraction. Pain 1998; 77(2): 191-9.
       [http://dx.doi.org/10.1016/S0304-3959(98)00100-6] [PMID: 9766837]

[84]   Jerjes W, El-Maaytah M, Swinson B, *et al.* Experience *versus* complication rate in third molar surgery.

Head Face Med 2006; 2(1): 14.
[http://dx.doi.org/10.1186/1746-160X-2-14] [PMID: 16725024]

[85]   Jones TA, Garg T, Monaghan A. Removal of a deeply impacted mandibular third molar through a sagittal split ramus osteotomy approach. Br J Oral Maxillofac Surg 2004; 42(4): 365-8.
[http://dx.doi.org/10.1016/j.bjoms.2004.02.022] [PMID: 15225962]

[86]   Homze EJ, Harn SD, Bavitz BJ. Extraoral ligation of the lingual artery: an anatomic study. Oral Surg Oral Med Oral Pathol Oral Radiol Endod 1997; 83(3): 321-4.
[http://dx.doi.org/10.1016/S1079-2104(97)90236-5] [PMID: 9084192]

[87]   Almendros-Marqués N, Alaejos-Algarra E, Quinteros-Borgarello M, Berini-Aytés L, Gay-Escoda C. Factors influencing the prophylactic removal of asymptomatic impacted lower third molars. Int J Oral Maxillofac Surg 2008; 37(1): 29-35.
[http://dx.doi.org/10.1016/j.ijom.2007.06.008] [PMID: 17913461]

[88]   Karaca I, Simşek S, Uğar D, Bozkaya S. Review of flap design influence on the health of the periodontium after mandibular third molar surgery. Oral Surg Oral Med Oral Pathol Oral Radiol Endod 2007; 104(1): 18-23.
[http://dx.doi.org/10.1016/j.tripleo.2006.11.049] [PMID: 17448707]

[89]   Golusińska-Kardach E, Sobieszczyk M, Sokalski J. A Rare Case of Concrescence of Impacted Maxillary Molars. Dental and Medical Problems 2016; 53(2): 291-5.
[http://dx.doi.org/10.17219/dmp/61348]

[90]   Kim J-C, Choi S-S, Wang S-J, Kim S-G. Minor complications after mandibular third molar surgery: type, incidence, and possible prevention. Oral Surgery, Oral Medicine, Oral Pathology, Oral Radiology, and Endodontology 2006; 102(2): e4-e11.
[http://dx.doi.org/10.1016/j.tripleo.2005.10.050]

[91]   Chossegros C, Guyot L, Cheynet F, Belloni D, Blanc JL. Is lingual nerve protection necessary for lower third molar germectomy? A prospective study of 300 procedures. Int J Oral Maxillofac Surg 2002; 31(6): 620-4.
[http://dx.doi.org/10.1054/ijom.2002.0236] [PMID: 12521318]

[92]   Humphris GM, O'Neill P, Field EA. Knowledge of wisdom tooth removal: influence of an information leaflet and validation of a questionnaire. Br J Oral Maxillofac Surg 1993; 31(6): 355-9.
[http://dx.doi.org/10.1016/0266-4356(93)90190-8] [PMID: 8286288]

[93]   Faber J, Berto PM, Quaresma M. Rapid prototyping as a tool for diagnosis and treatment planning for maxillary canine impaction. Am J Orthod Dentofacial Orthop 2006; 129(4): 583-9.
[http://dx.doi.org/10.1016/j.ajodo.2005.12.015] [PMID: 16627189]

[94]   Gharaibeh TM, Al-Nimri KS. Postoperative pain after surgical exposure of palatally impacted canines: closed-eruption *versus* open-eruption, a prospective randomized study. Oral Surg Oral Med Oral Pathol Oral Radiol Endod 2008; 106(3): 339-42.
[http://dx.doi.org/10.1016/j.tripleo.2007.12.025] [PMID: 18547839]

[95]   González-Sánchez MA, Berini-Aytés L, Gay-Escoda C. Transmigrant impacted mandibular canines: a retrospective study of 15 cases. J Am Dent Assoc 2007; 138(11): 1450-5.
[http://dx.doi.org/10.14219/jada.archive.2007.0080] [PMID: 17974641]

[96]   Lappin MM. Practical management of the impacted maxillary cuspid. Am J Orthod 1951; 37(10): 769-78.
[http://dx.doi.org/10.1016/0002-9416(51)90048-6] [PMID: 14877988]

[97]   Morris DO. Management of the unerupted maxillary canine. Br Dent J 1990; 169(5): 113-4.
[http://dx.doi.org/10.1038/sj.bdj.4807292] [PMID: 2206663]

[98]   Jacobs SG. Localization of the unerupted maxillary canine: how to and when to. Am J Orthod Dentofacial Orthop 1999; 115(3): 314-22.
[http://dx.doi.org/10.1016/S0889-5406(99)70335-5] [PMID: 10066981]

[99]   Almendros-Marqués N, Berini-Aytés L, Gay-Escoda C. Evaluation of intraexaminer and interexaminer agreement on classifying lower third molars according to the systems of Pell and Gregory and of Winter. J Oral Maxillofac Surg 2008; 66(5): 893-9.
[http://dx.doi.org/10.1016/j.joms.2007.09.011] [PMID: 18423277]

[100] Henry CB. Trans-antral approach for the removal of misplaced maxillary third molars in suitable cases. Br J Oral Surg 1972; 10(2): 205-10.
[http://dx.doi.org/10.1016/S0007-117X(72)80038-6] [PMID: 4509983]

[101] Browne WG. Lingual flap retractor for surgery in third molar area. Br J Oral Surg 1982; 20(2): 151-2.
[http://dx.doi.org/10.1016/0007-117X(82)90025-7] [PMID: 6954983]

SUBJECT INDEX

A

Acetylcholine 36, 144

Aching 39, 40, 158, 160

Acids, arachidonic 40, 183, 201

Action Potentials (AP) 26, 27, 30, 32

Activated protein C (APC) 184, 186

Acute inflammation 69, 70, 71, 72, 74, 75, 76, 77, 78, 79, 80, 81

Adequate hemostasis 122, 123, 124, 125, 126, 127, 128, 129, 130, 131, 132, 133, 134, 135

Adjacent teeth 206, 212, 274, 311, 313, 314, 316, 317

Adrenaline 56, 57, 59, 61, 85, 86, 87, 89, 144, 176, 177, 192, 198, 202

Adrenal vasoconstrictors 177

Afterload, cardiac 154, 155

Allergens 197, 199

Allergic reactions 94, 99, 196, 201, 202

Alveolar bone 115, 118, 122, 123, 124, 125, 126, 127, 128, 129, 130, 131, 132, 133, 134, 135, 138, 209, 213, 216, 271, 309

Alveolar nerve 16, 17, 21, 22, 23, 80, 272
inferior 21, 22, 80, 272
superior 16, 17, 23

Alveolar process 75, 118, 138, 209, 213, 233, 284, 294, 307, 311

American board of oral and maxillofacial surgery (ABOMS) 286, 299

American college of cardiology (ACC) 241, 243

Anaesthesia 83, 84, 85, 91, 98, 99, 101, 102, 276

Analgesics 35, 46, 100, 103, 188, 236
adjuvant 46, 47

Analgesic system, endogenous 25, 43, 45

Anaphylaxis 99, 175, 176, 197, 198, 199, 200, 201

Anesthesia 55, 57, 66, 67, 69, 70, 71, 73, 74, 75, 77, 78, 79, 80, 81, 82, 90, 91, 124, 177, 178, 237, 276

failure of 69, 70, 71, 72, 74, 75, 77, 78, 79, 80, 81, 82, 91

Anesthetic solution 65, 69, 70, 71, 72, 74, 75, 76, 77, 78, 79, 80, 82, 92, 178
depositing 69, 75

Angiotensin 164, 165, 168, 171, 172
converting enzyme (ACE) 164, 171, 172
receptor blockers (ARBs) 168, 172

Ankylosed tooth 209, 210

Ankyloses 203, 204, 206, 207, 209, 210

Anterior superior alveolar nerve infilteration 70

Antibiotic prophylaxis 242, 243, 244, 245

Anticoagulation therapy 189, 191

Anti-hemophilic factor (AHF) 184

Apical force 122, 123, 124, 125, 126, 127, 128, 129, 130, 131, 132, 133, 134, 135

Apply pressure gauze 122, 123, 124, 125, 126, 127, 128, 129, 130, 131, 132, 133, 134, 135

Arch, zygomatic 20, 284, 290, 295, 303, 308

Area, bifurcation 218, 222

Areas Anesthetized 69, 70, 71, 72, 73, 74, 75, 76, 77, 79, 80, 81, 82

Arrhythmias 55, 93, 96, 158, 160, 166, 179, 180
supraventricular 158, 160, 179

Arterial pressures 86, 164, 165, 167, 168

Arteries 154, 155, 161, 162, 165, 293, 294, 305
coronary 154, 155
posterior superior alveolar 284, 293, 305, 306

Aspiration 61, 62, 63, 67, 68, 79, 82, 87, 178, 271
positive 67, 68

Aspiration results 100, 101

Atherosclerosis 93, 154, 155, 238

Atrial fibrillation 93, 158, 160, 179, 180, 190

Axon 3, 12, 27, 31, 32, 33, 34, 35, 43

Axon hillock 26, 31, 32, 33, 34

Axon terminals 45, 47

Masticatory fat pad 284, 292, 293
Maxilla 15, 73, 118, 213, 235, 254, 272, 283,
      284, 285, 288, 290, 291, 292, 293, 294,
      295, 296, 297, 299, 300, 303, 304, 307,
      308, 311, 313, 316
Maxillary canine 310, 312, 313, 314
Maxillary cuspids 310, 311
Maxillary nerve 1, 13, 14, 15, 16, 17
Maxillary nerve branches 13, 15
Maxillary sinus 16, 124, 125, 126, 127, 128,
      207, 283, 285, 286, 290, 291, 292, 295,
      303, 304, 305, 306, 307, 308, 311, 314,
      316, 317
Maxillary sinus approximation 283
Maxillary third molar 264, 281, 285
Maxillary third molar removal 286
Maxillary tooth 109, 284
Maxillary tooth results 69, 75
Maxillary tuberosity 73, 80, 285, 293, 296,
      298, 308
Maxillofacial surgeons 256, 286, 299, 304
Mean arterial pressure (MAP) 161
Mechanical advantage 214, 215, 216, 217
Mediators 163, 199, 200, 201, 202
   inflammatory 41, 198, 199, 200, 202
   preformed 199, 200
Medications 35, 37, 41, 46, 47, 51, 85, 91, 94,
      97, 149, 152, 153, 170, 173, 174, 193,
      234, 236, 238, 250, 253, 255, 315
   antiangiogenic 250, 253
   antiresorptive 250, 253
Medulla, adrenal 59, 164, 166, 167
Menorrhagia 184, 185, 186
Mental foramen 21, 22, 74, 78, 80, 81, 132,
      133
Mesiobuccal corner 277
Metformin 149, 152
Middle superior alveolar nerve infilteration 71
Modified ward's incision 276, 277
Molar, distal aspect of second 266
Mucobuccal fold 69, 70, 72, 73, 81
Mucous membrane 9, 11, 15, 19, 21, 22, 23,
      43, 59, 66, 69, 74, 77, 78, 79, 81
Muscles 10, 11, 21, 32, 33, 59, 97, 100, 101,
      146, 203, 267, 284, 285, 294, 295, 297
   skeletal 33, 59, 97, 146

superior constrictor 21, 284, 285, 294, 297
temporalis 203, 295
Myelinated axon 31, 33, 34
Myocardial infarction 92, 93, 154, 156, 157,
      158, 159, 160, 161, 173, 174, 175, 176,
      184
Myocardial infarction (MI) 92, 93, 154, 156,
      157, 158, 159, 160, 161, 172, 173, 174,
      175, 176, 184

N

Nasopalatine nerves 15, 16, 17, 76
Necrotic bone 248, 256
Needle 77, 293, 305
   local anesthetic injection 293, 305
   long dental 77
Nerve 1, 3, 4, 5, 6, 8, 9, 10, 11, 13, 18, 19, 21,
      23, 35, 36, 53, 69, 73, 90, 91, 92, 100,
      103, 163, 213, 294, 316
   glossopharyngeal 3, 4, 6, 21
   infra-orbital 13
   lacrimal 10
   nasociliary 11
   ophthalmic 9, 10
   trochlear 9, 10
Nerve block 74, 75, 76, 81, 134, 135
   incisive 74, 81
   mental 81
   nasopalatine 74, 75, 76
Nerve fibers 31, 32, 33, 39, 42
Nerve injury 47, 91
Nerve of lateral pterygoid muscle 19
Nervus intermedius 3, 5, 6, 16, 23
Neurotransmitters 31, 36, 41, 42, 45
Neurovascular bundle 271, 272
Neutrophils 201, 202
Nifedipine 173, 174, 175
Nitroglycerin 154, 157, 158, 161, 174, 175
Nociceptors 35, 38, 39, 40, 41, 46
   mechanical 38, 39, 40
   thermal 38, 39
Norepinephrine 58, 147, 164, 165, 166, 167,
      170, 171

www.ingramcontent.com/pod-product-compliance
Lightning Source LLC
Chambersburg PA
CBHW050807220326
41598CB00006B/137